MW00604085

Atlas of Oral and Maxillofacial Radiology

Atlas of Oral and Maxillofacial Radiology

Bernard Koong

BDSc (UWA), MSc (OMR)(Toronto), FICD, FADI, FPFA
Oral and Maxillofacial Radiologist, Envision Medical Imaging;
Clinical Professor, University of Western Australia
Perth, Western Australia

WILEY Blackwell

This edition first published 2017 © 2017 by John Wiley & Sons Ltd

Registered Office
John Wiley & Sons Ltd, The Atrium, Southern Gate, Chichester, West Sussex, PO19 8SQ, UK

Editorial Offices
9600 Garsington Road, Oxford, OX4 2DQ, UK
The Atrium, Southern Gate, Chichester, West Sussex, PO19 8SQ, UK
1606 Golden Aspen Drive, Suites 103 and 104, Ames, Iowa 50010, USA

For details of our global editorial offices, for customer services and for information about how to apply for permission to reuse the copyright material in this book please see our website at www.wiley.com/wiley-blackwell

The right of the author to be identified as the author of this work has been asserted in accordance with the UK Copyright, Designs and Patents Act 1988.

Library of Congress Cataloging-in-Publication Data

Names: Koong, Bernard, 1962– , editor.
Title: Atlas of oral and maxillofacial radiology / edited by Bernard Koong.
Description: Chichester, West Sussex ; Ames, Iowa : John Wiley & Sons Inc., 2017. |
    Includes bibliographical references and index.
Identifiers: LCCN 2016007778 | ISBN 9781118939642 (cloth) | ISBN 9781118939635 (Adobe PDF) |
    ISBN 9781118939628 (epub)
Subjects: | MESH: Stomatognathic Diseases–radiography | Stomatognathic Diseases–diagnosis |
    Radiography, Dental | Atlases
Classification: LCC RK309 | NLM WU 17 | DDC 617.52/2075722–dc23
LC record available at http://lccn.loc.gov/2016007778

A catalogue record for this book is available from the British Library.

Wiley also publishes its books in a variety of electronic formats. Some content that appears in print may not be available in electronic books.

Cover image: © Bernard Koong

Set in 9.5/12pt Minion by SPi Global, Pondicherry, India
Printed and bound in Malaysia by Vivar Printing Sdn Bhd

1   2017

Contents

List of Contributors

Michael Bynevelt BHB, MBChB, FRANZCR
Consultant Neuroradiologist
Neurological Intervention and Imaging Service of Western Australia
Royal Perth, Sir Charles Gairdner and Princess Margaret Hospitals;
Neuroradiologist, Envision Medical Imaging;
Clinical Associate Professor, University of Western Australia
Perth, Western Australia

Tom Huang BDSc, DClinDent (DMFR)
Oral and Maxillofacial Radiologist
Envision Medical Imaging
Perth, Western Australia

Andrew Thompson FRANZCR, MBBS
Consultant Neuroradiologist
Neurological Intervention and Imaging Service Western Australia
Royal Perth, Sir Charles Gairdner and Princess Margaret Hospitals
Perth, Western Australia

Preface

Radiological interpretation of anomalies affecting the jaws is primarily based upon an understanding of the pathophysiology, including how a lesion behaves within a specific anatomical constraint. While an understanding of anatomy and pathology is essential, the knowledge of key radiological features and the ability to identify and weight these features is critical in interpretation.

The impetus for this atlas came from colleagues, students and audiences at speaking engagements. The request was for a radiological atlas dedicated to conditions affecting the jaws and teeth which would assist them in daily practice. They wanted an atlas that is easy to use and based upon tried and true key radiological features that are used in my daily radiological practice.

This problem-solving-style atlas fulfils the wishes of these clinicians, radiologists, surgeons and students. It is much more than a summary of radiological features that have been identified in the published literature. This atlas highlights the key features of jaw lesions which have been learnt, identified, analysed, validated and weighted over the course of personally reporting over 200 000 radiological examinations of the jaws. Multiple examples of common conditions are demonstrated with a variety of techniques to demonstrate the variation in the radiological features and also assist the reader in the application of the optimal modality. There is a focus on conditions where diagnostic imaging often substantially contributes to diagnosis. Less common and many rare conditions are also covered. The 'differential diagnosis' sections highlight radiological features which assist in differentiating the lesion in question from conditions which may otherwise appear similar. A summarised description of every condition focuses on the clinically important points.

This atlas includes a chapter dedicated to the temporomandibular joint. Panoramic radiograph and orofacial cone beam CT radiological anatomy are also covered in detail. The nasal cavity, paranasal sinuses, upper aerodigestive tract morphological alterations, base of skull and cervical spine are often seen in dentofacial imaging, especially cone beam CT. These are also covered in specific chapters.

Students of dentistry, radiology and surgery have also been very much kept in mind in the writing of this atlas. While nothing is better than one-to-one hands-on training in a clinical–radiology environment, I believe that a thorough study of this atlas would substantially improve a student's interpretive skill set and also prepare them well for any examination.

I would like to acknowledge the training I received from Dr Michael Pharoah of the University of Toronto, which started my journey in interpretive radiology. I am also extremely thankful to the contributing authors. These highly respected and experienced full-time radiologists have substantially contributed to making this a truly clinically relevant atlas.

I sincerely hope that you will find this atlas relevant and useful. Ultimately, it is my hope that the use or study of this atlas will contribute positively to your patients' wellbeing.

Bernard Koong

Acknowledgements

This atlas is dedicated to Seok Leng, Swee Yen, Angelina, Chrysten and Danielle. You are my strength and my inspiration.

A sincere thank you to all my colleagues in dentistry and medicine. Your trust in me over many years to care for the radiological needs of your patients has allowed me to continually grow and develop, culminating in the writing of this atlas.

A special thank you to all my colleagues at Envision Medical Imaging, Australia. You are the most wonderful team of people I have ever had the pleasure to work with.

A heartfelt thank you to Dr Michael Pharoah. Your generosity, kindness and contribution to my career in radiology will never be forgotten.

Bernard Koong

How to Use This Atlas

- As a book for the study of radiological interpretation:
  - A study of this entire atlas would prepare any student of dentistry, radiology and surgery well for any examination on interpretive diagnostic imaging of the jaws and related structures.
- As a reference atlas for lesions affecting the jaws:
  - Using the 'problem solving' method:
    1. Go to the relevant 'problem solving' page(s) in Chapter 1, depending on whether the lesion is considered to be opaque/largely opaque, lucent or demonstrates mixed density internal appearances.
       - It should be noted that some conditions can present differently depending on the modality employed. For example, a lesion which presents as a unilocular lucency on a panoramic radiograph may demonstrate internal opacities on a CBCT or MDCT scan. In these instances, the reader is encouraged to refer to more than one 'problem solving' page.
    2. Check the lists of possible conditions, beginning with the common conditions. Also refer to the diagrams which identify conditions that have a predilection for a specific region of the jaw.
    3. Refer to the relevant section for a description of the possible condition and images highlighting the key features.
  - The more experienced reader may wish to go directly to the relevant chapters or refer to specific conditions listed in the index.
- For conditions affecting the temporomandibular joint, sinonasal structures, upper aerodigestive tract morphology, skull base and cervical spine, refer to the specific chapters.

CHAPTER 1
Problem Solving Diagrams

1.1 Opaque and largely opaque conditions related to the jaws

For conditions affecting the temporomandibular joint (TMJ), nasal cavity, paranasal sinuses, upper airway morphology, skull base and cervical spine, please refer to the dedicated chapters.

On plain films, including panoramic and cephalometric radiographs, soft tissue calcifications may be projected over the jaws (see Chapter 16).

Common conditions

- Reactive sclerosis related to a periapical inflammatory lesion (see section 5.1)
- Bone island (see section 7.4)
- Exostoses (see section 7.3)
- Torus palatinus (see section 7.1)
- Torus mandibularis (see section 7.2)
- Ectopic teeth (see section 3.4)
- Chronic pericoronitis (see section 5.3)
- Supernumerary teeth (see section 3.1)
- Cemento-osseous dysplasia including periapical osseous dysplasia (see section 9.2)
- Pulp stones (see section 3.21)
- Hypercementosis (see section 3.22)
- Odontoma (see section 10.3)
- Dens invaginatus (see section 3.11)
- Fibrous dysplasia (see section 9.1)
- Enamel pearl (see section 3.9)
- Talon cusp (see section 3.10)

Less common conditions

- Osteoma (see section 10.10)
- Malignant lesions including metastatic disease (see sections 11.1–11.3)
- Chronic osteomyelitis (see section 5.4)
- Ossifying fibroma (see section 9.3)
- Cementoblastoma (see section 10.9)
- Osteoblastoma (see section 10.14)
- Osteoid osteoma (see section 10.15)
- Paget disease of bone (see section 13.5)
- Osteopetrosis (see section 15.2)

(a)

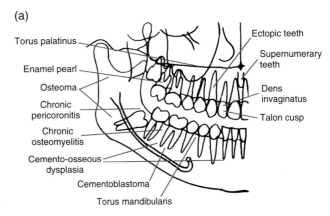

(b)

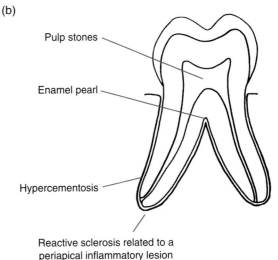

Figure 1.1 (a) Representation of the jaws and teeth and (b) larger representation of the fully erupted tooth. Conditions that have a predilection for certain regions of the jaws and teeth are shown. Note: (1) These lesions are not necessarily more common than other conditions. See the text for lists of common and less common conditions. (2) Most of these lesions also occur elsewhere within the jaws. (3) The pointers identify a region, not a specific site.

Atlas of Oral and Maxillofacial Radiology, First Edition. Bernard Koong.
© 2017 John Wiley & Sons Ltd. Published 2017 by John Wiley & Sons Ltd.

1.2 Lucent lesions of the jaws

For conditions affecting the TMJ, nasal cavity, paranasal sinuses, upper airway morphology, skull base and cervical spine, please refer to the dedicated chapters.

Common conditions

- Caries (see section 4.1)
- Periodontal bone loss (see section 5.2)
- Tooth abrasion (see section 4.3)
- Periapical inflammatory lesion (see section 5.1)
- Root resorption (see sections 4.5–4.6)
- Radicular cyst (see section 8.1)
- Dentigerous cyst (see section 8.3)
- Stafne defect (see section 14.4)
- Simple bone cyst (see section 8.9)
- Keratocystic odontogenic tumour (see section 8.5)
- Nasopalatine duct cyst (see section 8.10)
- Residual cyst (see section 8.2)
- Cemento-osseous dysplasia (see section 9.2)

Less common conditions

- Osteoradionecrosis (see section 6.1)
- Osteonecrosis of the jaws (see section 6.2)
- Buccal bifurcation cyst (see section 8.4)
- Lateral periodontal cyst (see section 8.7)
- Osteomyelitis (see section 5.4)
- Malignant lesions including metastatic disease (see sections 11.1–11.3)
- Vascular anomalies (see sections 12.1–12.4)
- Cleft lip and palate (see section 14.5)
- Ameloblastoma (see section 10.1)
- Schwannoma (see section 10.13)
- Langerhans cell histiocytosis (see section 13.4)
- Nasolabial cyst (see section 8.11)
- Glandular odontogenic cyst (see section 8.8)
- Ameloblastic fibroma (see section 10.4)

(a)

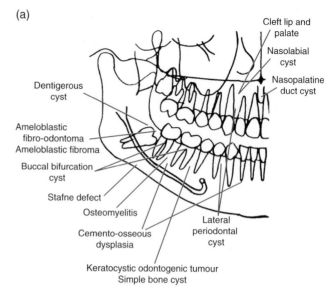

(b)

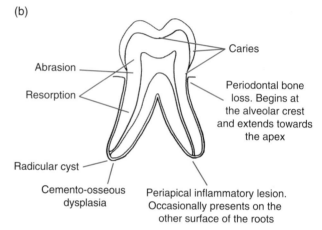

Figure 1.2 (a) Representation of the jaws and teeth and (b) larger representation of the fully erupted tooth. Conditions that have a predilection for certain regions of the jaws are shown. Note: (1) These lesions are not necessarily more common than other conditions. Refer to the text for lists of common and less common conditions. (2) Most of these lesions also occur elsewhere within the jaws. (3) The pointers identify a region, not a specific site.

1.3 Mixed density lesions of the jaws

For conditions affecting the TMJ, nasal cavity, paranasal sinuses, upper airway morphology, skull base and cervical spine, please refer to the dedicated chapters.

Common conditions

- Chronic pericoronitis (see section 5.3)
- Cemento-osseous dysplasia (see section 9.2)
- Odontoma (see section 10.3)
- Fibrous dysplasia (see section 9.1)

Less common conditions

- Osteoradionecrosis (see section 6.1)
- Osteonecrosis of the jaws (see section 6.2)
- Osteomyelitis (see section 5.4)
- Ameloblastoma (see section 10.1)
- Central giant cell granuloma (see section 13.1)
- Odontogenic myxoma (see section 10.8)
- Ossifying fibroma (see section 9.3)
- Vascular anomalies (see sections 12.1–12.4)
- Malignant lesions including metastatic disease (see sections 11.1–11.3)
- Aneurysmal bone cyst (see section 13.3)
- Ameloblastic fibro-odontoma (see section 10.5)
- Adenomatoid odontogenic tumour (see section 10.6)
- Calcifying cystic odontogenic tumour (see section 10.7)
- Paget disease of bone (see section 13.5)
- Calcifying epithelial odontogenic tumour (Pindborg) (see section 10.2)
- Osteoblastoma (see section 10.14)
- Osteoid osteoma (see section 10.15)
- Desmoplastic fibroma (see section 10.16)
- Cherubism (see section 13.2)

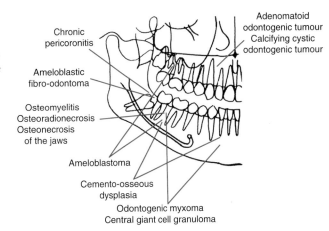

Figure 1.3 Representation of the jaws and teeth. Conditions that have a predilection for certain regions of the jaws are shown. Note: (1) These lesions are not necessarily more common than other conditions. Refer to the text for lists of common and less common conditions. (2) Most of these lesions also occur elsewhere within the jaws. (3) The pointers identify a region, not a specific site.

CHAPTER 2
Radiological Anatomy

2.1 The panoramic radiograph

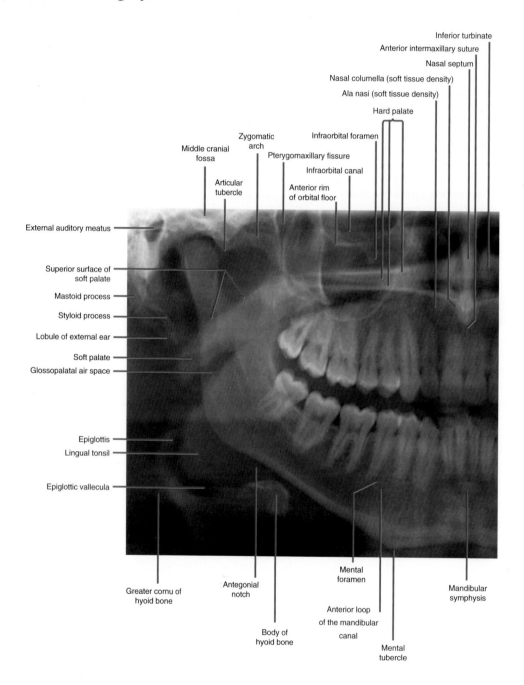

Figure 2.1

Atlas of Oral and Maxillofacial Radiology, First Edition. Bernard Koong.
© 2017 John Wiley & Sons Ltd. Published 2017 by John Wiley & Sons Ltd.

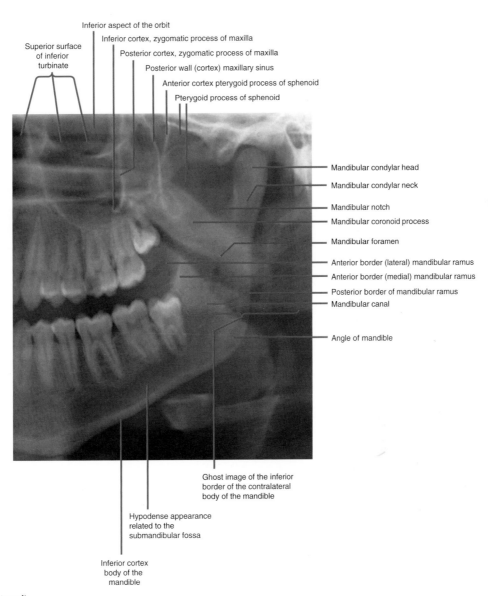

Superior surface
of inferior
turbinate

Inferior aspect of the orbit

Inferior cortex, zygomatic process of maxilla

Posterior cortex, zygomatic process of maxilla

Posterior wall (cortex) maxillary sinus

Anterior cortex pterygoid process of sphenoid

Pterygoid process of sphenoid

Mandibular condylar head

Mandibular condylar neck

Mandibular notch

Mandibular coronoid process

Mandibular foramen

Anterior border (lateral) mandibular ramus

Anterior border (medial) mandibular ramus

Posterior border of mandibular ramus

Mandibular canal

Angle of mandible

Ghost image of the inferior
border of the contralateral
body of the mandible

Hypodense appearance
related to the
submandibular fossa

Inferior cortex
body of the
mandible

Figure 2.1 (Continued)

Figure 2.2

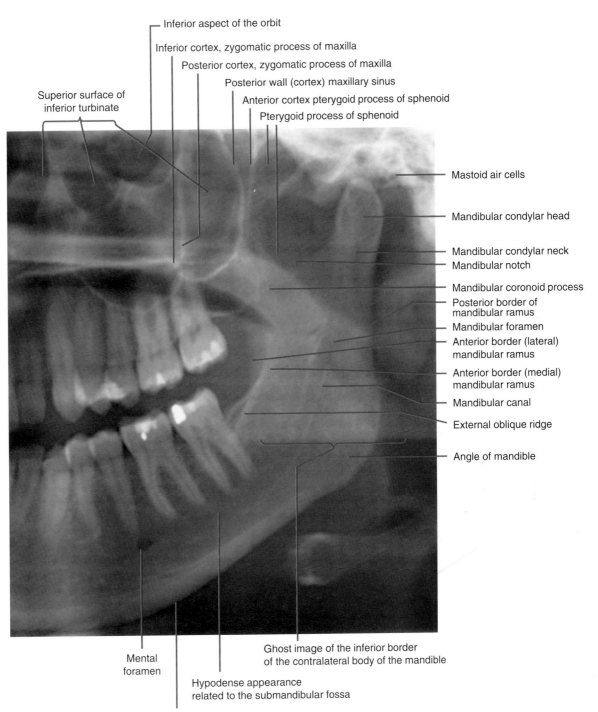

Inferior aspect of the orbit

Inferior cortex, zygomatic process of maxilla

Posterior cortex, zygomatic process of maxilla

Posterior wall (cortex) maxillary sinus

Anterior cortex pterygoid process of sphenoid

Pterygoid process of sphenoid

Superior surface of
inferior turbinate

Mastoid air cells

Mandibular condylar head

Mandibular condylar neck

Mandibular notch

Mandibular coronoid process

Posterior border of
mandibular ramus

Mandibular foramen

Anterior border (lateral)
mandibular ramus

Anterior border (medial)
mandibular ramus

Mandibular canal

External oblique ridge

Angle of mandible

Mental
foramen

Ghost image of the inferior border
of the contralateral body of the mandible

Hypodense appearance
related to the submandibular fossa

Inferior cortex body
of the mandible

Figure 2.2 (Continued)

2.2 Identification of teeth – FDI (Fédération Dentaire Internationale) World Dental Federation notation

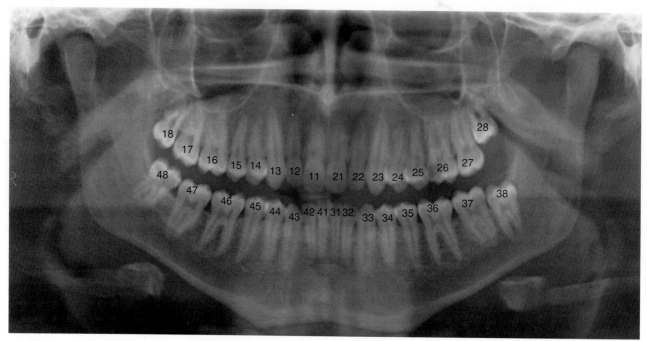

Figure 2.3

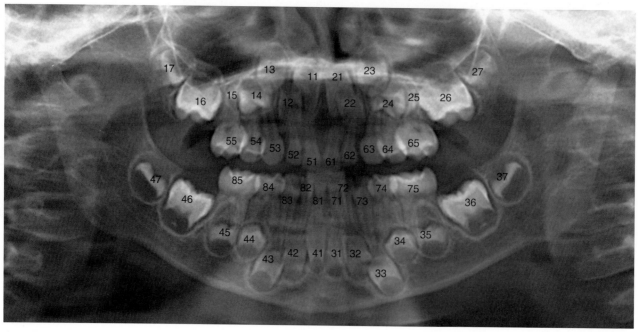

Figure 2.4

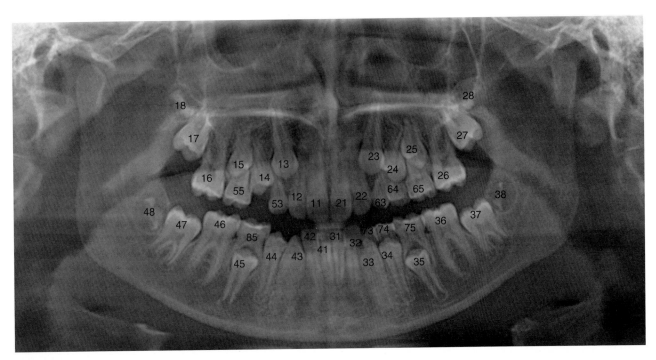

Figure 2.5

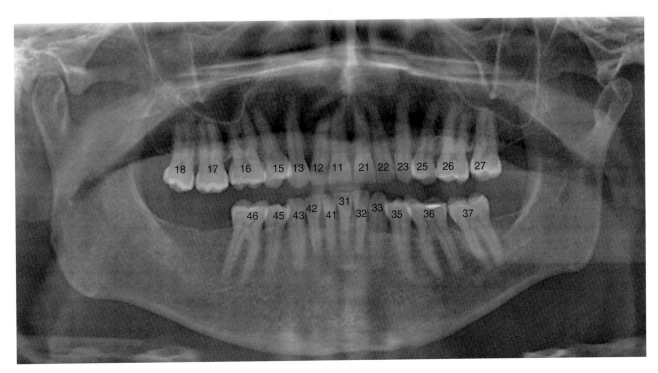

Figure 2.6

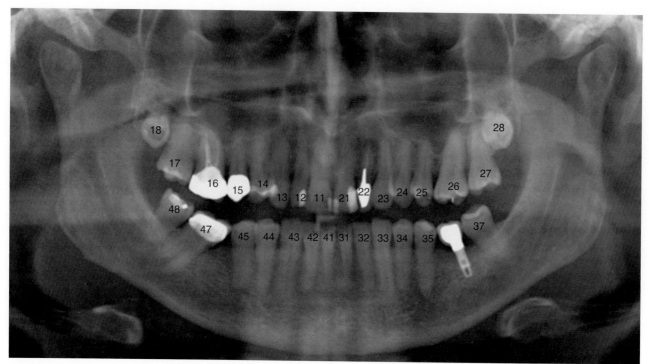

Figure 2.7

2.3 Cone beam computed tomography

Axial

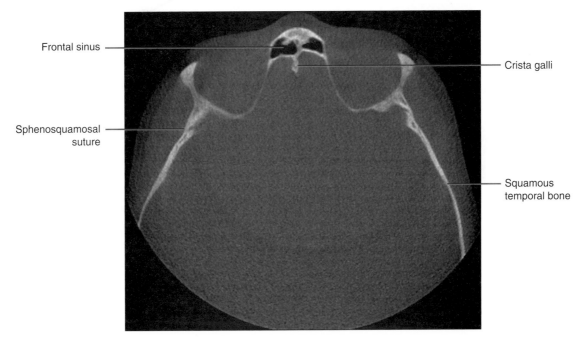

Frontal sinus —

— Crista galli

Sphenosquamosal
suture —

— Squamous
temporal bone

Figure 2.8

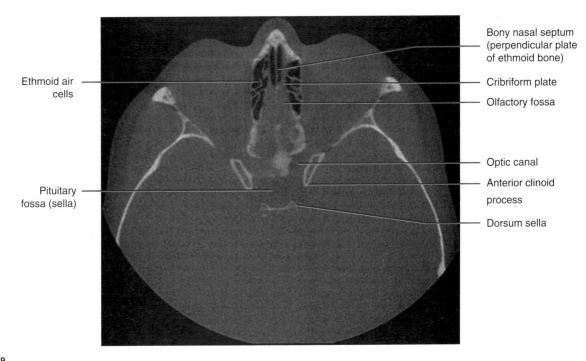

— Bony nasal septum
(perpendicular plate
of ethmoid bone)

Ethmoid air
cells —

— Cribriform plate

— Olfactory fossa

— Optic canal

Pituitary
fossa (sella) —

— Anterior clinoid
process

— Dorsum sella

Figure 2.9

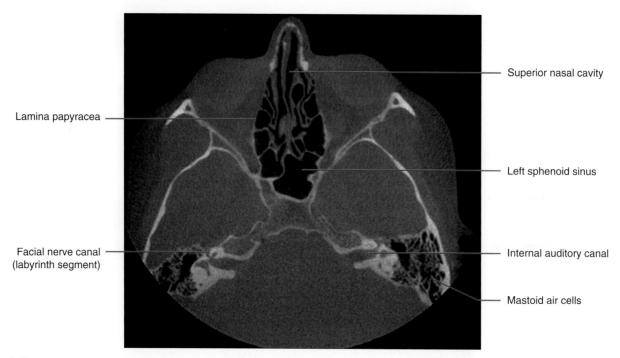

Superior nasal cavity

Lamina papyracea

Left sphenoid sinus

Facial nerve canal
(labyrinth segment)

Internal auditory canal

Mastoid air cells

Figure 2.10

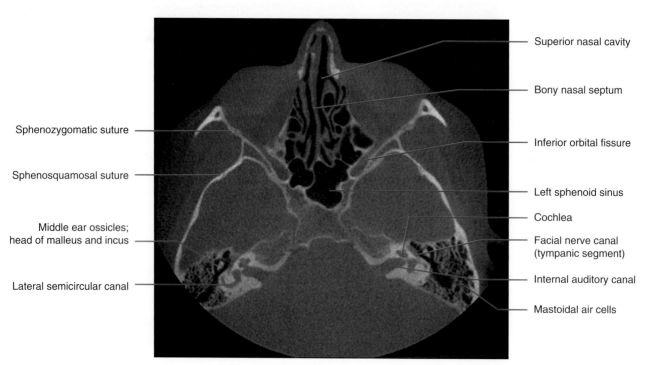

Superior nasal cavity

Bony nasal septum

Sphenozygomatic suture

Inferior orbital fissure

Sphenosquamosal suture

Left sphenoid sinus

Cochlea

Middle ear ossicles;
head of malleus and incus

Facial nerve canal
(tympanic segment)

Lateral semicircular canal

Internal auditory canal

Mastoidal air cells

Figure 2.11

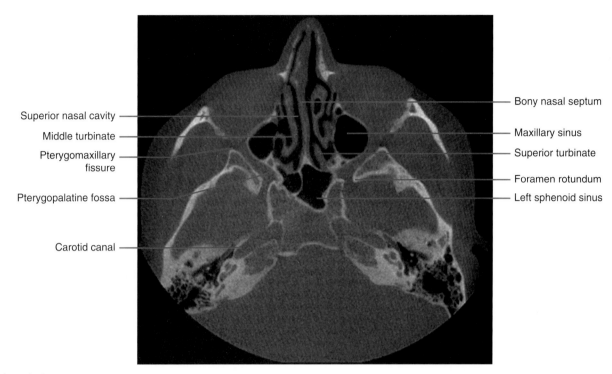

Superior nasal cavity

Middle turbinate

Pterygomaxillary fissure

Pterygopalatine fossa

Carotid canal

Bony nasal septum

Maxillary sinus

Superior turbinate

Foramen rotundum

Left sphenoid sinus

Figure 2.12

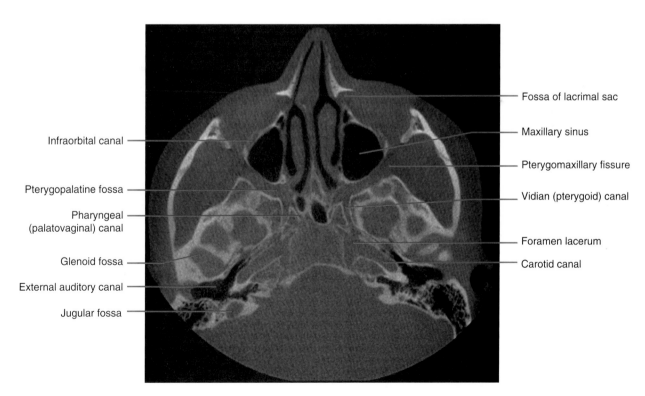

Infraorbital canal

Pterygopalatine fossa

Pharyngeal (palatovaginal) canal

Glenoid fossa

External auditory canal

Jugular fossa

Fossa of lacrimal sac

Maxillary sinus

Pterygomaxillary fissure

Vidian (pterygoid) canal

Foramen lacerum

Carotid canal

Figure 2.13

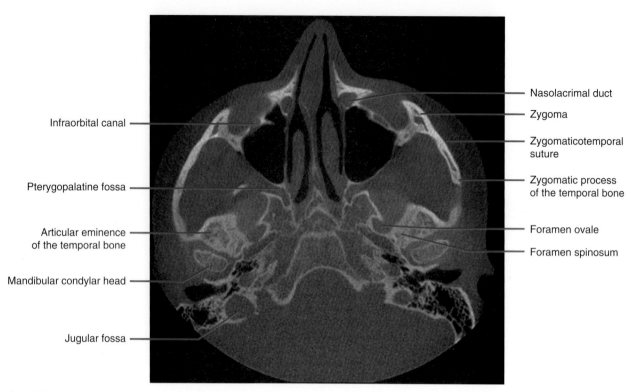

Nasolacrimal duct

Zygoma

Zygomaticotemporal suture

Zygomatic process of the temporal bone

Foramen ovale

Foramen spinosum

Infraorbital canal

Pterygopalatine fossa

Articular eminence of the temporal bone

Mandibular condylar head

Jugular fossa

Figure 2.14

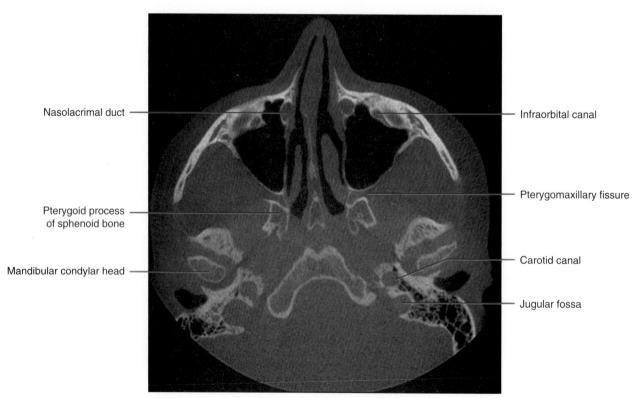

Nasolacrimal duct

Infraorbital canal

Pterygoid process of sphenoid bone

Pterygomaxillary fissure

Mandibular condylar head

Carotid canal

Jugular fossa

Figure 2.15

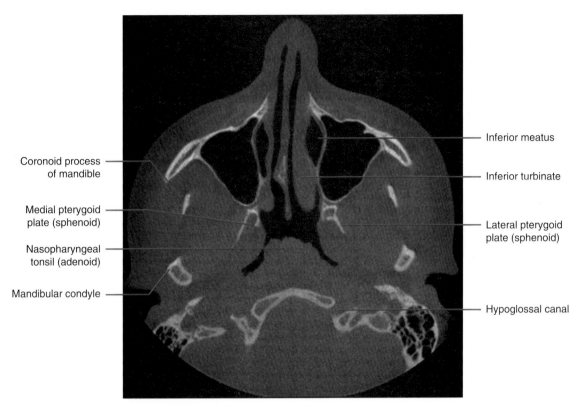

Coronoid process of mandible

Medial pterygoid plate (sphenoid)

Nasopharyngeal tonsil (adenoid)

Mandibular condyle

Inferior meatus

Inferior turbinate

Lateral pterygoid plate (sphenoid)

Hypoglossal canal

Figure 2.16

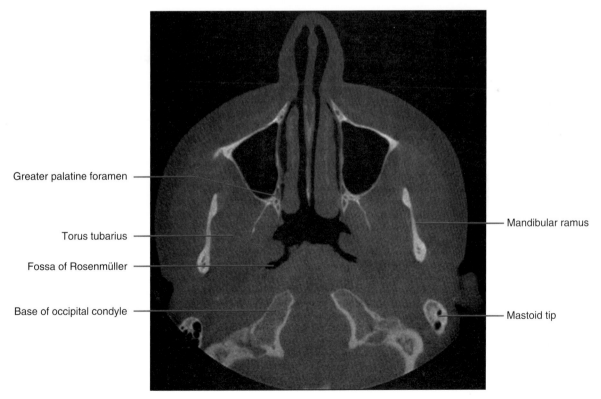

Greater palatine foramen

Torus tubarius

Fossa of Rosenmüller

Base of occipital condyle

Mandibular ramus

Mastoid tip

Figure 2.17

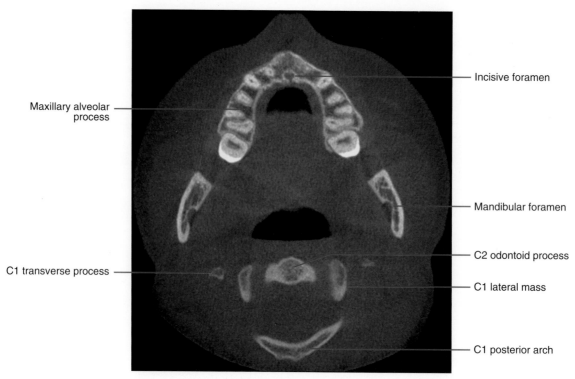

Maxillary alveolar process

Incisive foramen

Mandibular foramen

C2 odontoid process

C1 transverse process

C1 lateral mass

C1 posterior arch

Figure 2.18

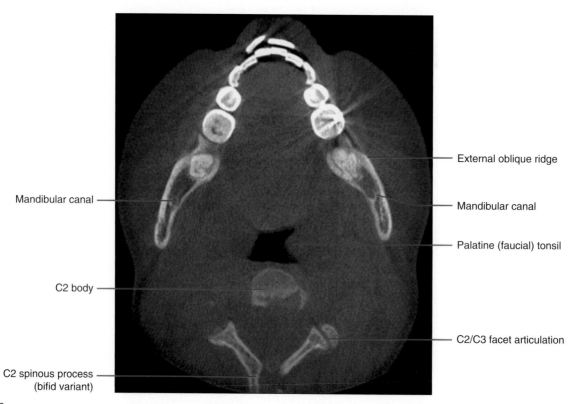

External oblique ridge

Mandibular canal

Mandibular canal

Palatine (faucial) tonsil

C2 body

C2/C3 facet articulation

C2 spinous process (bifid variant)

Figure 2.19

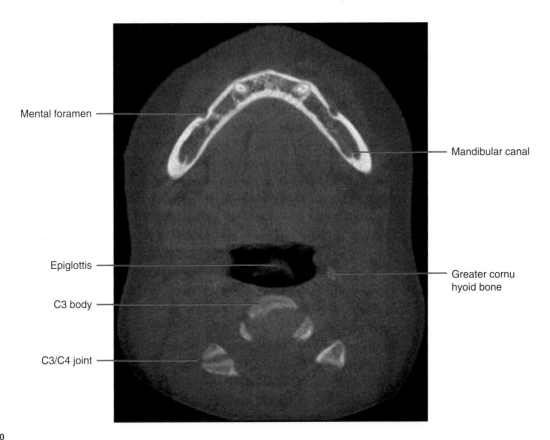

Mental foramen

Mandibular canal

Epiglottis

Greater cornu hyoid bone

C3 body

C3/C4 joint

Figure 2.20

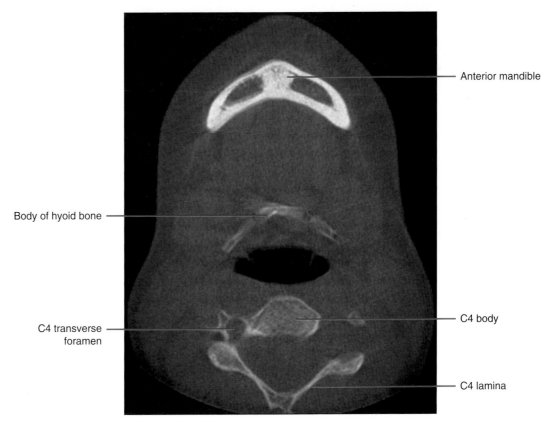

Anterior mandible

Body of hyoid bone

C4 transverse foramen

C4 body

C4 lamina

Figure 2.21

Sagittal

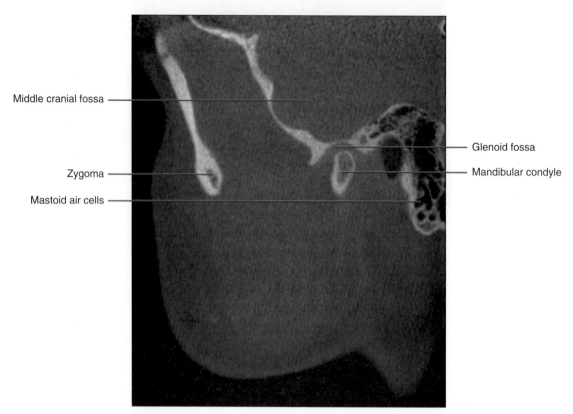

Middle cranial fossa ⎯⎯

Glenoid fossa ⎯⎯

Zygoma ⎯⎯

Mandibular condyle ⎯⎯

Mastoid air cells ⎯⎯

Figure 2.22

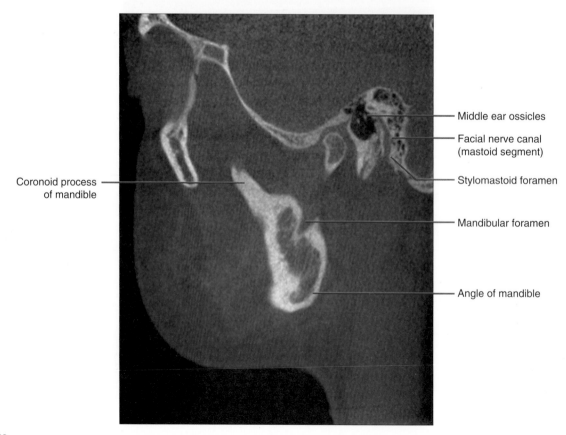

Coronoid process of mandible ⎯⎯

Middle ear ossicles ⎯⎯

Facial nerve canal (mastoid segment) ⎯⎯

Stylomastoid foramen ⎯⎯

Mandibular foramen ⎯⎯

Angle of mandible ⎯⎯

Figure 2.23

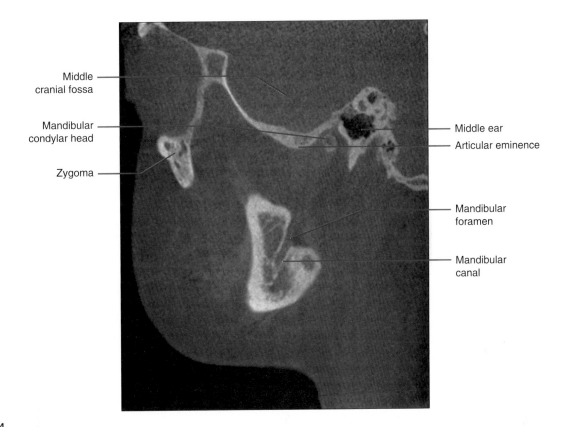

Middle cranial fossa

Mandibular condylar head

Zygoma

Middle ear

Articular eminence

Mandibular foramen

Mandibular canal

Figure 2.24

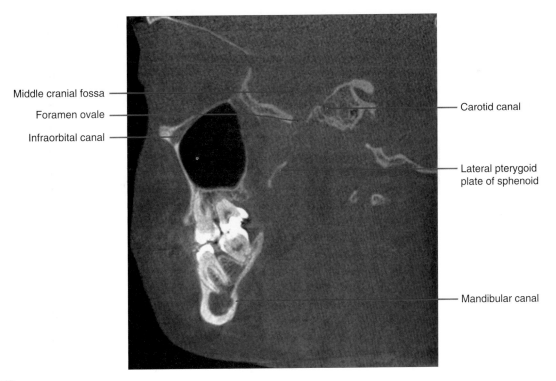

Middle cranial fossa

Foramen ovale

Infraorbital canal

Carotid canal

Lateral pterygoid plate of sphenoid

Mandibular canal

Figure 2.25

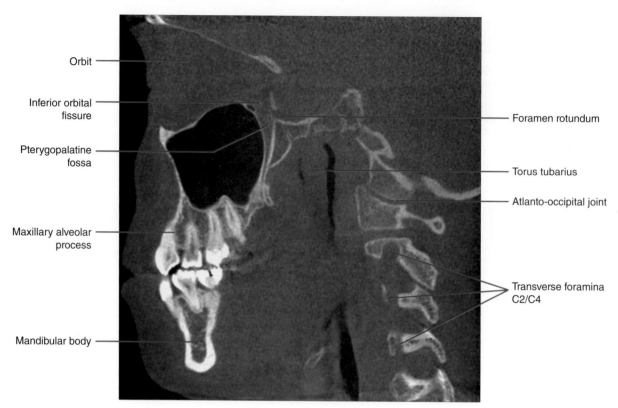

Orbit

Inferior orbital fissure

Pterygopalatine fossa

Maxillary alveolar process

Mandibular body

Foramen rotundum

Torus tubarius

Atlanto-occipital joint

Transverse foramina C2/C4

Figure 2.26

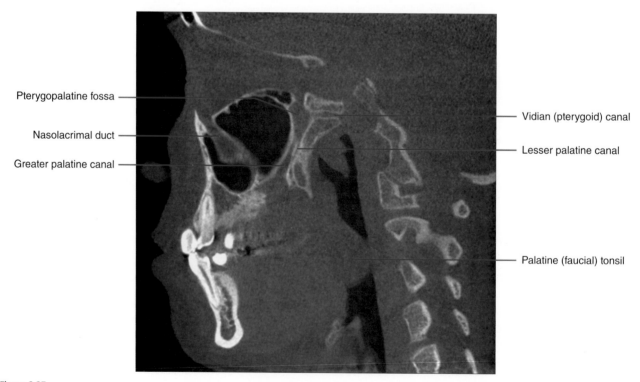

Pterygopalatine fossa

Nasolacrimal duct

Greater palatine canal

Vidian (pterygoid) canal

Lesser palatine canal

Palatine (faucial) tonsil

Figure 2.27

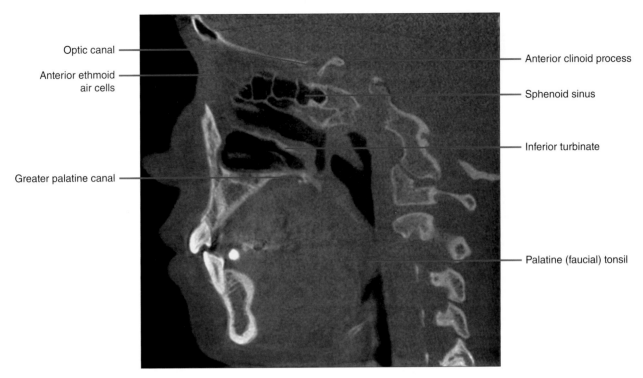

Optic canal

Anterior ethmoid air cells

Greater palatine canal

Anterior clinoid process

Sphenoid sinus

Inferior turbinate

Palatine (faucial) tonsil

Figure 2.28

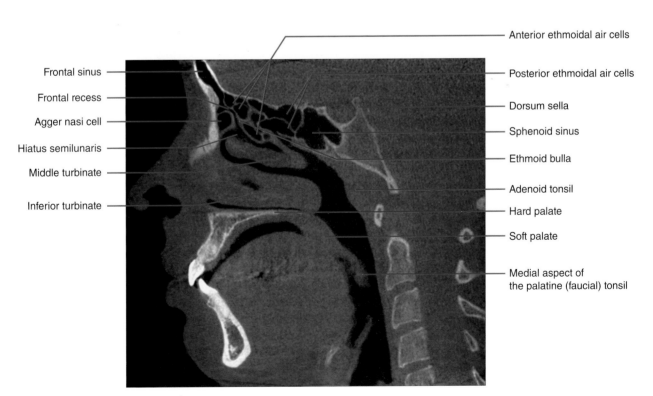

Frontal sinus

Frontal recess

Agger nasi cell

Hiatus semilunaris

Middle turbinate

Inferior turbinate

Anterior ethmoidal air cells

Posterior ethmoidal air cells

Dorsum sella

Sphenoid sinus

Ethmoid bulla

Adenoid tonsil

Hard palate

Soft palate

Medial aspect of the palatine (faucial) tonsil

Figure 2.29

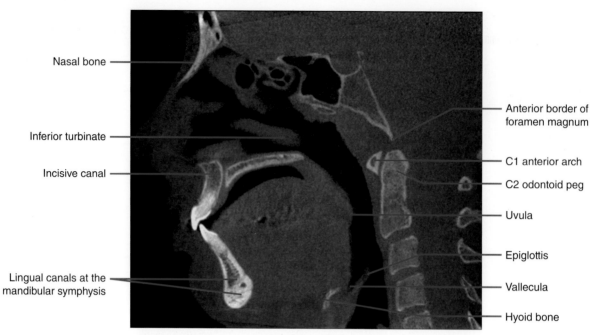

Nasal bone

Inferior turbinate

Incisive canal

Lingual canals at the
mandibular symphysis

Anterior border of
foramen magnum

C1 anterior arch

C2 odontoid peg

Uvula

Epiglottis

Vallecula

Hyoid bone

Figure 2.30

Coronal

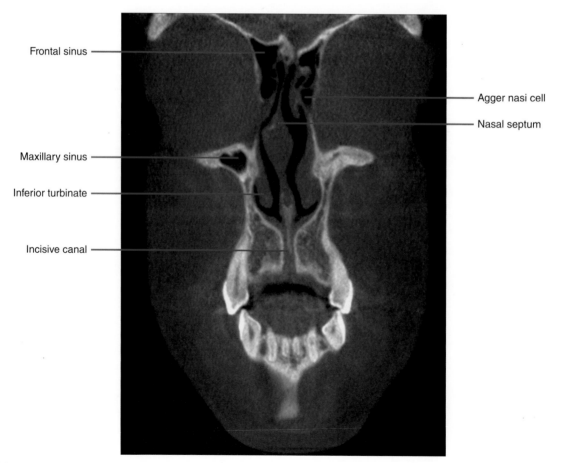

Frontal sinus

Maxillary sinus

Inferior turbinate

Incisive canal

Agger nasi cell

Nasal septum

Figure 2.31

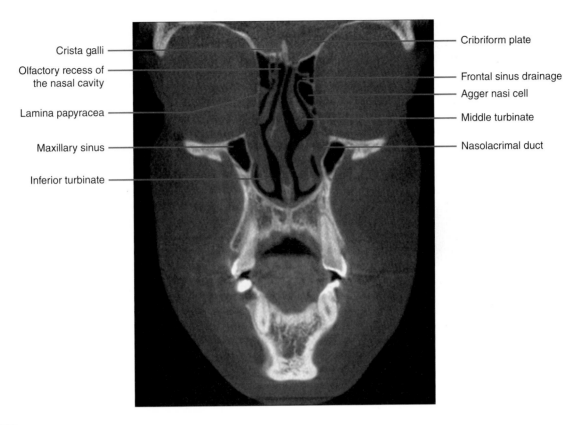

Crista galli — Cribriform plate

Olfactory recess of the nasal cavity — Frontal sinus drainage

— Agger nasi cell

Lamina papyracea — Middle turbinate

Maxillary sinus — Nasolacrimal duct

Inferior turbinate

Figure 2.32

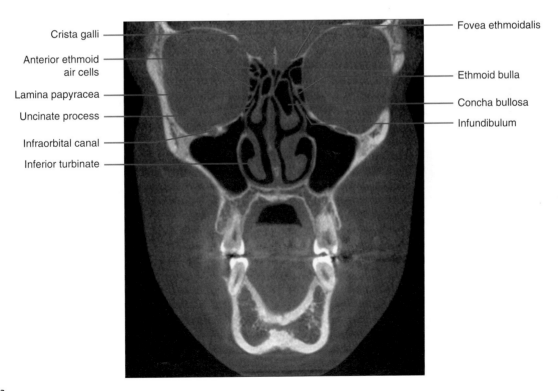

Crista galli — Fovea ethmoidalis

Anterior ethmoid air cells

— Ethmoid bulla

Lamina papyracea — Concha bullosa

Uncinate process — Infundibulum

Infraorbital canal

Inferior turbinate

Figure 2.33

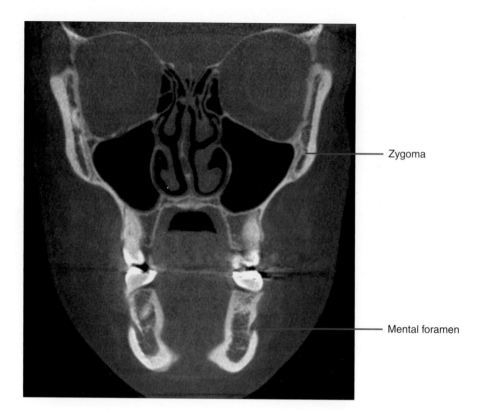

Zygoma

Mental foramen

Figure 2.34

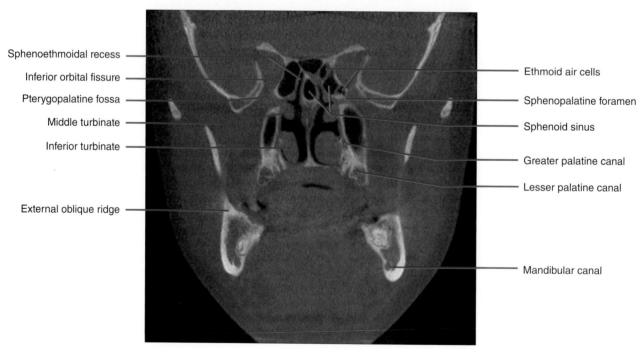

Sphenoethmoidal recess

Inferior orbital fissure

Pterygopalatine fossa

Middle turbinate

Inferior turbinate

External oblique ridge

Ethmoid air cells

Sphenopalatine foramen

Sphenoid sinus

Greater palatine canal

Lesser palatine canal

Mandibular canal

Figure 2.35

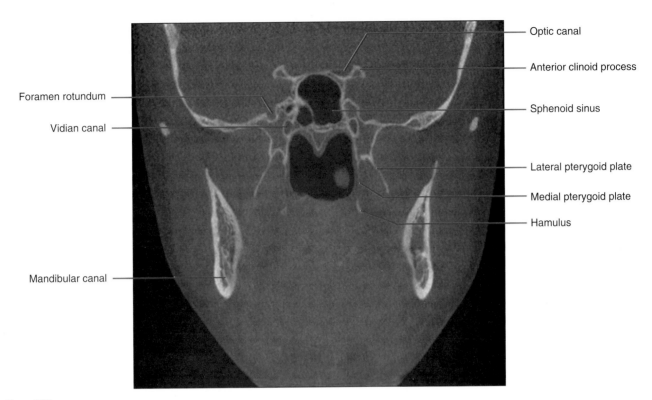

Optic canal

Anterior clinoid process

Foramen rotundum

Sphenoid sinus

Vidian canal

Lateral pterygoid plate

Medial pterygoid plate

Hamulus

Mandibular canal

Figure 2.36

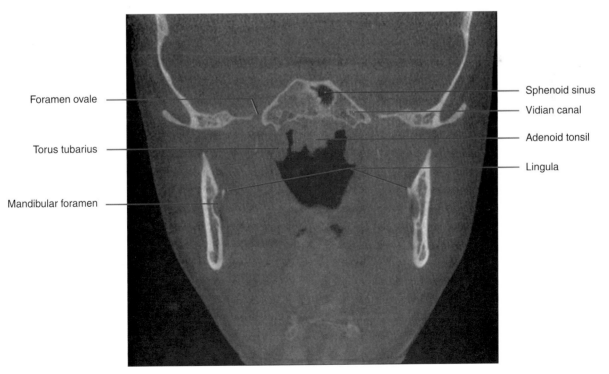

Foramen ovale

Sphenoid sinus

Vidian canal

Torus tubarius

Adenoid tonsil

Lingula

Mandibular foramen

Figure 2.37

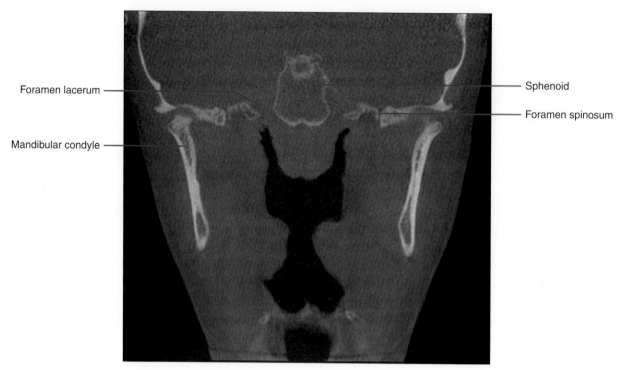

Foramen lacerum

Mandibular condyle

Sphenoid

Foramen spinosum

Figure 2.38

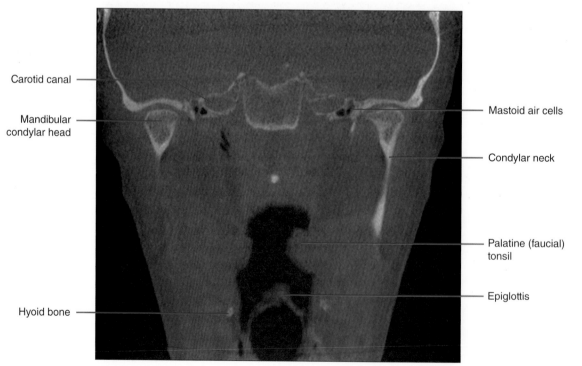

Carotid canal

Mandibular condylar head

Hyoid bone

Mastoid air cells

Condylar neck

Palatine (faucial) tonsil

Epiglottis

Figure 2.39

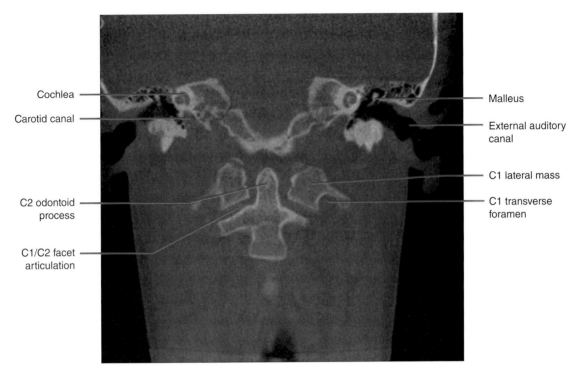

Cochlea

Carotid canal

C2 odontoid process

C1/C2 facet articulation

Malleus

External auditory canal

C1 lateral mass

C1 transverse foramen

Figure 2.40

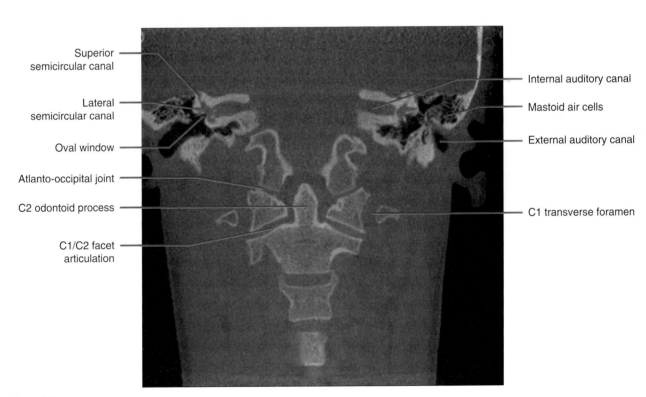

Superior semicircular canal

Lateral semicircular canal

Oval window

Atlanto-occipital joint

C2 odontoid process

C1/C2 facet articulation

Internal auditory canal

Mastoid air cells

External auditory canal

C1 transverse foramen

Figure 2.41

CHAPTER 3

Anomalies Related to the Teeth

3.1 Supernumerary teeth (Figures 3.1–3.5)

- *Synonyms*: hyperdontia, supplemental teeth, mesiodens, paramolars.
- Teeth developing in addition to the normal 32 permanent and 20 deciduous teeth.
- 1–4% of population.
- More common in the permanent dentition. The anterior maxilla and mandibular premolar regions are quite common locations.
- Multiple supernumerary teeth may be associated with some syndromes.
- May affect the normal dentition. For example, crowding, impaction and, less commonly, resorption of the normal teeth.

- Ultra-low-dose cone beam computed tomography (CBCT) or multidetector computed tomography (MDCT) may be required to accurately locate these teeth for removal and also to assess the effects on the adjacent teeth.

Radiological features
- Resemble teeth but the size and morphology may or may not resemble the normal dentition.

Differential diagnosis

	Key radiological differences
Compound odontoma	Dental tissue arrangements are not as close to normal tooth architecture, often demonstrating a clump of multiple tooth-like structures.

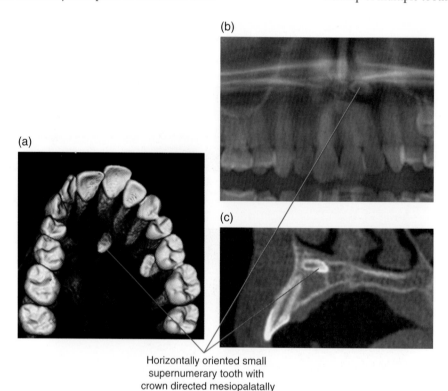

(b)

(a)

(c)

Horizontally oriented small
supernumerary tooth with
crown directed mesiopalatally

Figure 3.1 Supernumerary tooth left premaxilla: surface-rendered CBCT (a), cropped panoramic radiograph (b) and corrected sagittal CBCT (c) images.

Atlas of Oral and Maxillofacial Radiology, First Edition. Bernard Koong.
© 2017 John Wiley & Sons Ltd. Published 2017 by John Wiley & Sons Ltd.

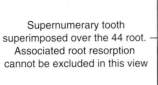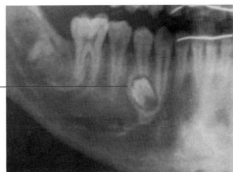

Supernumerary tooth superimposed over the 44 root. Associated root resorption cannot be excluded in this view

Figure 3.2 Supernumerary tooth: cropped panoramic radiograph.

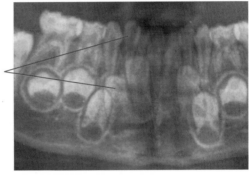

Right anterior mandibular supernumerary deciduous and permanent teeth resembling incisors

Figure 3.3 Supernumerary teeth: cropped panoramic radiograph.

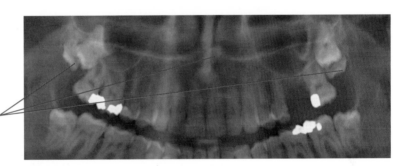

Supernumerary teeth in the 18, 11/21 and 28 regions. The anterior supernumerary tooth is not well demonstrated, being at the edge of the focal trough

Figure 3.4 Supernumerary teeth: cropped panoramic radiograph.

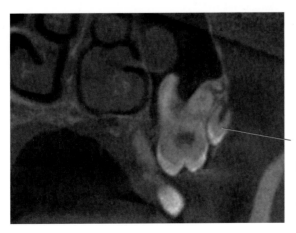

Supernumerary tooth contributes to the impaction of the molar

Figure 3.5 Supernumerary tooth left maxilla: coronal CBCT image.

3.2 Congenital absence (Figures 3.6 and 3.7)

- *Synonyms*: hypodontia, partial or complete anodontia, oligodontia.
- Third molars are most commonly affected, followed by second premolars, maxillary lateral incisors and mandibular central incisors.
- May be seen in ectodermal dysplasia.
- Occasionally, ultra-low-dose CBCT or MDCT may be required to confirm absence where there is suspicion that the tooth is ectopic and may not be visualised within the field of view of the intraoral radiograph or is outside of the focal trough of the panoramic radiograph.

Radiological features
- Absence of normal dentition.

Differential diagnosis

	Key radiological differences
Delayed development	This is occasionally challenging as there is a large variation in the chronology of tooth development and contralateral teeth may also be absent.
Ectopic teeth	Present but not located in the normal position.

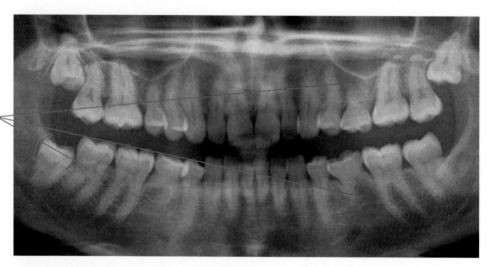

Congenital absence of 25, 35 and 45; 65, 75 and 85 are retained

Figure 3.6 Congenital absence: cropped panoramic radiograph.

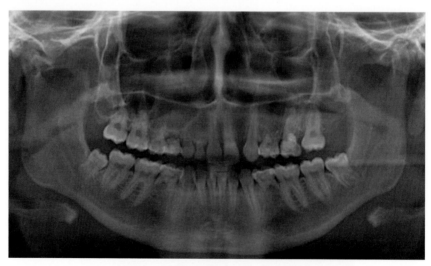

Several congenitally absent permanent teeth. Note several retained deciduous teeth with variable resorption

Figure 3.7 Partial anodontia: panoramic radiograph.

3.3 Delayed and early development/eruption

- Many tables identifying the mean development/eruption times of teeth in relation to chronological age are widely available. However, the wide variation in the chronology of tooth development and eruption is noted.
- Eruption is when a tooth is seen in the oral cavity.
- Several local conditions, including impactions, presence of supernumerary teeth and pathology, can delay tooth eruption and alter development. Ultra-low-dose CBCT or MDCT may be useful for these cases.

Radiological features

- Radiological investigations are often performed to evaluate whether all the teeth are present, and whether entities are present that may interfere with the development and eruption of the teeth.

3.4 Ectopic development and eruption
(Figures 3.8–3.16)

- When a tooth develops and erupts away from its expected native location.
- Transposition is where two adjacent teeth have exchanged positions, most commonly involving the maxillary canines and first premolars.
- It is noted that pathological entities, such as cysts and tumours, can displace teeth.

Radiological features

- A key radiological role in the evaluation of ectopic teeth is to ensure that the ectopic position is developmental in nature and not related to tooth displacement by a pathological entity.
- Ultra-low-dose CBCT or MDCT should be considered, especially if the precise location is required or if there is concern for possible associated abnormality which is not clearly depicted on intraoral and/or panoramic radiography.

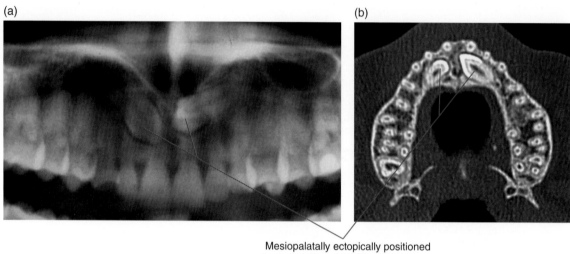

(a) (b)

Mesiopalatally ectopically positioned impacted 13 and 23. The MDCT scan demonstrates no root resorption, which cannot be excluded with the panoramic radiograph

Figure 3.8 Impacted 13 and 23: cropped panoramic radiograph (a) and axial MDCT image (b).

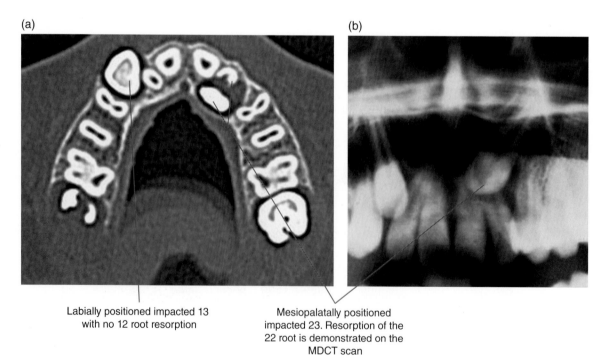

(a) (b)

Labially positioned impacted 13 with no 12 root resorption

Mesiopalatally positioned impacted 23. Resorption of the 22 root is demonstrated on the MDCT scan

Figure 3.9 Impacted 13 and 23: axial MDCT image (a) and cropped panoramic radiograph (b).

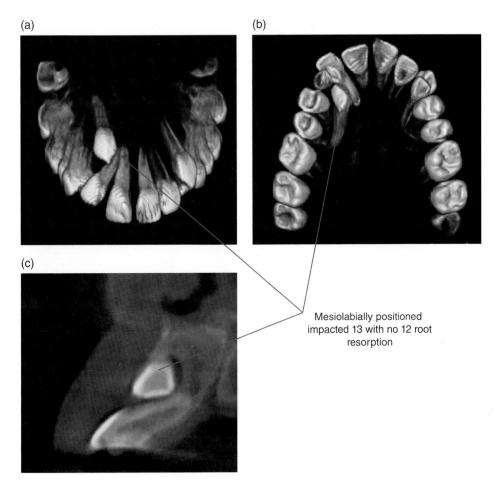

(a)

(b)

(c)

Mesiolabially positioned impacted 13 with no 12 root resorption

Figure 3.10 Impacted 13: surface-rendered (a,b) and cross-sectional (para-axial) (c) CBCT images.

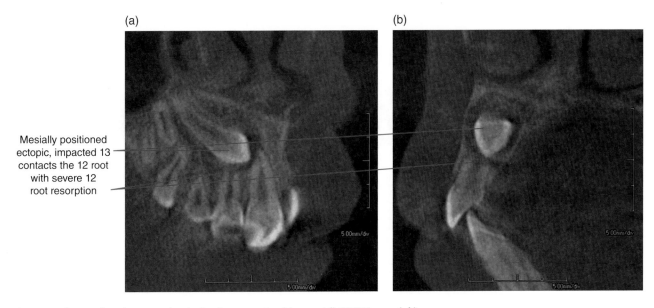

(a)

(b)

Mesially positioned ectopic, impacted 13 contacts the 12 root with severe 12 root resorption

Figure 3.11 Impacted tooth: corrected sagittal and cross-sectional (para-axial) CBCT images (a,b).

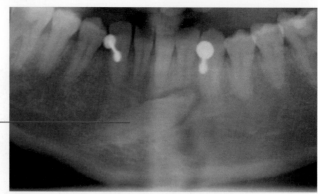

Ectopic 43 with the crown superimposed over the 32 apex where root resorption cannot be excluded

Figure 3.12 Ectopic 43: cropped panoramic radiograph.

(a)

(b)

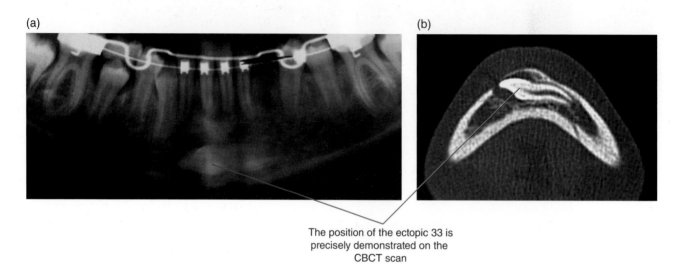

The position of the ectopic 33 is precisely demonstrated on the CBCT scan

Figure 3.13 Ectopic 33: cropped panoramic radiograph (a) and axial CBCT image (b).

(a)

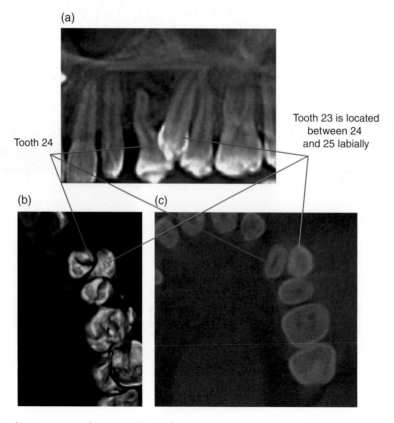

Tooth 24

Tooth 23 is located between 24 and 25 labially

(b)

(c)

Figure 3.14 Transposition 23 and 24: reconstructed panoramic (a), surface-rendered (b) and axial CBCT (c) images.

(a)

(b)

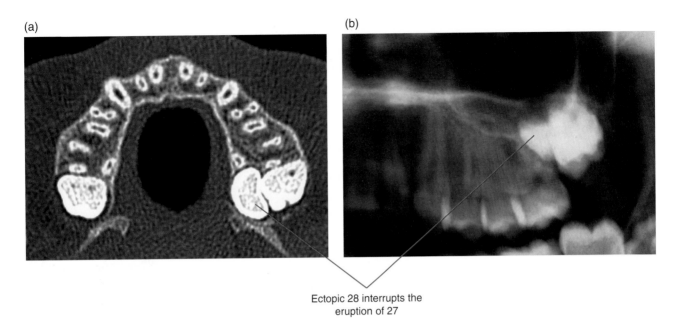

Ectopic 28 interrupts the
eruption of 27

Figure 3.15 Ectopic 28: axial MDCT image (a) and cropped panoramic radiograph (b).

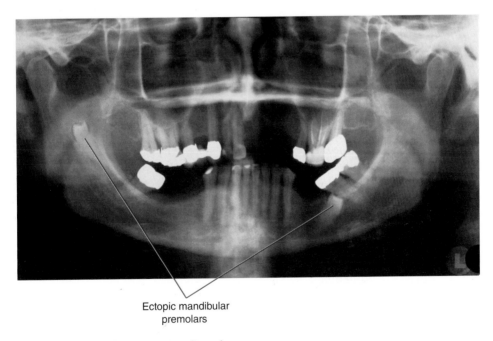

Ectopic mandibular
premolars

Figure 3.16 Two ectopic mandibular premolars: panoramic radiograph.

3.5 Impaction (Figures 3.17–3.23)

- Usually refers to failure of eruption of a tooth where there is a physical obstruction, such as another tooth, dense bone or occasionally soft tissue.
  - The term non-eruption is sometimes used to refer to teeth which do not erupt but do not demonstrate any particular dense physical barrier or pathology obstructing the eruption pathway.
- Most commonly affecting the third molars (especially the mandibular), followed by the maxillary canines. Impacted teeth may be ectopic and/or abnormal in morphology. Supernumerary teeth are often impacted.
- May be associated with:
  - Pericoronitis (refer to Chapter 5).
  - Periodontal bone loss of the adjacent teeth (refer to Chapter 5).
  - Caries (refer to Chapter 4).
  - Root resorption.
  - Cystic and odontogenic tumours (refer to Chapters 8 and 10).
- Like any surgical procedure, extraction of the impacted teeth is associated with potential complications. A particular potential risk associated with the removal of mandibular third molars is damage to the inferior alveolar nerve.

Radiological features

- Ultra-low-dose CBCT and MDCT are the imaging techniques of choice for:
  - Precise location and orientation of the impacted tooth and when the relationship with adjacent anatomical structures is required. Useful features demonstrated by these techniques include the number of roots, root morphology, mandibular and incisive canals, mental foramen, preservation of jaw cortices over the roots and relationship with the maxillary sinus.
  - Evaluation of associated pathology, such as root resorption of the adjacent teeth.
- Third molars:
  - Panoramic radiograph is often employed initially. While it does not depict these impacted teeth as accurately and with as much detail as CBCT and MDCT, it may provide sufficient information. Based upon the appearances in this view, ultra-low-dose CBCT and MDCT are sometimes indicated. Indications include:
    - Mandibular canal appears projected over the third molar roots in the panoramic view.
      - There are radiological criteria (on panoramic radiographs) which have been used. Examples include darkening, narrowing, deviation of the canal and absence of the canal borders when projected over the third molar root. However, the absence of these criteria does not mean that there is no contact of the mandibular canal with the third molar.
    - Complex root anatomy including root dilacerations.
    - Suspicion for substantial cortical fenestrations over the roots.
    - Concern for possible resorption of adjacent teeth. For example, it is not uncommon that impacted teeth are projected over the adjacent teeth on panoramic and dental intraoral radiographs. Root resorption cannot be fully excluded in these views.
    - Suspicion for associated pathology.
  - Classification:
    - Assists in identifying the orientation and relative complexity in extracting the tooth, usually applied to the impacted mandibular third molars.
    - The most commonly used classification describes the orientation of the long axis third molar in relation to those of the adjacent molars.
      - Mesioangular impaction: third molar is mesially inclined.
      - Vertical impaction: third molar demonstrates a similar mesiodistal orientation to the other molars.
      - Distoangular impaction: third molar is distally inclined.
      - Horizontal impaction: third molar is essentially horizontally oriented, with the crown directed mesially.
    - Other additional descriptors sometimes used refer to the direction in which the crown is inclined in the other planes, namely buccal and lingual.
- Impacted canines and supernumerary teeth:
  - Many of these cases are eventually examined with CBCT as it is often difficult to plan the surgical extraction/exposure with panoramic and intraoral radiography, e.g. whether the surgical approach should be buccal or palatal for an impacted maxillary canine. Also, root resorption cannot be excluded nor the extent reliably evaluated with 2D radiography.

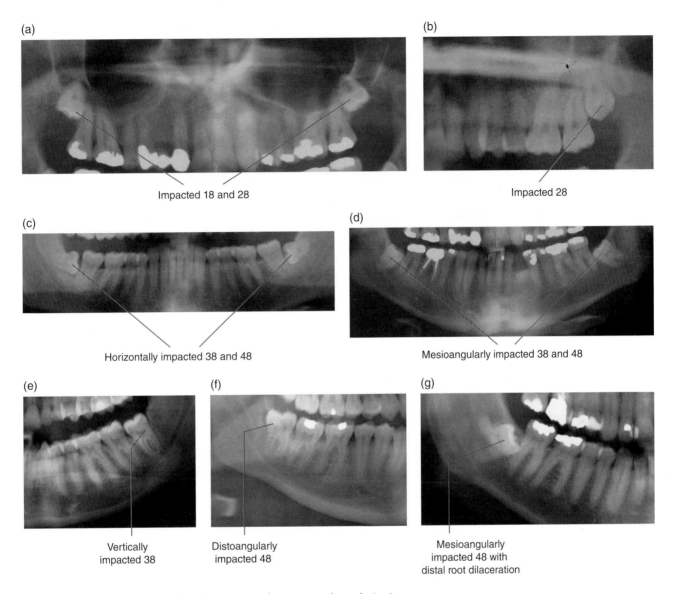

Figure 3.17 Impacted third molars of several cases: cropped panoramic radiographs (a–g).

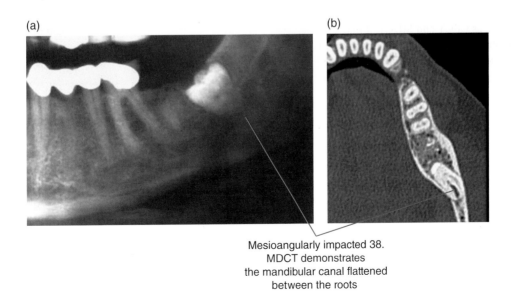

Figure 3.18 Impacted 38: cropped panoramic radiograph (a) and axial MDCT image (b).

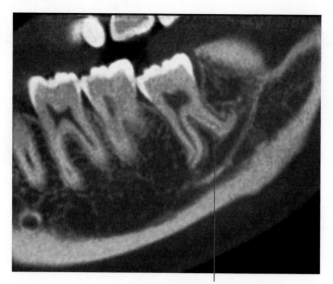

Mesioangularly impacted 38 with
severely dilacerated roots.
Mandibular canal contacts the
inferior surfaces

Figure 3.19 Impacted 38: corrected sagittal CBCT image.

(a)　　　　　　　　　　　　　　　(b)

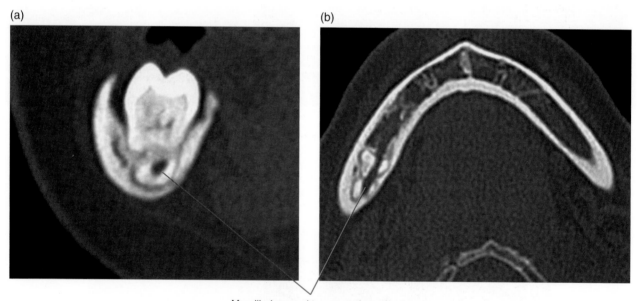

Mandibular canal traverses through
('perforates') the roots of the
impacted 48

Figure 3.20 Impacted 48: corrected coronal (a) and axial (b) MDCT images.

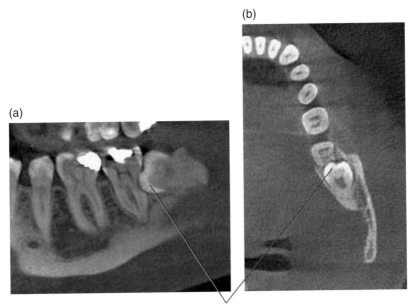

Mesioangularly impacted 38 contributes to
the resorption of 37. Note also the associated
distal periodontal bone loss of 37

Figure 3.21 Impacted 38: corrected sagittal (a) and axial (b) CBCT images.

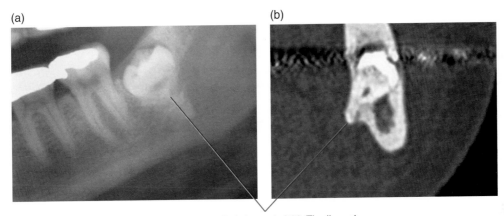

Mesioangularly impacted 38. The lingual
position of the root 'external' to the body of
the mandible, with lingual cortical fenestration,
is demonstrated on the MDCT image

Figure 3.22 Impacted 38: cropped panoramic radiograph (a) and corrected coronal MDCT image (b).

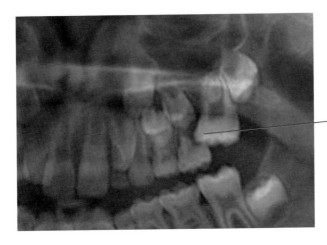

26 is impacted against the distal
aspect of 65 with associated
resorption of the deciduous molar

Figure 3.23 Impacted 26: cropped panoramic radiograph.

3.6 Macrodontia (Figure 3.24)

- Larger than normal teeth.
- Most are likely to be developmental in nature.
- Occasionally seen in association with a vascular malformation or haemangioma.

Radiological features
- Larger than normal tooth.
- Most demonstrate essentially normal morphology.
- May contribute to impactions and crowding.

Differential diagnosis

	Key radiological differences
Gemination	May demonstrate morphology suggesting attempted division of a tooth into two, e.g. grooving of the crown/root.
Fusion	A tooth should be absent.

(a)   (b)

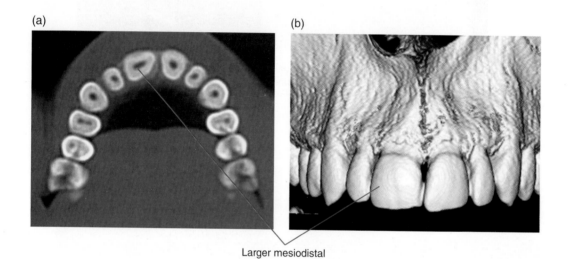

Larger mesiodistal
dimension of 11
compared with 21

Figure 3.24 Macrodontic 11: axial (a) and surface-rendered (b) CBCT images.

3.7 Microdontia (Figures 3.25–3.27)

- Smaller than normal teeth.
- Most are likely to be developmental in nature. May be familial.
- Most commonly affecting third molars and maxillary lateral incisors.
- Occasionally related to childhood incident, e.g. chemotherapy.

Radiological features
- Smaller than normal tooth.
- Often demonstrates altered morphology, e.g. a microdontic lateral incisor often has a conical crown.

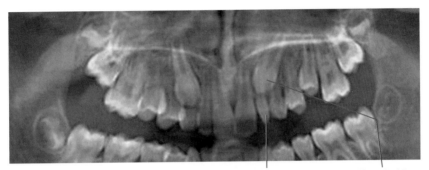

Small 22 with conical ('pegged') coronal morphology   Ectopic 23

Figure 3.25 Microdontic 22: cropped panoramic radiograph.

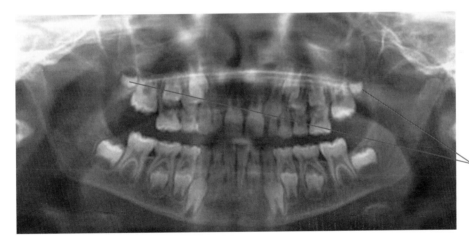

Small crowns of maxillary second molars

Figure 3.26 Microdontic 17 and 27: cropped panoramic radiograph.

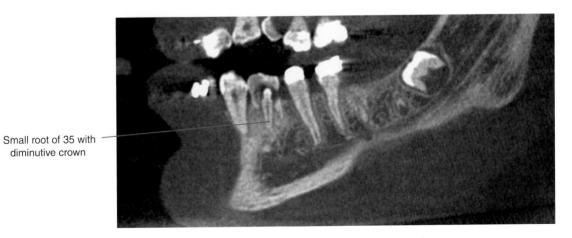

Small root of 35 with diminutive crown

Figure 3.27 Microdontic 35 related to chemotherapy: corrected sagittal CBCT.

3.8 Dilaceration (Figure 3.28)

- A distinct bend of a tooth crown or root. Root dilacerations are much more common.
- Most are likely to be developmental in nature. Some may be related to trauma during tooth development.
- May interfere with orthodontic tooth movement.

Radiological features
- Appearance of a distinct bend in the crown or root of a tooth.
- This may not be appreciated on 2D intraoral or the panoramic radiograph or it may appear as a focal increased density.
- CBCT or MDCT more accurately identify and demonstrate the precise morphology of dilacerations.

(a)

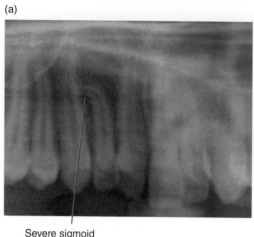

Severe sigmoid
dilaceration of the 22 root

(b)

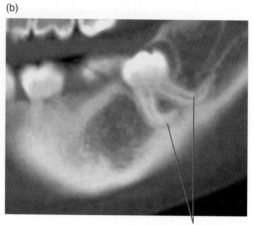

Severe root dilacerations of 38,
with root apices directed
posterosuperiorly

Figure 3.28 Root dilacerations of two separate cases: cropped panoramic radiograph (a) and corrected sagittal CBCT image (b).

3.9 Enamel pearl (Figure 3.29)

- *Synonym*: enameloma.
- A small focal enamel prominence on the root, usually less than 3 mm, developmental in nature. Larger pearls may demonstrate a small amount of dentin at the base centrally.
- Almost all are seen on molar roots, often at the cervical and furcation regions.
- May have relevance to the progression and management of plaque-related inflammatory periodontal disease.

Radiological features
- Smooth, round, well-defined enamel density focus.
- May not be detected with 2D intraoral or panoramic radiographs.

Differential diagnosis

	Key radiological differences
Pulp stone	Within the pulp chamber or root canal of the tooth. The enamel pearl is more opaque than the pulp stone.

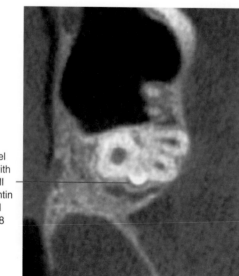

Focal enamel
prominence with
central small
amount of dentin
at the distal
surface of 28
cervically

Figure 3.29 Enamel pearl 28: axial CBCT image.

3.10 Talon cusp (Figure 3.30)

- An additional cusp of an incisor, thought to be related to an extremely prominent cingulum.
- Developmental in nature.

Radiological features

- Appearance of an opaque cusp-like structure over the incisor crown on 2D intraoral or panoramic radiographs. Clinically obvious when erupted.

Differential diagnosis

	Key radiological differences
Supernumerary tooth	May require volumetric imaging (CBCT or MDCT) to clarify.
Odontoma	May require volumetric imaging (CBCT or MDCT) to clarify.

(a)   (b)

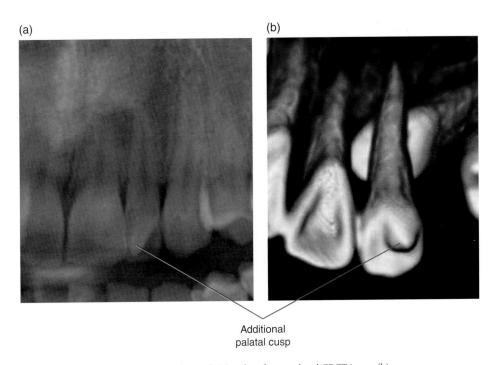

Additional
palatal cusp

Figure 3.30 Talon cusp of two cases: cropped panoramic radiograph (a) and surface-rendered CBCT image (b).

3.11 Dens invaginatus (Figures 3.31 and 3.32)

- *Synonym*: dens in dente.
- Invagination of enamel into the crown, to varying extents.
- Occurs most frequently in the maxillary lateral incisors.
- Associated with increased risk of pulpal and periapical inflammatory disease:
  - Infolded enamel is often defective, including canals which lead to the pulp.
  - Usually, a deep pit connects this with the oral cavity, with resultant increased caries risk.

- Radicular invaginations are rare, and involve infolding of cementum.

Radiological features

- Variable invagination of the pit or incisal edge.
- Larger invaginations are associated with altered crown morphology.
- There may be incomplete root development and/or periapical inflammatory lesions, related to the death of the pulp tissues.

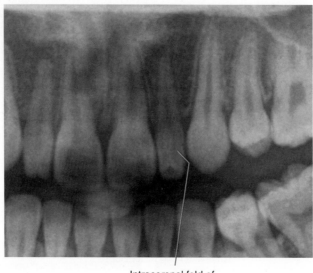

Intracoronal fold of
enamel with central
lucency

Figure 3.31 Dens invaginatus 22: cropped panoramic radiograph.

(a) (b)

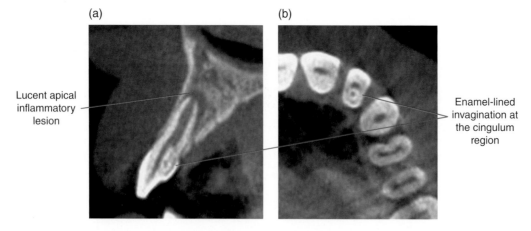

Lucent apical
inflammatory
lesion

Enamel-lined
invagination at
the cingulum
region

Figure 3.32 Dens invaginatus 22: cross-sectional (para-axial) (a) and axial (b) CBCT images.

3.12 Dens evaginatus (Figure 3.33)

- Small focal enamel prominence at the occlusal surfaces of posterior teeth or lingual surfaces of anterior teeth.
- Often demonstrates dentin centrally and there may be an associated pulp horn.
- More commonly affecting premolars and lateral incisors.
- Associated with increased risk of pulpal and periapical inflammatory disease.

Radiological features

- Focal enamel prominence, usually with dentin centrally. A fine pulp horn is often only visualised in volumetric (CBCT or MDCT) imaging.
- There may be incomplete root development and/or periapical inflammatory lesions, related to the death of the pulp tissues.

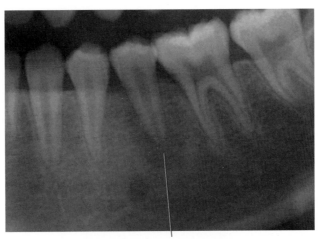

While evagination is (typically) not well demonstrated on this image, a patient will sometimes present with an apical inflammatory lesion, with no other identifiable potential cause (e.g. substantial caries or a deep restoration)

Figure 3.33 Dens evaginatus: cropped panoramic radiograph.

3.13 Taurodontism (Figure 3.34)

- Longer body of the tooth with shorter roots.
- Likely to be a normal variant in most cases. Reported to occur more frequently in trisomy 21 syndrome.

Radiological features

- Appearance of a longer body with short roots, and a normal crown.

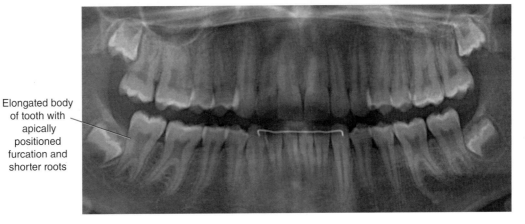

Elongated body of tooth with apically positioned furcation and shorter roots

Figure 3.34 Taurodontic first and second molars: cropped panoramic radiograph.

3.14 Fusion (Figures 3.35 and 3.36)

- Union of two normally separate tooth germs, to varying extents.
- More common in the deciduous dentition.
- More commonly associated with anterior teeth.

Radiological features

- Appearance of the two fused teeth varies depending on the stage and anatomic relationship.

- Effectively, one tooth is absent. Rarely, there may be fusion of a normal tooth with a supernumerary tooth.

Differential diagnosis

	Key radiological differences
Gemination	No missing teeth.

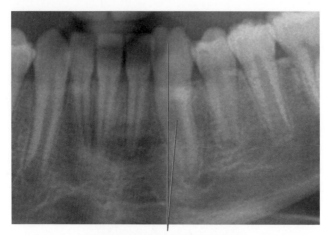

Large appearance of the fused root.
Note the residual cleft at the incisal
edge, related to the incomplete fusion

Figure 3.35 Fusion 33 and 32: cropped panoramic radiograph.

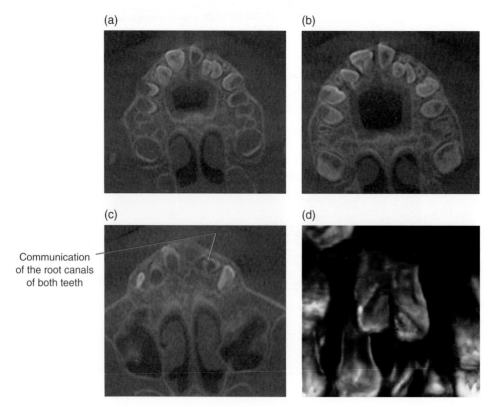

(a)   (b)

(c)   (d)

Communication
of the root canals
of both teeth

Figure 3.36 Fusion 22 and 23: axial (a–c) and surface-rendered (d) CBCT images.

3.15 **Gemination** (Figure 3.37)

- Incomplete division of a single tooth bud, to varying extents.
- More common in the deciduous dentition.

Radiological features
- Appearances vary depending on the degree of division.

Differential diagnosis

Key radiological differences

Fusion   One tooth is absent, unless there is fusion with a supernumerary tooth.

3.16 **Concrescence** (Figure 3.38)

- The joining of roots of normally separate teeth with cementum.
- Most commonly affects the maxillary molars.

- May interfere with tooth eruption.
- Extraction of these teeth can be challenging.

Radiological features
- Definite identification of concrescence with 2D intraoral and panoramic radiography is difficult.
- CBCT or MDCT is more accurate; absence of the periodontal ligament space is often a key feature.
  - However, it is sometimes difficult to fully exclude root contact with no cemental bridging, where the periodontal ligament space is present but extremely narrow and subresolution.

Differential diagnosis

Key radiological differences

Fusion   Can be difficult to differentiate when fusion is limited to the roots. It is difficult to radiologically identify whether the roots are connected with cementum (concrescence) or dentin (fusion).

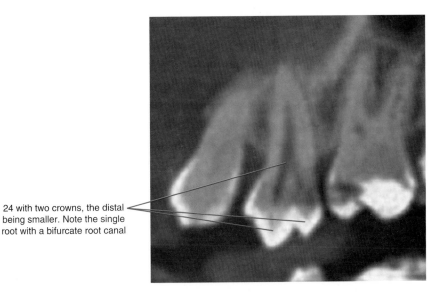

24 with two crowns, the distal being smaller. Note the single root with a bifurcate root canal

Figure 3.37 Gemination: corrected sagittal CBCT image.

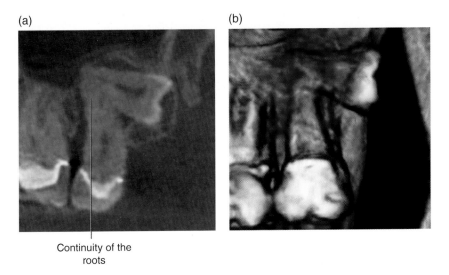

(a)   (b)

Continuity of the roots

Figure 3.38 Concrescence 27 and 28: corrected sagittal (a) and surface-rendered (b) CBCT images.

3.17 Amelogenesis imperfecta (Figure 3.39)

- Inherited abnormal enamel formation not associated with other diseases.
- Related to malfunction of the proteins which form the largely mineral content of enamel.
- Many variants with variable enamel abnormalities. Four main types have been described: hypoplasia, hypomaturation, hypocalcification and hypomaturation/hypocalcification. The clinical appearances are well described.
- Rare.
- May be more susceptible to caries.

Radiological features

Compared with normal enamel

Hypoplasia	Thinner but normal density. Flatter occlusal surfaces, especially when fully erupted (attrition), contribute to a square appearance of the crowns. Focal lucent defects may be seen. The anterior teeth may demonstrate the 'picket fence' appearance.
Hypomaturation	Normal thickness but decreased density, usually isodense with dentin. Post eruption attrition and enamel fractures are often seen.
Hypocalcification	Normal thickness but decreased density, hypodense to dentin. Post eruption attrition and enamel fractures are often seen.
Hypomaturation/ hypocalcification	Usually isodense with dentin. The enamel may be thin.
All four types	The dentin and the roots are normal. Pulpal obliteration (opacification) may occur when there is severe attrition.

Differential diagnosis

Key radiological differences

Dentinogenesis imperfecta	Bulbous crowns and narrow roots are features of dentinogenesis imperfecta.

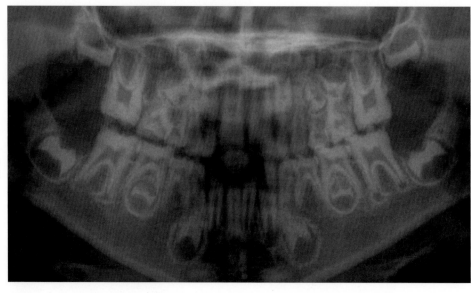

The enamel is not visualised. Square appearance of the crowns noted

Figure 3.39 Amelogenesis imperfecta: cropped panoramic radiograph.

3.18 Dentinogenesis imperfecta (Figure 3.40)

- Hereditary abnormal dentin formation.
- Three types (types I, II and III), each associated with specific genetic defects.
- Can be associated with osteogenesis imperfecta (type I).
- Clinical appearances are well described.
- Dental restorative management is often challenging.

Radiological features
- Narrow cervical aspect of the crown, resulting in a bulbous crown appearance.
- There is often substantial attrition of erupted teeth.
- Usually short and narrow roots.

- Varying degrees of pulpal obliteration (opacification), although some may demonstrate large pulp chambers early in development.

Differential diagnosis

	Key radiological differences
Dentin dysplasia	Can be similar in appearance.
	Type I dentin dysplasia: presence of crescent-shaped pulp morphology favours dentin dysplasia.
	Type II dentin dysplasia: bulbous crown morphology is a feature of dentinogenesis imperfecta.

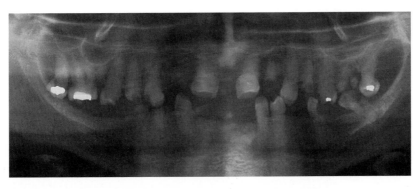

Bulbous crown appearances. Marked pulpal opacification

Figure 3.40 Dentinogenesis imperfecta: cropped panoramic radiograph.

3.19 Dentin dysplasia (Figures 3.41 and 3.42)

- Hereditary dentin abnormality.
- Similar appearance to dentinogenesis imperfecta but rarer.
- Two types: type I (radicular) and type II (coronal).
- There may be misalignment of teeth and abnormal exfoliation.

Radiological features

- Type I (radicular):
  - Short and/or abnormal (often conical) root morphology. Usually normal crown morphology.
  - Pulps are largely obliterated (opacified) pre-eruption. A residual crescent-shaped pulp chamber may be seen.
  - Higher risk of non-caries-related periapical inflammatory lesions.
- Type II (coronal):
  - Normal roots. Usually normal crown morphology.
  - Obliteration (opacification) of the pulp occurs post eruption.
  - 'Thistle tube' pulp morphology of the permanent teeth (usually single-rooted teeth) may be seen, sometimes with pulp stones.
  - Higher risk of non-caries-related periapical inflammatory lesions.

Differential diagnosis

	Key radiological differences
Dentinogenesis imperfecta	Can be similar in appearance.
	Type I dentin dysplasia: presence of crescent-shaped pulp morphology favours dentin dysplasia.
	Type II dentin dysplasia: bulbous crown morphology is a feature of dentinogenesis imperfecta.

Opacification and reduction in the size of coronal pulp chambers and the root canals

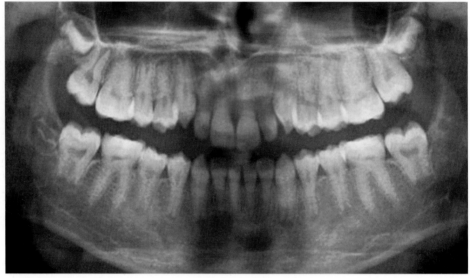

Figure 3.41 Dentin dysplasia: cropped panoramic radiograph.

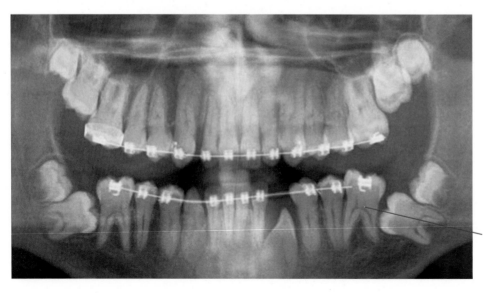

Opacification and reduction in the size of the pulp chambers, some demonstrating 'thistle tube' morphology. Decrease in the dimension of the root canals

Figure 3.42 Dentin dysplasia: cropped panoramic radiograph.

3.20 Secondary and tertiary dentin

(Figures 3.43 and 3.44)

- Secondary dentin is considered as the physiological continued laying down of dentin post completion of root development.
- Tertiary dentin (reparative or sclerotic dentin) usually refers to the dentin which is laid down as a response to a specific stimulus, e.g. caries.

Radiological features

- Secondary and tertiary dentin are isodense with primary dentin (dentin formed during tooth development).
- Secondary dentin formation reduces the size of the pulp. The pulp morphology is generally maintained but the pulp chamber often appears to be relatively smaller than the root canals with age, especially the pulp horns.
- The morphology of tertiary dentin can vary, depending on the stimulus, usually altering the morphology of the pulp chamber.

Differential diagnosis

Key radiological differences

Pulpal sclerosis (diffused pulpal calcifications)

With age, substantial secondary dentin formation (± tertiary dentin) may almost or completely obliterate the pulp and this can appear similar to pulpal sclerosis, especially on intraoral and panoramic radiography.

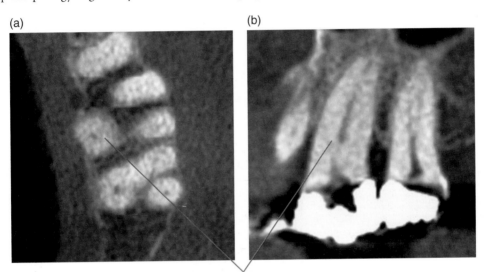

(a)   (b)

Reduction in the size of root canals in the visualised teeth

Figure 3.43 Secondary dentin: axial (a) and corrected sagittal (b) CBCT images.

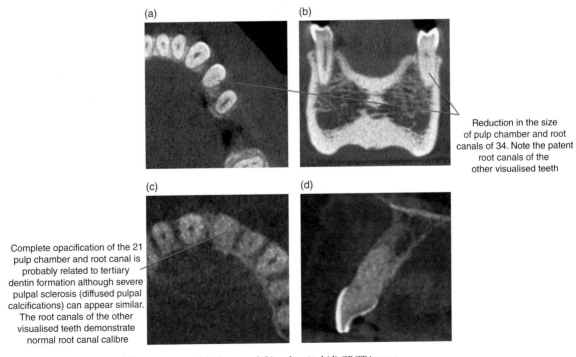

(a)   (b)

Reduction in the size of pulp chamber and root canals of 34. Note the patent root canals of the other visualised teeth

(c)   (d)

Complete opacification of the 21 pulp chamber and root canal is probably related to tertiary dentin formation although severe pulpal sclerosis (diffused pulpal calcifications) can appear similar. The root canals of the other visualised teeth demonstrate normal root canal calibre

Figure 3.44 Tertiary dentin of two different cases: axial (a,c), coronal (b) and sagittal (d) CBCT images.

3.21 **Pulp stones** (Figure 3.45)

- Relatively common calcific foci within the pulp.
- Generally considered idiopathic, possibly a normal variant.
- May be seen in type II dentin dysplasia.

Radiological features
- Opaque foci within the pulp chamber and/or root canal. Variable in numbers and morphology.
- Many pulp stones are subresolution or insufficiently dense to be identified radiologically.

Differential diagnosis

Pulpal sclerosis (diffused pulpal calcifications)

Enamel pearl

Key radiological differences

Multiple extremely small pulp stones can appear similar to pulpal sclerosis, especially on intraoral and panoramic radiography.

Can appear similar on intraoral and panoramic radiography if the enamel pearl is projected over the pulp. The enamel pearl is denser.

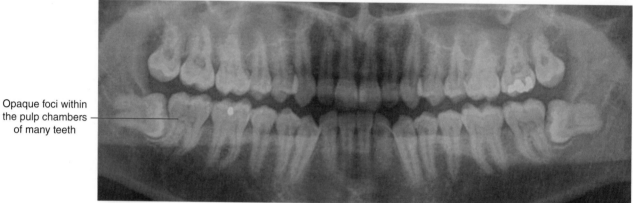

Opaque foci within the pulp chambers of many teeth

Figure 3.45 Pulp stones: cropped panoramic radiograph.

3.22 Hypercementosis (Figures 3.46 and 3.47; see also Figure 5.39)

- Non-neoplastic excessive deposition of cementum over tooth roots.
- Most cases are idiopathic.
- May be seen in association with increased/decreased occlusal loading, chronic periapical inflammatory lesions, Paget disease and hyperpituitarism.
- Asymptomatic and the hypercementosis itself does not require treatment. A primary cause, if present, may require management.
- Extraction can be more difficult.

Radiological features

- Bulbous enlargement of the root with preservation of the periodontal ligament space. Occasionally irregular morphology.
- The excessive cementum often appears slightly hypodense to dentin.

Differential diagnosis

Key radiological differences

Other opaque entities	May be projected over a root on 2D intraoral and panoramic radiography. CBCT or MDCT may be required to clarify.
Ankylosis	It can be difficult to identify the presence and location of the periodontal ligament space. Therefore, it can be difficult to differentiate hypercementosis from ankylosis with dense periradicular bone. CBCT or MDCT may be useful although the periodontal ligament space may be present but thin and subresolution.

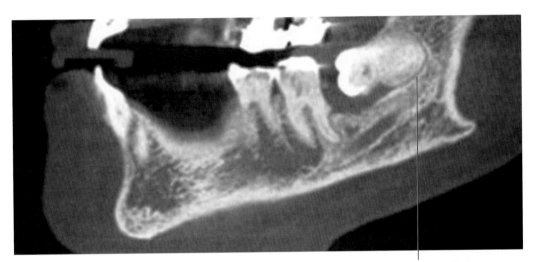

Prominent bulbous radicular appearance isodense with cementum. Note the classically preserved periodontal ligament space surrounding this prominence

Figure 3.46 Hypercementosis 38: corrected sagittal MDCT image.

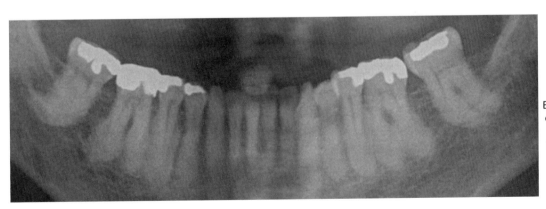

Bulbous prominences of the posterior tooth roots with slightly variable morphology

Figure 3.47 Hypercementosis posterior teeth: cropped panoramic radiograph.

CHAPTER 4
Conditions Related to Loss of Tooth Structure

Tom Huang and Bernard Koong

4.1 Caries (Figures 4.1–4.12)

- Bacterial demineralisation of tooth structure.
- Related to bacterial dental plaque formation and presence of simple sugars.
- The clinical features are well described.
- Usually asymptomatic until the lesion approximates or involves the pulp.
- Most common direct and indirect cause of pulpal pathology and associated periapical inflammatory lesions.
- Several factors contribute to the presence of caries, notably xerostomia.
- Treatment varies from improved oral hygiene, topical fluoride to a range of restorative ('fillings') procedures as well as the management of contributing factors, when present.
- Recurrent caries are lesions which occur at the margins of restorations (Figure 4.12).
- Clinical and radiological diagnosis of caries can be challenging.
  - Radiological identification of a carious lesion, unless obvious, should be verified clinically.
    - While not without limitations, intraoral 2D radiography remains the imaging modality of choice.
    - Caries cannot be fully excluded with the panoramic radiograph, although many lesions can be identified, especially moderate and large lesions.
    - Although the precise morphology and extent of carious lesions can be well demonstrated with cone beam computed tomography (CBCT) and multidetector computed tomography (MDCT), the application of these techniques in caries diagnosis requires further clarification. There has been concern with specificity. When present, artefacts related to restorations substantially reduce the ability to identify carious lesions.

Interproximal caries (Figures 4.1–4.7)

- Originate at the mesial and distal surfaces of the crowns, usually between the contact point and the gingival margin.

Radiological features

- Within the enamel, the early lesion presents as a relatively well-defined triangular-shaped lucency with the base at the enamel surface. This triangular morphology is lost as the lesion enlarges. Enamel lesions can also present with a more linear morphology.
- When the lesion reaches the dentinoenamel junction (DEJ), it spreads out along the DEJ, resulting in the appearance of a relatively ill-defined triangular lucency within the dentin. The base of this second triangular lucency is at the DEJ with the apex directed towards the pulp. However, other presentations, such as more linear or rounded appearances, are possible.
- As the lesion progresses, it takes on a generally rounded morphology, usually progressing quicker within the dentin than within the enamel. Large lesions usually present with more substantial dentin involvement, undermining the overlying enamel, which may fracture. Extremely large lesions often contribute to complete or near complete loss of the entire tooth crown.
- On CBCT and MDCT, the lucent lesions usually demonstrate a more well-defined appearance than is seen on intraoral or panoramic radiographs, especially the lesions within dentin.

Differential diagnosis

	Key radiological differences
Cervical burnout	Artefactual and seen on intraoral and panoramic radiographs. Present as lucencies in the interproximal regions but usually extends from the cementoenamel junction to the interdental alveolar crest.
Lucent or absent (lost) restoration	Usually more well defined and may demonstrate sharp surgically prepared angles.

Pit and fissure caries (Figures 4.8–4.10; see also Figure 5.4)

- Caries originating at developmental pits and fissures, usually at the occlusal, buccal and palatal aspects of the crown, most common at the occlusal pit or fissure.

Atlas of Oral and Maxillofacial Radiology, First Edition. Bernard Koong.
© 2017 John Wiley & Sons Ltd. Published 2017 by John Wiley & Sons Ltd.

Radiological features

- 2D radiographs: the dentin lucency is usually seen first, subjacent to enamel. The enamel lesion is usually not seen unless large. It is difficult to identify if these lesions are buccal, lingual or occlusal although the occlusal dentin lesion appears more centred against the occlusal enamel.
- On CBCT and MDCT: the dentin lucency is usually more well defined and the location is better demonstrated. The enamel lesion may be seen.
- When large, cavitation often occurs.

Differential diagnosis

	Key radiological differences
Deep pits and fissures	It is often difficult to differentiate these from carious lesions. Clinical correlation is important.

Root caries (Figure 4.11)

- Caries involving the root surface, usually accompanied with gingival recession.

Radiological features

- Seen as lucent lesions apical to the cementoenamel junction.
- Usually coronal to the alveolar crest. Occasionally extend beyond the alveolar crest.

Differential diagnosis

	Key radiological differences
Cervical burnout	Artefactual and seen on bitewings or periapical radiographs. Present as lucencies in the interproximal regions but usually extends from the cementoenamel junction to the interdental alveolar crest.

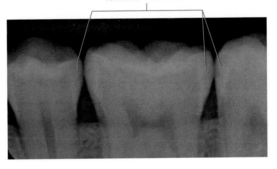

Well-defined triangular-shaped lucency within the enamel with the apex directed towards the DEJ

Figure 4.1 Proximal (mesial and distal) enamel caries: cropped intraoral bitewing radiograph.

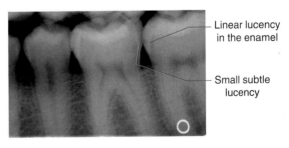

Linear lucency in the enamel

Small subtle lucency

Figure 4.2 Proximal enamel caries, 36 and 37: cropped intraoral bitewing radiograph.

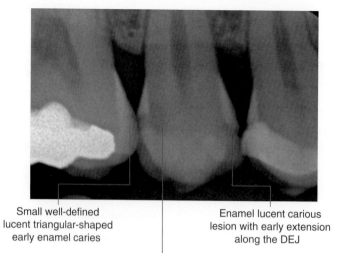

Small well-defined
lucent triangular-shaped
early enamel caries

Enamel lucent carious
lesion with early extension
along the DEJ

Ill-defined triangular-shaped
lucency in the dentin
with the apex directed
towards the pulp

Figure 4.3 Proximal enamel and dentin caries: intraoral bitewing radiograph.

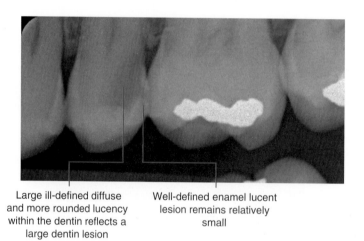

Large ill-defined diffuse
and more rounded lucency
within the dentin reflects a
large dentin lesion

Well-defined enamel lucent
lesion remains relatively
small

Figure 4.4 Caries within distal enamel and dentin, 25: cropped intraoral bitewing radiograph.

(a) (b)

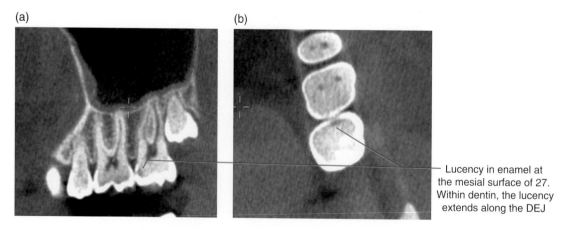

Lucency in enamel at
the mesial surface of 27.
Within dentin, the lucency
extends along the DEJ

Figure 4.5 Caries in mesial enamel and dentin, 27: corrected sagittal (a) and axial (b) CBCT images.

(a)

(b)

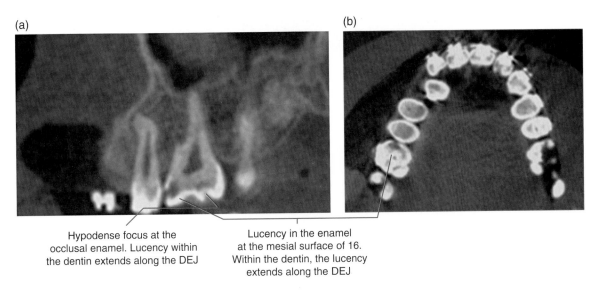

Hypodense focus at the
occlusal enamel. Lucency within
the dentin extends along the DEJ

Lucency in the enamel
at the mesial surface of 16.
Within the dentin, the lucency
extends along the DEJ

Figure 4.6 Caries in mesial and occlusal enamel and dentin, 16: corrected sagittal (a) and axial (b) CBCT images.

(a)

(b)

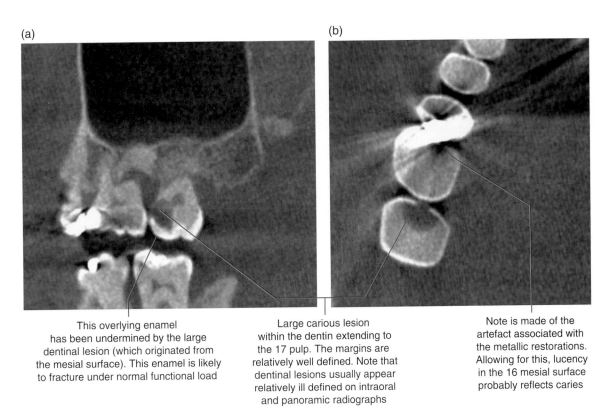

This overlying enamel
has been undermined by the large
dentinal lesion (which originated from
the mesial surface). This enamel is likely
to fracture under normal functional load

Large carious lesion
within the dentin extending to
the 17 pulp. The margins are
relatively well defined. Note that
dentinal lesions usually appear
relatively ill defined on intraoral
and panoramic radiographs

Note is made of the
artefact associated with
the metallic restorations.
Allowing for this, lucency
in the 16 mesial surface
probably reflects caries

Figure 4.7 Caries in mesial enamel and dentin, 17 and 16: corrected sagittal (a) and axial (b) CBCT images.

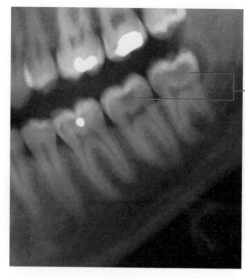

Relatively large ill-defined lucency within the dentin centred at the occlusal DEJ of the 38 and 37 crowns. The enamel lesions are not demonstrated

Figure 4.8 Occlusal caries, 37 and 38: cropped panoramic radiograph.

(a)

(b)

Large ill-defined lucent occlusal caries within 47

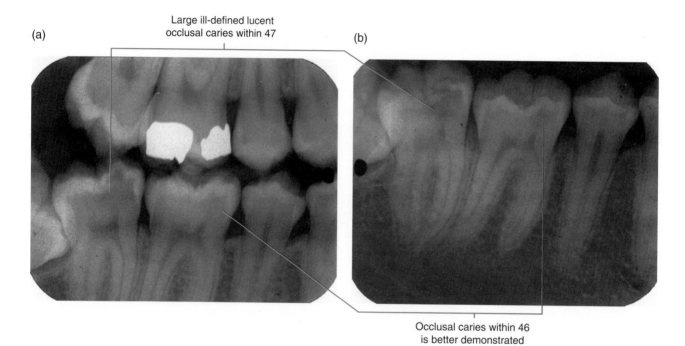

Occlusal caries within 46 is better demonstrated on the periapical radiograph, with a slight negative angulation

Figure 4.9 Occlusal caries: intraoral bitewing (a) and periapical (b) radiographs.

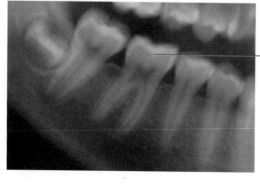

Small round lucency at the centre of 46 at the DEJ reflects the buccal pit, a normal anatomical feature

Figure 4.10 Buccal pit: cropped panoramic radiograph.

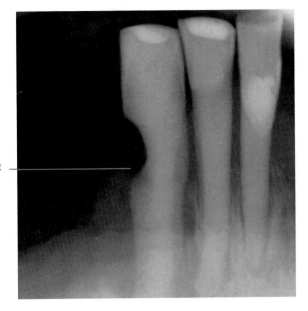

The cervical aspect of this lucent defect demonstrates the typically ill-defined border of root caries. The well-defined border superiorly is related to toothbrush abrasion. Note the periodontal bone loss

Figure 4.11 Root caries at abrasion defect, 43: intraoral periapical radiograph.

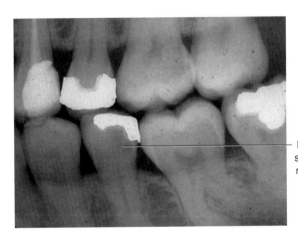

Ill-defined lucency subjacent to the 35 restoration reflects recurrent caries

Figure 4.12 Recurrent caries: intraoral bitewing radiograph.

4.2 Attrition (Figure 4.13)

- Gradual loss of tooth structure from contact of teeth; related to mechanical forces.
- Most often seen at the incisal and occlusal surfaces where opposing teeth contact. Occasionally at the interproximal surfaces.
- May eventually involve the dentin.
- When the degree of attrition is age appropriate, it is usually considered physiological.
- Parafunctional activities, including clenching and bruxism ('grinding'), are common causes of excessive or pathological attrition.
- Other factors, including diet, saliva and resistance of the tooth crown to mechanical wear, may influence the rate of attrition.
- Only affects erupted teeth, so this condition is clinically observable.

- Not uncommonly seen in the deciduous teeth in children, presumably related to bruxism, which often ceases as permanent teeth erupt.
- May require management if excessive for age.

Radiological features

- Flattened appearance of the incisal edges of the anterior teeth and occlusal surfaces of the posterior teeth. Where more severe, the crowns appear short.
- Flattened interproximal surfaces are much less common.
- Reduction in the size of the pulp chamber is usually evident in moderate to severe attrition, related to increased formation of secondary/tertiary dentin. Narrowing of the root canals is sometimes seen.

Flattening of the incisal edges and
the occlusal surfaces

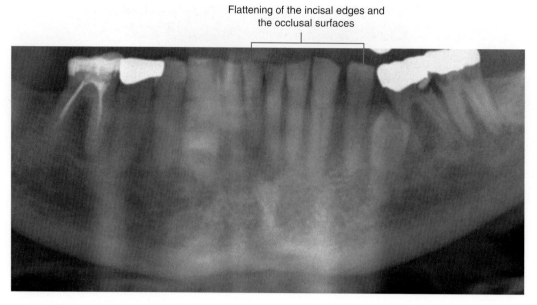

Figure 4.13 Attrition: cropped panoramic radiograph.

4.3 Abrasion (Figure 4.14)

- Non-physiological gradual loss of tooth structure related to repeated contact of teeth with a foreign object.
- Most commonly related to excessive incorrect tooth brushing and, less commonly, flossing. Occasionally seen in association with repeated biting of hard items such as pins, pipes, etc.
- May expose dentin and contribute to tooth hypersensitivity.
- Clinically evident.

Radiological features

- Most commonly presents as a V-shaped groove defect or a concave dish-shaped defect at the cervical aspects of the teeth, usually the buccal/labial surfaces. Sometimes seen interproximally, related to dental flossing.
- Usually appears as a relatively well-defined lucency on 2D intraoral and panoramic radiographs. The morphology is appreciated on CBCT and MDCT.
- Focal narrowing of the cervical pulp chamber and root canals is often seen with moderate and severe lesions, related to tertiary dentin formation.

(a) (b)

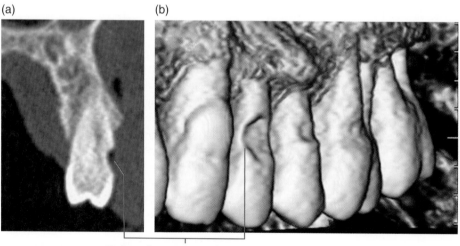

V-shaped groove/concave defects
centred at the cervical aspects of 24,
25 and 26

Figure 4.14 Abrasion: cross-sectional (para-axial) (a) and surface-rendered (b) CBCT images.

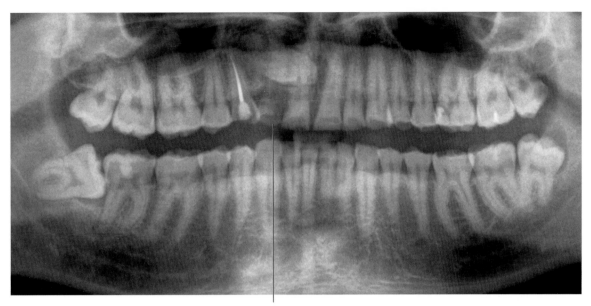

Flattening of the incisal
edge of the with a
'cupping' appearance

Figure 4.15 Erosion: cropped panoramic radiograph.

Differential diagnosis

Key radiological differences

Caries   Differentiation can be difficult. Abrasion lesions demonstrate more well-defined margins. The V- or concave-shaped morphology is typical, better demonstrated on CBCT and MDCT. However, abrasion lesions are usually clinically obvious.

4.4 Erosion (Figure 4.15)

- Non-microbial chemical-related gradual loss of tooth structure.
- Most commonly related to acidic foods and drinks.
- Gastric acids can also cause erosion. For example, acid reflux and chronic vomiting.
- Usually seen in the younger person.
- Clinically observable and the location of the erosive lesions may provide clues to the probable cause.

Radiological features

- These defects appear lucent on 2D intraoral/panoramic radiographs and often demonstrate a concave 'cupping' morphology at the incisal/palatal surfaces of the crowns. The margins often appear 'feathered' on intraoral and panoramic radiographs.
- Most commonly affects anterior teeth, usually several teeth.

Differential diagnosis

Key radiological differences

Abrasion   Abrasion lesions usually demonstrate the typical morphology and the margins are more well defined.

4.5 Internal resorption (Figures 4.16 and 4.17)

- Resorption of the pulpal walls (dentin) by activation of odontoclastic cells.
- Often idiopathic. May be related to insult to the pulp/tooth. For example, trauma and pulpotomies. Also not infrequently seen within longstanding impacted third molars.
- If it involves the coronal pulp of an erupted tooth and is of sufficient size, a pink hue may be clinically observed. Enamel fracture may occur with large coronal lesions.
- Larger radicular lesions may extend to the cemental surface. There is also an associated risk for pathological root fracture.
- More cervically positioned radicular lesions involving the root surface may be associated with periodontal bone loss.

Radiological features

- Identification and evaluation of the extent/morphology of these lesions are more accurately performed with CBCT or MDCT.
- Usually presents as a focal lucent/hypodense widening of the pulp chamber or root canal with a well-defined, sometimes scalloped or irregular, margin.
- May extend to the root surface, where it can be difficult to differentiate from external resorption. Can range from minimal to extensive lesions.

Differential diagnosis

Key radiological differences

Caries   The margins of carious lesions are usually less well defined. Caries begins at the tooth surface.

External resorption   Usually larger at the tooth surface, as the resorption begins at the surface.

(a)

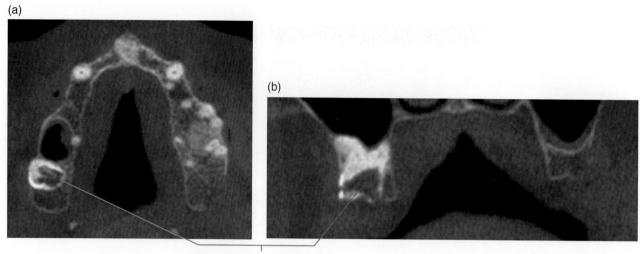

(b)

Well-defined lucency within the
crown and root breaching the tooth
surface at a few sites

Figure 4.16 Internal root resorption, 18: axial (a) and coronal (b) CBCT images.

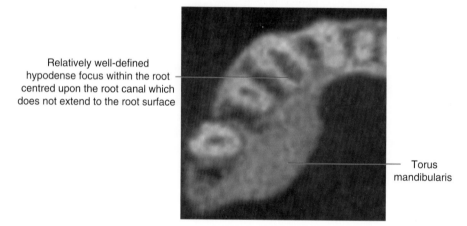

Relatively well-defined
hypodense focus within the root
centred upon the root canal which
does not extend to the root surface

Torus
mandibularis

Figure 4.17 Internal root resorption, 43: axial CBCT image.

4.6 External resorption (Figure 4.18; see also
Figures 3.9, 3.11, 3.21, 3.23, 5.8, 5.39, 7.13, 7.16–7.18, 8.15, 10.1,10.5, 10.6, 12.9)

- Resorption of the external surface of the tooth, more commonly affecting the root. Associated with activation of osteo/odontoclastic cells.
  ○ Physiological:
    ▪ Exfoliation process of deciduous teeth, as permanent successors erupt.
  ○ Pathological:
    ▪ Often seen in association with pressure exerted upon the tooth. For example, orthodontic forces, impacted teeth, cysts and benign tumours.
    ▪ Also seen in association with chronic periapical inflammatory lesions.

- Can be idiopathic.
- Larger lesions may extend to the pulp. There is associated risk for pathological root fracture.
- More cervically positioned radicular lesions may be associated with periodontal bone loss.

Radiological features
- Identification and evaluation of the extent/morphology of these lesions are more accurately performed with CBCT or MDCT.
- Well-defined focal absence of tooth structure, with variable morphology. Begins at the tooth surface.
- Radicular lesions are most commonly seen at the apex and cervically.
- Apical lesions often result in a blunted appearance of the residual apex.

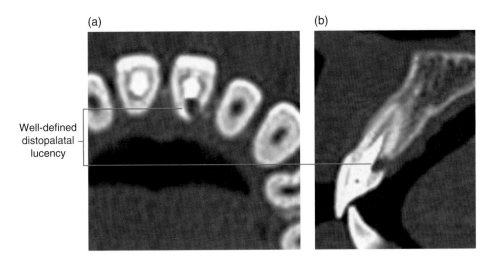

Figure 4.18 Invasive cervical root resorption, 21: axial (a) and sagittal (b) MDCT images.

- The adjacent periodontal ligament space and lamina dura are almost always preserved, unless the resorption is related to a chronic inflammatory lesion or an entity (e.g. impacted tooth, cyst or tumour) which is in contact with the root surface.
- When the resorption is related to direct pressure (e.g. impacted tooth, cyst or tumour) the morphology of the resorptive defect often matches the surface of the entity exerting the pressure (e.g. impacted third molar or canine, cysts and benign tumours).
- Can be severe, where an entire tooth root is largely absent. For example, resorption of a lateral incisor, related to an ectopic impacted canine.

Differential diagnosis

	Key radiological differences
Internal resorption	It may be difficult to differentiate with intraoral and panoramic radiography. These are much better demonstrated with CBCT or MDCT although it can be occasionally difficult to differentiate large lesions where much of the root structure is resorbed.

4.7 Fracture related to trauma

- Refer to Chapter 17.

CHAPTER 5
Inflammatory Lesions of the Jaws

5.1 Periapical inflammatory lesions
(Figures 5.1–5.17)

- *Synonyms*: apical periodontitis, periapical rarefying osteitis, periapical condensing or sclerosing osteitis, periapical granuloma.
- Periradicular inflammatory lesions related to pulpal pathology are mostly seen at the apical aspect of the tooth root(s), centred at the apical foramen, i.e. periapical inflammatory lesion. However, these lesions are sometimes centred upon the root surface away from the apical foramen, most of which are related to lateral canals and foramina (normal variant) or root fractures. The term osteomyelitis is reserved for more extensive infection of bone.
- Clinical presentation varies substantially, from an asymptomatic low-grade chronic picture to severe infections with substantial local and systemic manifestations.
- Osteomyelitis (see section 5.4), the radicular cyst (see Chapter 8) and involvement of the soft tissues including cellulitis and abscess collections (see section 5.5) are possible sequelae.

Radiological features
- Cone beam computed tomography (CBCT) and multidetector computed tomography (MDCT) are more sensitive for periapical lesions than 2D intraoral and panoramic radiography although 2D radiography is usually the first modality of choice. Where indicated, soft tissue involvement is best examined with MDCT, often with intravenous contrast.
- Magnetic resonance imaging (MRI) may be useful:
  ○ For identification of early lesions.
  ○ Where 2D radiography, MDCT and CBCT are equivocal and there remains clinical suspicion for periapical inflammatory disease.
  ○ Where there are unusual symptoms.
- It should be noted that, even when the clinical presentation is that of an acute periapical inflammatory lesion, it often reflects an acute phase of a chronic lesion (acute-on-chronic) and the bony changes seen radiologically reflect the chronic features. The acute features are often only demonstrated with multislice CT or MRI.

- Early or lower grade lesions often present as widened apical periodontal ligament space with preservation of the lamina dura.
- Very early or acute lesions may not demonstrate bony changes detectable with 2D radiography, CBCT or MDCT. MRI may demonstrate periapical inflammatory marrow oedema.
- With some progression, it usually presents as a lucency or hypodense focus centred at the apex of a root with effacement of the lamina dura.
- Sometimes, these lesions are centred elsewhere on the root surface, related to accessory lateral pulp canals and foramina (normal variant) or root fractures. Lateral canals and root fractures may not be radiologically detectable.
- Margins can be ill defined or relatively well defined.
  ○ Many of these lesions identified radiologically are longstanding and are either acute-on-chronic or solely chronic in nature. Therefore, the margins are often relatively well defined.
  ○ More acute lesions tend to demonstrate less or poorly defined margins.
- Adjacent reactive sclerosis is a common feature since many lesions demonstrated radiologically are chronic in nature.
  ○ The degree of sclerosis is variable. It can be focal and mild or dense, extensive and diffused, related to the degree of chronicity.
  ○ Occasionally, the sclerosis can be extremely focal and dense where the widened apical periodontal ligament space or small apical lucency is not apparent. Some refer to these as periapical condensing/sclerosing osteitis. However, MDCT and CBCT almost always demonstrate subtle widening of the periodontal space or a small periapical hypodense or lucent focus, which may not be appreciated on panoramic or periapical radiography.
- Apical root resorption may be seen with chronic lesions.
- The pulp chamber and root canals of the involved tooth may appear larger/wider than the contralateral tooth, related to arrested deposition of dentin.
- Larger lesions may efface the jaw cortices.

Atlas of Oral and Maxillofacial Radiology, First Edition. Bernard Koong.
© 2017 John Wiley & Sons Ltd. Published 2017 by John Wiley & Sons Ltd.

- There may be periosteal response (periosteal new bone formation).
- Lesions approximating the maxillary antral bases:
  - Commonly stimulate variable reactive mucosal thickening at the antral floor.
  - Focal reactive periosteal response (focal periostitis) is also quite commonly seen, appearing as a dome-shaped opaque lamina.
  - There may be focal effacement of the antral cortical floor, often not appreciated with 2D radiography.
  - Occasionally, there is variable inflammatory disease affecting the ipsilateral paranasal sinuses, secondary to the periapical inflammatory lesion. This is usually limited to the maxillary sinus.
  - These features are better appreciated with MDCT or CBCT.

Differential diagnosis

Key radiological differences

Periapical osseous dysplasia	Presence of internal opaque deposits or homogeneous 'ground-glass' appearance. Early lesions without internal opacities can appear similar to chronic periapical inflammatory lesions. The periapical osseous dysplasia is usually multiple. CBCT or MDCT is more sensitive in demonstrating subtle internal increased densities.
Radicular cyst	It can be difficult to differentiate from chronic periapical inflammatory lesions. The radicular cyst tends to demonstrate corticated borders although this may not be evident in early cystic change. Expansion and displacement of structures (e.g. mandibular canal) are cystic features. As a rule of thumb, lesions larger than 10 mm have been considered to be more likely to be radicular cysts but other features must be taken into account. CBCT/MDCT can better differentiate these lesions.
Bone island	May resemble the adjacent chronic reactive sclerosis but bone islands are usually well defined and homogeneous internally, isodense with cortical bone. In addition, there is almost always a periapical lucent/hypodense appearance or widening of the apical periodontal ligament space with apical inflammatory lesions.
Fibrous healing	Postendodontic therapy fibrous healing can appear similar and differentiation is often difficult. Fibrous healing tends to demonstrate a well-defined thick cortex, which may be slightly irregular. CBCT and MDCT may better demonstrate these features and may also be used to evaluate the integrity of the endodontic treatment.
Malignant lesions	Demonstrate aggressive borders. Metastatic and infiltrative malignant lesions often demonstrate other and/or adjacent lesions, e.g. periradicular lucencies elsewhere on the same or adjacent teeth, with absence of lamina dura.
Osteomyelitis	A periapical inflammatory lesion rarely progresses to osteomyelitis. Osteomyelitis involves a much larger region of bone and may not be centred upon the root apex. Sequestra and periosteal new bone formation are features of osteomyelitis.

Post-treatment appearances of periapical lesions
(Figures 5.15–5.17)

After successful endodontic therapy or extraction, apical appearances include re-establishment of normal periapical structures, variant trabecular architecture, fibrous healing and periapical osseous prominence at the maxillary sinus base, as follows.

Re-establishment of normal periapical structures
Radiological features

- New bone formation begins at the periphery of the periapical lucency. This new bone is usually relatively homogeneous in appearance initially and eventually remodels.
- Re-establishment of the lamina dura and periodontal ligament space, if the tooth has not been extracted (i.e. endodontically treated).

Variant trabecular architecture (Figure 5.16)

- Bony healing and remodelling following successful treatment may result in a trabecular appearance that is different from the trabecular bone typical of that region of the jaws.

Radiological features

- A variety of altered trabecular bone pattern is seen.
- There is usually re-establishment of normal periodontal ligament space and lamina dura.

Fibrous healing (Figure 5.17)
Radiological features

- The classical periapical fibrous healing presents as a lucency with a well-defined relatively thick corticated border which is sometimes irregular.
- This may also present as a widened apical periodontal ligament space. Classically, the lamina is thicker than is usually seen and may be slightly irregular.
- It is often difficult to definitively differentiate between periapical fibrous healing and an inflammatory lesion and clinical correlation is required.

Periapical osseous prominence at the maxillary sinus base (Figure 5.15)

- Occasionally, following extraction or endodontic management, healing of a maxillary posterior periapical inflammatory lesion or radicular cyst can result in the appearance of a bony prominence at the sinus floor. This is related to osseous infill of the previously elevated mucoperiosteal lining by the inflammatory lesion (focal periostitis) or radicular cyst prior to 'collapse' of this elevated mucoperiosteum.

Radiological features

- When other opaque prominences at the maxillary sinus base cannot be excluded with 2D radiography, MDCT or CBCT is recommended.
- Appearance of a bony prominence at the maxillary floor centred at the apex of an endodontically treated root apex or at an edentulous site corresponding with the previous site of the apex of the extracted tooth.

- This bony prominence is of variable size, morphology and density.

Differential diagnosis

Any opaque prominence at the maxillary sinus base may resemble periapical osseous healing

Key radiological differences

Examples include osteoma, exostoses, septae at the sinus floor, calcifications related to chronic inflammatory sinus disease and root remnants. Post-treatment periapical healing is usually centred at an apical region (even if the tooth has been extracted) and internally demonstrates the appearances of variable stages of bone formation and remodelling. These features are better demonstrated with MDCT or CBCT.

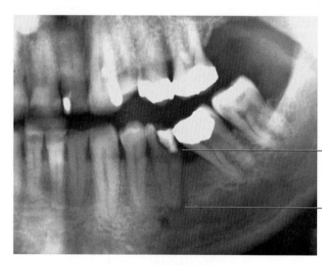

Caries at the margins of the restoration, which probably involves the pulp

Apical lucency with effaced lamina dura and surrounding reactive sclerosis

Figure 5.1 Periapical chronic inflammatory lesion: cropped panoramic radiograph.

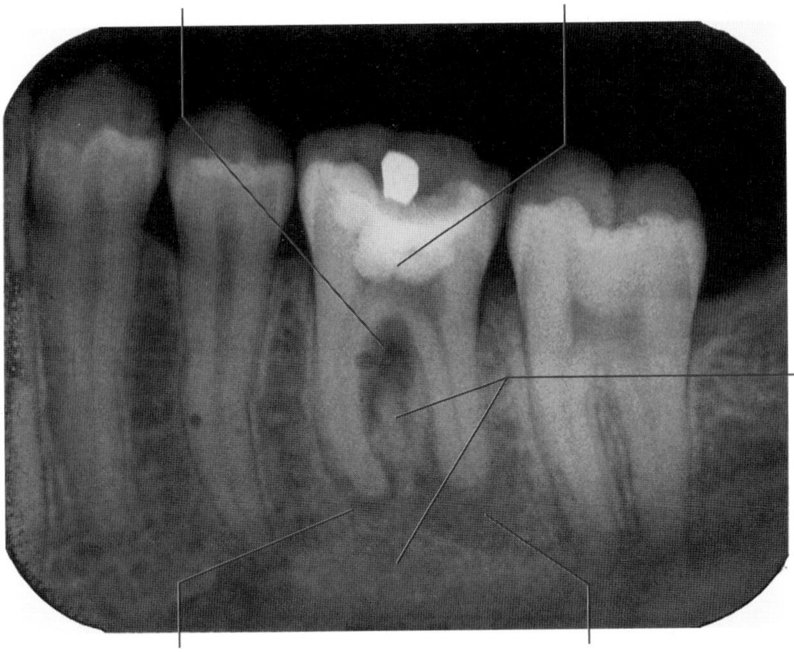

Furcation hypodense inflammatory lesion, probably centred bucally or lingually (note the trabecular bone projected over the lesion). This is probably related to a lateral canal at the furcation

Dressing and temporary restoration related to endodontic management

Reactive sclerosis related to chronicity

Inflammatory widening of the apical periodontal ligament space, with early effacement of the lamina dura

Periapical hypodense inflammatory lesion with effacement of the lamina dura. This lesion is not completely lucent in appearance, related to preservation of trabecular bone buccal and/or lingual to the lesion and also the mandibular cortices

Figure 5.2 Periapical and furcation inflammatory lesions: periapical radiograph. (Courtesy of Koong B. Diagnostic imaging of the periodontal and implant patient. In: Lindhe J, Lang NP, editors. Clinical Periodontology and Implant Dentistry. 6th ed. Wiley Blackwell; 2015. Reproduced with permission from Wiley.)

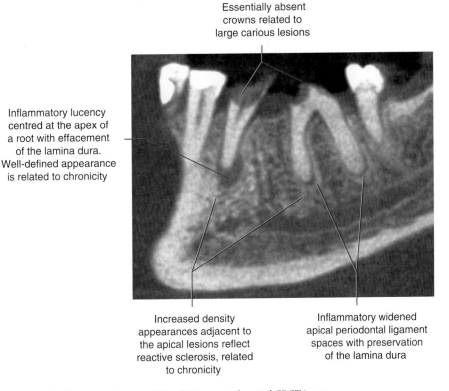

Essentially absent crowns related to large carious lesions

Inflammatory lucency centred at the apex of a root with effacement of the lamina dura. Well-defined appearance is related to chronicity

Increased density appearances adjacent to the apical lesions reflect reactive sclerosis, related to chronicity

Inflammatory widened apical periodontal ligament spaces with preservation of the lamina dura

Figure 5.3 Periapical inflammatory lesions of 35 and 36: corrected sagittal CBCT image.

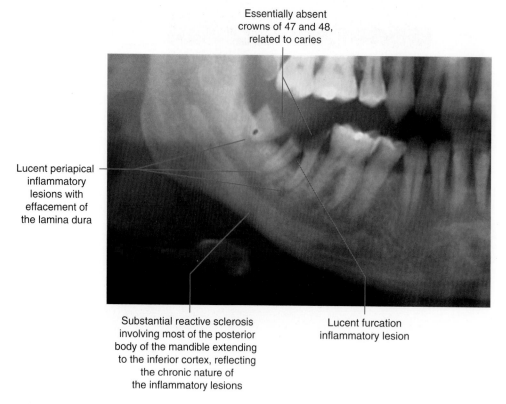

Essentially absent crowns of 47 and 48, related to caries

Lucent periapical inflammatory lesions with effacement of the lamina dura

Substantial reactive sclerosis involving most of the posterior body of the mandible extending to the inferior cortex, reflecting the chronic nature of the inflammatory lesions

Lucent furcation inflammatory lesion

Figure 5.4 Chronic periapical and furcation inflammatory lesions of 48 and 47: cropped panoramic radiograph.

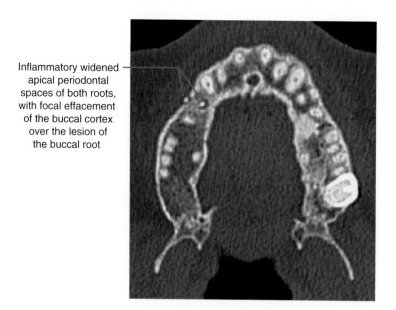

Inflammatory widened apical periodontal spaces of both roots, with focal effacement of the buccal cortex over the lesion of the buccal root

Figure 5.5 Periapical inflammatory lesion (apical periodontitis) of 14: axial MDCT image.

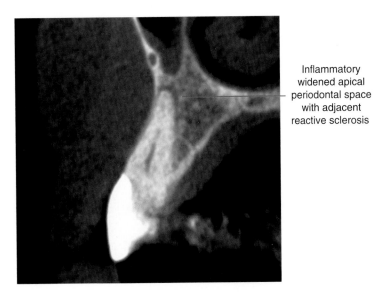

Figure 5.6 Periapical inflammatory lesion (apical periodontitis) of 13: corrected coronal CBCT image.

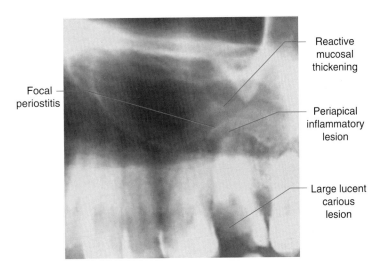

Figure 5.7 Periapical inflammatory lesion of carious 27 with reactive changes at the maxillary antral base: cropped panoramic radiograph.

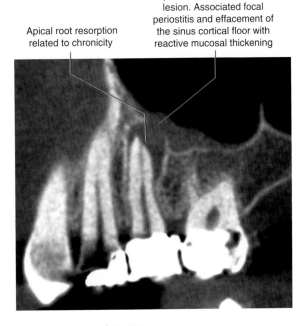

Figure 5.8 Periapical inflammatory lesion of 25: corrected sagittal CBCT image.

Apical lucent inflammatory lesion of the distobuccal root, with effacement of the lamina dura and also focal effacement of the cortical floor of the right maxillary sinus. Note is made of the reactive mucosal thickening. These findings are not appreciated on the panoramic radiograph, related to projection of the inferior cortex of the zygomatic process of the maxilla

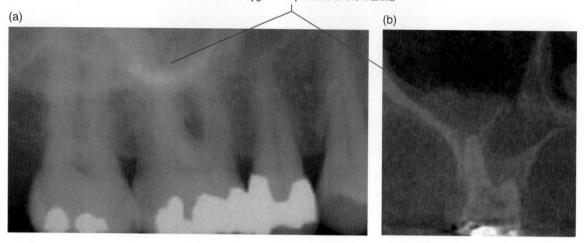

Figure 5.9 Periapical inflammatory lesion of 16: cropped panoramic radiograph (a) and coronal CBCT image (b).

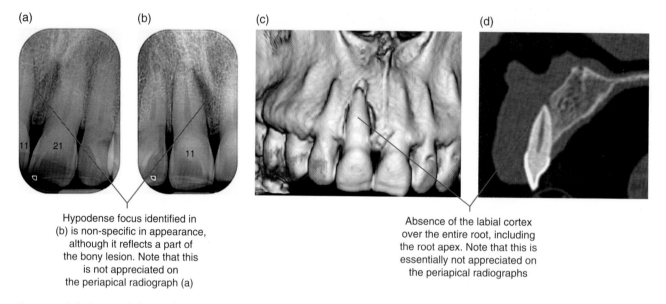

Hypodense focus identified in (b) is non-specific in appearance, although it reflects a part of the bony lesion. Note that this is not appreciated on the periapical radiograph (a)

Absence of the labial cortex over the entire root, including the root apex. Note that this is essentially not appreciated on the periapical radiographs

Figure 5.10 Labial perioendo lesion of 11: periapical radiographs (a,b) and surface-rendered (c) and corrected sagittal (d) MDCT images.

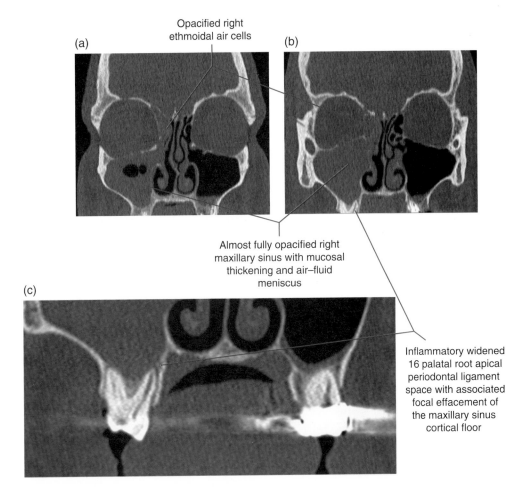

Opacified right
ethmoidal air cells

(a)

(b)

Almost fully opacified right
maxillary sinus with mucosal
thickening and air–fluid
meniscus

(c)

Inflammatory widened
16 palatal root apical
periodontal ligament
space with associated
focal effacement of
the maxillary sinus
cortical floor

Figure 5.11 Palatal root apical inflammatory lesion of 16 with secondary right-sided paranasal sinus inflammatory disease: coronal MDCT images (a–c).

Focal inflammatory lucent lesion centred
on the distal root surface with effacement
of the lamina dura, related to a lateral
canal. There is adjacent reactive sclerosis
related to chronicity

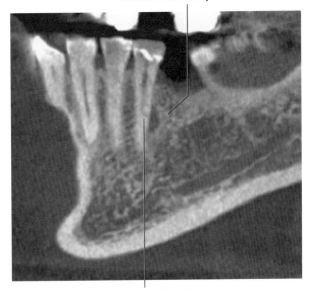

Lateral canal. Note that this is often
subresolution on CBCT and MDCT and
almost never demonstrated on plain 2D
radiography

Figure 5.12 Inflammatory lesion of 35 related to a lateral canal: corrected sagittal CBCT image.

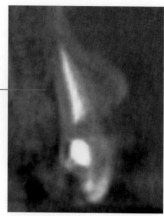

A palatally centred inflammatory lesion, with focal effacement of the lamina dura and adjacent reactive sclerosis. This is likely to be related to a lateral canal, which is subresolution

Figure 5.13 Endodontically treated 11 with ongoing chronic pain: corrected sagittal CBCT image.

(a)
(b)

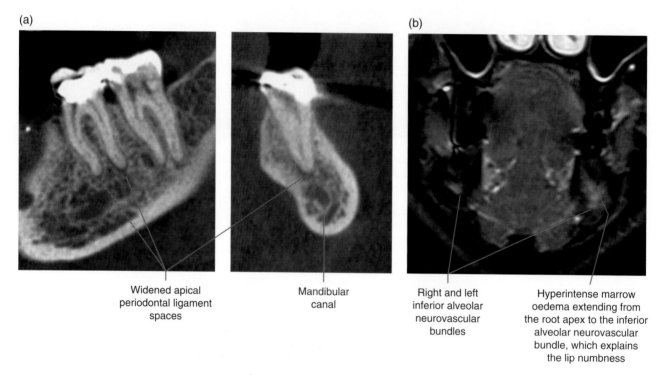

Widened apical periodontal ligament spaces

Mandibular canal

Right and left inferior alveolar neurovascular bundles

Hyperintense marrow oedema extending from the root apex to the inferior alveolar neurovascular bundle, which explains the lip numbness

Figure 5.14 Apical inflammatory lesions (apical periodontitis) of 36. The patient presented with 36 pain and numbness of the lip: corrected sagittal and coronal MDCT images (a) and MRI coronal STIR image (b).

Opaque bony prominence at the sinus
floor related to postendodontic therapy
healing of an apical inflammatory lesion

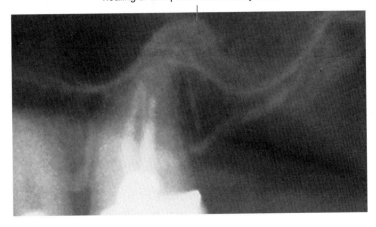

Figure 5.15 Postendodontic therapy healed apical lesion, 27: cropped panoramic radiograph.

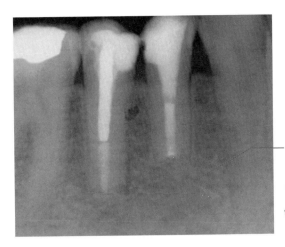

Postendodontic and apicectomy bony healing.
Note the re-establishment of the periodontal
ligament space and lamina dura at the residual
root apex. The new bone demonstrates a variant
architecture. This may resemble more 'normal'
trabecular bone after several years of remodelling
but may also remain different indefinitely

Figure 5.16 Postendodontic treatment and apicectomy: cropped periapical radiograph.

(a)   (b)

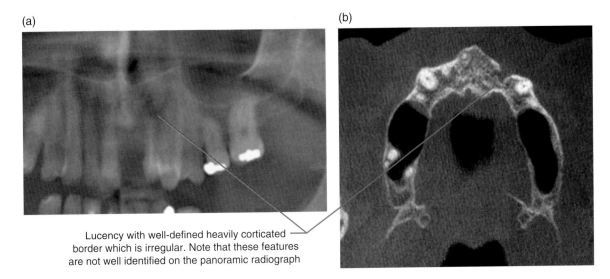

Lucency with well-defined heavily corticated
border which is irregular. Note that these features
are not well identified on the panoramic radiograph

Figure 5.17 Postendodontic treatment apical fibrous healing: cropped panoramic radiograph (a) and axial CBCT image (b).

5.2 Periodontal inflammatory disease
(Figures 5.18–5.34)

- *Synonyms*: periodontal disease, gum disease.
- Bacterial dental plaque-related inflammatory disease affecting the periodontium.
- Much of the injury is a result of the host response to the bacteria. However, some bacteria can also directly cause injury to the periodontium, with the release of toxins.
- Gingivitis refers to inflammation of the gingival tissues. Gingivitis precedes periodontitis but does not always progress to periodontitis.
- Periodontitis generally refers to the condition where the plaque-related inflammatory process affects the periodontal bone. The key clinical feature is periodontal pocket formation, detected with a periodontal probe. Other features include bleeding, periodontal bone loss, tooth mobility and purulent exudates, depending on the severity of the disease.
- There are several subtypes. More aggressive subtypes usually occur in younger patients (under 30 years).
- Apart from the aggressive varieties, periodontal disease is mostly chronic in nature, with acute episodes. A cyclical pattern, with periods of quiescence and active inflammation, is typical.
- Increased incidence with age.
- There are several factors which predispose or contribute to the progression of periodontal diseases.
  - Systemic factors including smoking, diabetes, some haematological diseases, some genetic/hereditary disorders and acquired immunodeficiency syndrome (AIDS).
  - Radiotherapy.
  - Xerostomia.
  - Local conditions which promote plaque formation. For example, overhangs, tooth crowding, dental calculus (calcified plaque), root fractures and dentures.

Radiological features
- General points:
  - Gingivitis is not radiologically detected.
  - Periodontal bone loss demonstrated at one radiological examination does not necessarily mean that there is ongoing active disease. That is, the bone loss may be related to previous disease activity where appropriate therapy has controlled the disease process. Clinical correlation is essential.
  - Imaging evidence of periodontal bone loss over a period of time probably reflects disease progression.
  - Following successful periodontal treatment and disease control, there may be periodontal bone regeneration but this is usually not the case. Therefore, no evidence of periodontal bone changes in postperiodontal treatment imaging can be compatible with successful treatment.

- MDCT and CBCT more accurately demonstrate the periodontal bone loss and morphology as well as the presence of furcation and perioendo defects. 2D intraoral and panoramic radiography typically underestimates the severity of periodontal bone loss and may not demonstrate furcation and perioendo defects but may be sufficient.
- The extent of periodontal bone loss including furcation and perioendo defects demonstrated radiologically may not correlate with the clinical findings (e.g. periodontal probing), related to:
  - Soft tissue attachment at the bony defects.
  - Difficult access to periodontal probing contributing to non-detection of an existing defect.
- Key radiological features
  - Lucent periodontal bone loss originates at the alveolar crest. The margins often appear relatively well defined as the periodontal bone loss is usually chronic in nature. Acute episodes and more aggressive subtypes may demonstrate more ill-defined margins.
  - Surrounding reactive sclerosis is usually a feature, related to the chronic nature of most cases. This sclerosis can be extensive, reflecting the degree of chronicity. This can persist, following successful treatment.
  - Can be focal, involving one or a few teeth, or generalised (widely distributed), involving most or all teeth.
  - Widened periodontal ligament spaces may reflect increased mobility of a tooth, related to loss of periodontal bone support. The widening can involve the entire root or be limited to the apical and cervical regions of the root. The lamina dura is sometimes thickened. It should be noted that many other conditions, including increased occlusal loading, can contribute to this.
  - MRI may demonstrate marrow oedema.
- Severity of periodontal bone loss.
  - More accurately demonstrated with MDCT and CBCT.
  - Normal: the periodontal alveolar crest is approximately 2–3 mm from the cementoenamel junction (CEJ).
  - Early bone loss includes:
    - Slight decrease in density and definition, blunting or loss of the alveolar crestal cortex.
    - Periodontal bone loss of up to 1 mm.
  - Moderate bone loss refers to periodontal bone loss of more than 1 mm, up to the midpoint of the root length.
  - Severe bone loss extends beyond the midroot or extends into a furcation.
- Morphology of periodontal bone loss.
  - More accurately demonstrated with CBCT and MDCT than 2D intraoral and panoramic radiography.
  - Horizontal bone loss.
    - Bone loss between two teeth is parallel with the CEJ, usually involving multiple teeth.
  - Vertical (angular) defects.
    - Refers to a focal vertical or oblique defect centred upon one tooth more than the adjacent tooth (in

relation to the CEJs of these adjacent teeth). Multiple teeth may demonstrate angular defects.

- Often not easily identified on 2D radiography when the buccal and/or lingual cortices remain preserved. Better demonstrated with CBCT/MDCT.
- Clinical detection of narrow defects, especially interdental lesions, can be challenging.
- Can be associated with a specific local contributing factor, such as a vertical root fracture or overhang.

◦ Infrabony defect. Focal periodontal bone loss, classified by the number of preserved bony walls:

- Three-walled: usually, the buccal and lingual cortices and one proximal wall are preserved.
- Two-walled: usually, the buccal or lingual cortex is effaced.
- Single-walled: usually, both buccal and lingual cortices are effaced. Only the one proximal wall remains.
- On 2D radiography, these appear as varying degrees of hypodense periodontal defects. Single-walled defects usually appear more lucent and well defined.

◦ Interdental crater defect.

- Concaved crestal bone loss between two teeth with relative preservation of the buccal and lingual cortices.

- Furcation defects.
  ◦ 2D intraoral and panoramic radiography:
  - Classically a hypodense focus or lucency is seen at the furcation, with effacement of the lamina dura. The degree of decreased density appreciated is dependent upon the severity, morphology, projection of the roots and the presence/absence of the adjacent buccal and lingual cortices.
  - The classical 'J-shaped' lucency is sometimes seen.
  - Early furcation involvement usually presents as a widened furcation periodontal ligament space.
  ◦ Bony furcation defects (especially maxillary molars) are often not appreciated with 2D radiography. MDCT and CBCT are much more accurate in identifying the presence, and in demonstrating the morphology, of these defects. In cases where the periodontal bone loss approaches the furcation regions, the presence of bony furcation defects cannot be fully excluded with 2D radiography.
  ◦ May be related to pulpal pathology with accessory pulpal canals extending to the furcation. May also be related to iatrogenic perforation of the roots at the furcation.

- Perioendo defect.
  ◦ Lucent periodontal bone absence extending from the crestal bone to the apex of a tooth root.
  ◦ Where there is severe periodontal bone loss, it is often difficult to identify the presence/absence of perioendo involvement on plain 2D imaging, related to the projection of the adjacent tooth and bony structures.

◦ May reflect contiguity of periodontal and periapical inflammatory lesions, where both lesions essentially merge to form one larger lesion. These may be primarily related to periodontal inflammatory disease or pulpal pathology.

◦ May be associated with a specific local contributing factor, for example a vertical root fracture.

- Acute periodontal abscess.
  ◦ These lesions are often an acute exacerbation of a chronic lesion. 2D radiography and CBCT usually only demonstrate the chronic bone defects.
  ◦ Abscess or inflammatory infiltrate often drain via the periodontal defect into the oral cavity. However, these may occasionally extend into the adjacent soft tissues. In these cases, MDCT (with intravenous contrast) may demonstrate the cellulitis, collections and airway patency.

- Severe inflammatory periodontal bone loss, including perioendo lesions, affecting the maxillary posterior teeth often induces a reactive mucosal thickening at the maxillary sinus bases (Figure 5.29; see also Figures 5.7–5.9). There may also be focal periosteal reaction (periostitis) at the sinus base, more often seen with perioendo lesions. Sometimes, there is associated focal effacement of the sinus floor. Not infrequently, there are variable degrees of ipsilateral paranasal sinus inflammatory disease secondary to severe periodontal defects, especially perioendo lesions (see also section 5.1, Figure 5.11).

- Related factors. There are many local factors which influence inflammatory periodontal disease that may be identified radiologically.
  ◦ Dental calculus.
  ◦ Dental restoration-related factors including overhangs, marginal deficiencies, incorrect contours and open contacts.
  ◦ Caries at the cervical region of the tooth or involving the roots.
  ◦ Root fractures.
  ◦ Perforations related to endodontic therapy and post preparations.

Differential diagnosis

	Key radiological differences
Malignant lesions	Infiltrative and invasive margins.
Langerhans cell histiocytosis	Centred at the midroot.
Benign tumours and cysts	More well-defined margins which may be corticated. Larger lesions may displace teeth and demonstrate expansion.

Overhang of the amalgam
restoration

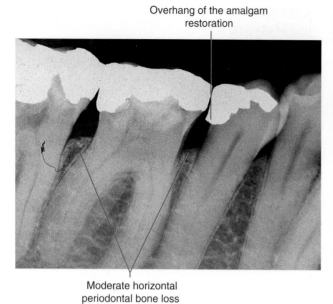

Moderate horizontal
periodontal bone loss

Figure 5.18 Moderate horizontal periodontal bone loss: periapical radiograph. (Courtesy of Koong B. Diagnostic imaging of the periodontal and implant patient. In: Lindhe J, Lang NP, editors. Clinical Periodontology and Implant Dentistry. 6th ed. Wiley Blackwell; 2015. Reproduced with permission from Wiley.)

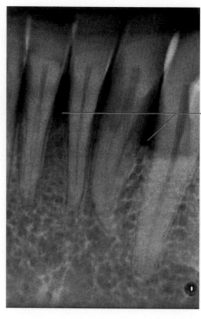

Absence of the crestal cortex suggests that the periodontal bone loss may be in an active/progressive phase

Figure 5.20 Moderate horizontal periodontal bone loss: periapical radiograph. (Courtesy of Koong B. Diagnostic imaging of the periodontal and implant patient. In: Lindhe J, Lang NP, editors. Clinical Periodontology and Implant Dentistry. 6th ed. Wiley Blackwell; 2015. Reproduced with permission from Wiley.)

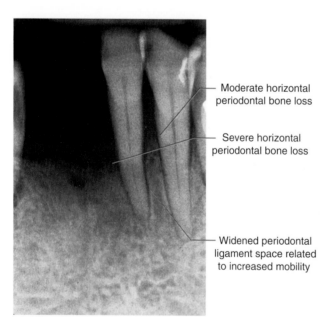

— Moderate horizontal
periodontal bone loss

— Severe horizontal
periodontal bone loss

— Widened periodontal
ligament space related
to increased mobility

Figure 5.19 Moderate to severe horizontal periodontal bone loss with increased mobility: periapical radiograph. (Courtesy of Koong B. Diagnostic imaging of the periodontal and implant patient. In: Lindhe J, Lang NP, editors. Clinical Periodontology and Implant Dentistry. 6th ed. Wiley Blackwell; 2015. Reproduced with permission from Wiley.)

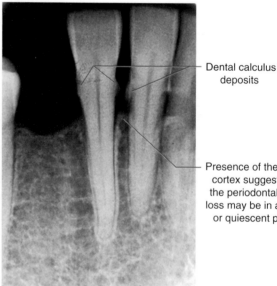

— Dental calculus
deposits

— Presence of the crestal
cortex suggests that
the periodontal bone
loss may be in a stable
or quiescent phase

Figure 5.21 Moderate horizontal periodontal bone loss and calculus deposits: periapical radiograph. (Courtesy of Koong B. Diagnostic imaging of the periodontal and implant patient. In: Lindhe J, Lang NP, editors. Clinical Periodontology and Implant Dentistry. 6th ed. Wiley Blackwell; 2015. Reproduced with permission from Wiley.)

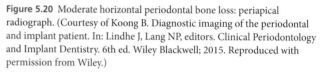

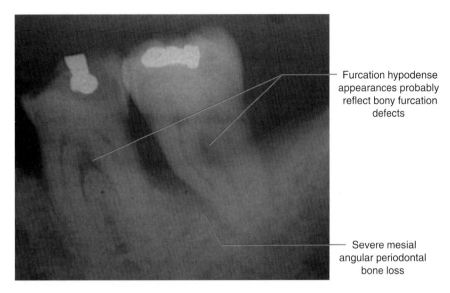

Furcation hypodense appearances probably reflect bony furcation defects

Severe mesial angular periodontal bone loss

Figure 5.22 Moderate to severe periodontal bone loss with probable furcation defects: periapical radiograph.

(a)

(b)

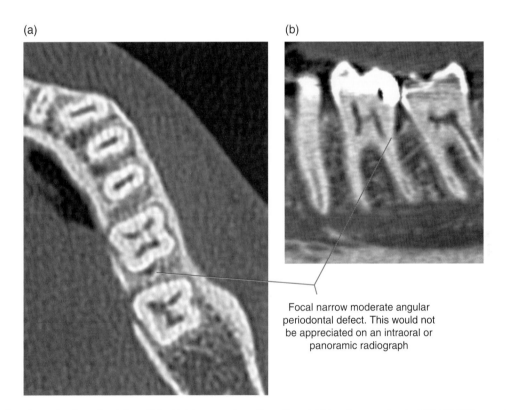

Focal narrow moderate angular periodontal defect. This would not be appreciated on an intraoral or panoramic radiograph

Figure 5.23 Focal moderate distal angular defect of 36, which is narrow buccolingually: axial (a) and corrected sagittal (b) MDCT images. (Courtesy of Koong B. Diagnostic imaging of the periodontal and implant patient. In: Lindhe J, Lang NP, editors. Clinical Periodontology and Implant Dentistry. 6th ed. Wiley Blackwell; 2015. Reproduced with permission from Wiley.)

(a)

(b)

Well-defined horizontal bone loss between 36 and 37 seen in the bitewing appears as an ill-defined hypodense focus on the periapical view, raising the possibility of a crater defect, or that the bone loss is more severe buccally or lingually, with absence of either cortex. This is related to the variation in the vertical projection angle

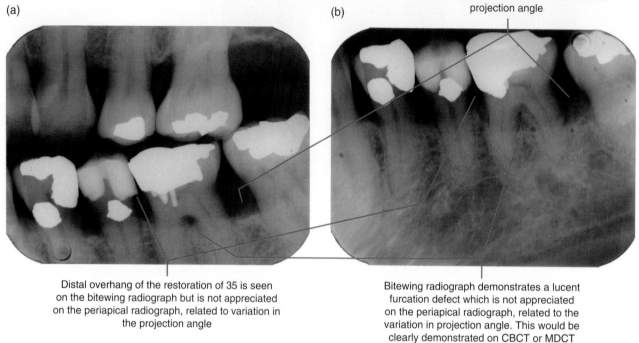

Distal overhang of the restoration of 35 is seen on the bitewing radiograph but is not appreciated on the periapical radiograph, related to variation in the projection angle

Bitewing radiograph demonstrates a lucent furcation defect which is not appreciated on the periapical radiograph, related to the variation in projection angle. This would be clearly demonstrated on CBCT or MDCT

Figure 5.24 Severe periodontal bone loss of 36 with bony furcation defect. Horizontal bone loss elsewhere: bitewing (a) and periapical (b) radiographs. (Courtesy of Koong B. Diagnostic imaging of the periodontal and implant patient. In: Lindhe J, Lang NP, editors. Clinical Periodontology and Implant Dentistry. 6th ed. Wiley Blackwell; 2015. Reproduced with permission from Wiley.)

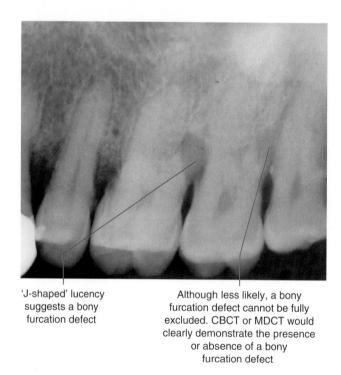

'J-shaped' lucency suggests a bony furcation defect

Although less likely, a bony furcation defect cannot be fully excluded. CBCT or MDCT would clearly demonstrate the presence or absence of a bony furcation defect

Figure 5.25 Appearances suggesting furcation defects: periapical radiograph. (Courtesy of Koong B. Diagnostic imaging of the periodontal and implant patient. In: Lindhe J, Lang NP, editors. Clinical Periodontology and Implant Dentistry. 6th ed. Wiley Blackwell; 2015. Reproduced with permission from Wiley.)

(a)

(b)

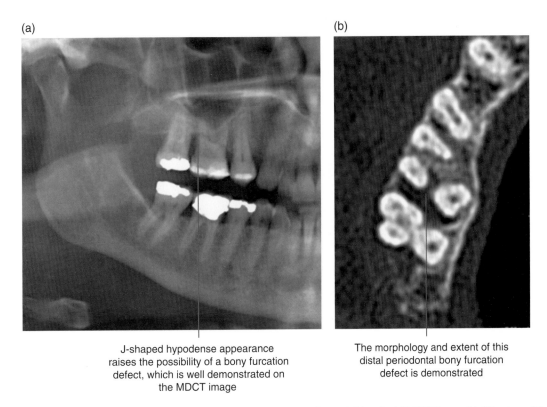

J-shaped hypodense appearance
raises the possibility of a bony furcation
defect, which is well demonstrated on
the MDCT image

The morphology and extent of this
distal periodontal bony furcation
defect is demonstrated

Figure 5.26 Distal periodontal bony furcation involvement, 17: cropped panoramic radiograph (a) and axial MDCT image (b). (Courtesy of Koong B. Diagnostic imaging of the periodontal and implant patient. In: Lindhe J, Lang NP, editors. Clinical Periodontology and Implant Dentistry. 6th ed. Wiley Blackwell; 2015. Reproduced with permission from Wiley.)

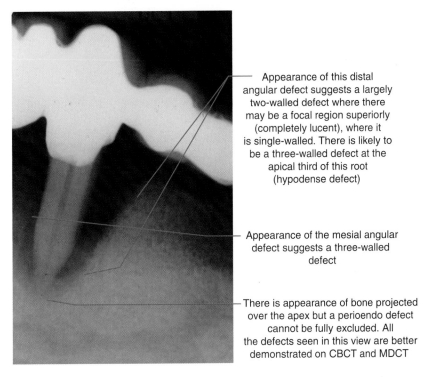

Appearance of this distal
angular defect suggests a largely
two-walled defect where there
may be a focal region superiorly
(completely lucent), where it
is single-walled. There is likely to
be a three-walled defect at the
apical third of this root
(hypodense defect)

Appearance of the mesial angular
defect suggests a three-walled
defect

There is appearance of bone projected
over the apex but a perioendo defect
cannot be fully excluded. All
the defects seen in this view are better
demonstrated on CBCT and MDCT

Figure 5.27 Angular periodontal bone loss with suspected perioendo defect of 33: periapical radiograph. (Courtesy of Koong B. Diagnostic imaging of the periodontal and implant patient. In: Lindhe J, Lang NP, editors. Clinical Periodontology and Implant Dentistry. 6th ed. Wiley Blackwell; 2015. Reproduced with permission from Wiley.)

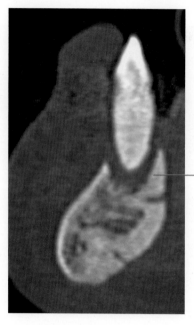

Perioendo defect is well demonstrated. A periapical or panoramic radiograph would probably project the residual cortical bone, especially the lingual cortex, over the apical third of the root, which may be misinterpreted for presence of periapical bone

Figure 5.28 Perioendo defect of 31: corrected sagittal (cross-sectional) MDCT image.

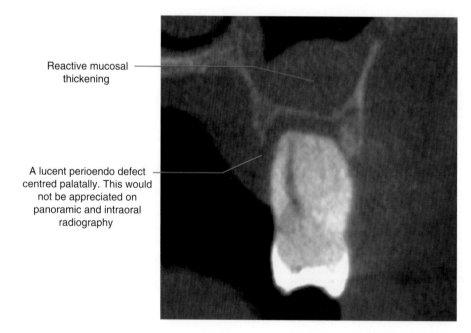

Reactive mucosal thickening

A lucent perioendo defect centred palatally. This would not be appreciated on panoramic and intraoral radiography

Figure 5.29 Perioendo lesion of 27: coronal CBCT image.

(a)

(b)

(c)

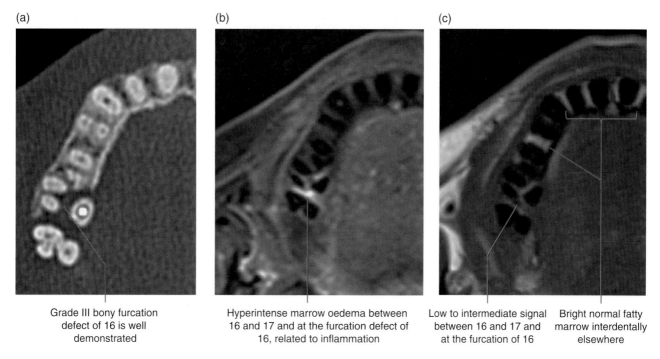

Grade III bony furcation
defect of 16 is well
demonstrated

Hyperintense marrow oedema between
16 and 17 and at the furcation defect of
16, related to inflammation

Low to intermediate signal
between 16 and 17 and
at the furcation of 16

Bright normal fatty
marrow interdentally
elsewhere

Figure 5.30 Grade III bony furcation defect of 16: axial MDCT image (a), axial MRI STIR (b) and T1 (c) images. (Courtesy of Koong B. Diagnostic imaging of the periodontal and implant patient. In: Lindhe J, Lang NP, editors. Clinical Periodontology and Implant Dentistry. 6th ed. Wiley Blackwell; 2015. Reproduced with permission from Wiley.)

Inflammatory vertical periodontal
defect associated with root fracture

(a)

(b)

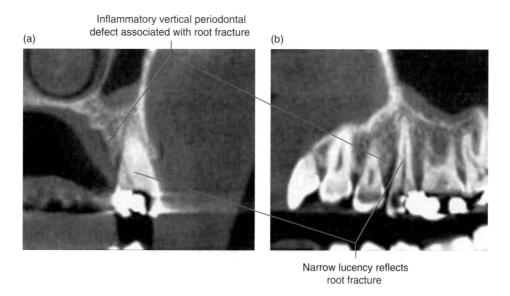

Narrow lucency reflects
root fracture

Figure 5.31 Periodontal defect associated with root fracture of 25: corrected coronal (a) and sagittal (b) CBCT images.

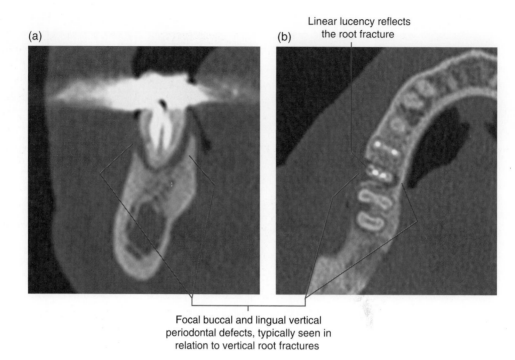

(a)

(b) Linear lucency reflects the root fracture

Focal buccal and lingual vertical periodontal defects, typically seen in relation to vertical root fractures

Figure 5.32 Endodontically treated 46 distal root fracture with periodontal bony defects: corrected coronal (a) and axial (b) CBCT image.

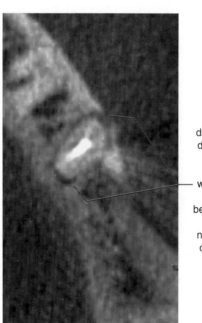

Focal buccal and distopalatal periodontal defects, highly likely to be associated with vertical root fracture which is subresolution. Note the substantial beam hardening artefact associated with the non-metallic obturation of this premolar, quite commonly seen with CBCT

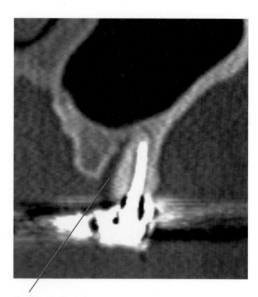

Severe focal vertical periodontal defect centred palatally. This is highly suspicious for a vertical root fracture which is subresolution. This would not be appreciated on panoramic and intraoral radiography

Figure 5.33 Focal periodontal defects related to root fracture of endodontically treated 35: axial CBCT image. (Courtesy of Koong B. Diagnostic imaging of the periodontal and implant patient. In: Lindhe J, Lang NP, editors. Clinical Periodontology and Implant Dentistry. 6th ed. Wiley Blackwell; 2015. Reproduced with permission from Wiley.)

Figure 5.34 Focal vertical periodontal defect of endodontically treated 25: coronal CBCT image. (Courtesy of Koong B. Diagnostic imaging of the periodontal and implant patient. In: Lindhe J, Lang NP, editors. Clinical Periodontology and Implant Dentistry. 6th ed. Wiley Blackwell; 2015. Reproduced with permission from Wiley.)

5.3 Pericoronitis (Figures 5.35–5.39)

- Inflammatory lesion involving the tissues adjacent to the crown of a partially erupted tooth.
- Related to food debris and/or bacterial accumulations below the gingival/mucosal margins around the partially erupted tooth. This is often related to the patient's inability to access and clean these regions.
- Most commonly associated with the mandibular third molars.
- Clinical presentation varies from the low-grade subclinical chronic pericoronitis to severe pain and/or swelling, sometimes with cellulitis. Symptomatic presentations are often acute-on-chronic in nature, although solely acute pericoronitis is sometimes seen.

Radiological features
- The radiological changes seen are often related to chronic pericoronitis.

- Pericoronal reactive sclerosis is the most commonly seen radiological feature, which can be extensive depending on the degree of chronicity.
- There may be slight widening of the pericoronal space. The margins are often relatively well defined with adjacent reactive sclerosis, related to the chronic nature of most cases. More acute cases may demonstrate ill-defined margins.
- Periosteal new bone formation is seen in more severe cases.
- Severe cases may result in cellulitis and abscess collections, which usually require further evaluation with MDCT (usually with intravenous contrast).

Differential diagnosis

	Key radiological differences
Any condition causing an increase in pericoronal density appearance	These may resemble the reactive sclerosis associated with chronic pericoronitis.
Dentigerous cyst	Corticated border. Larger lesions are expansile.

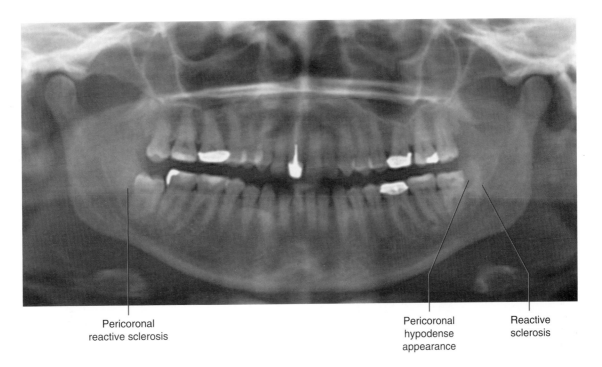

Pericoronal reactive sclerosis

Pericoronal hypodense appearance

Reactive sclerosis

Figure 5.35 Chronic pericoronitis related to 38 and 48: panoramic radiograph.

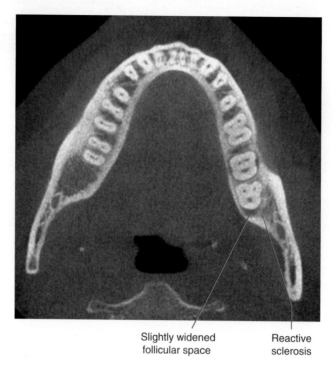

Slightly widened
follicular space

Reactive
sclerosis

Figure 5.36 Chronic pericoronitis related to 38: axial CBCT image.

(a)

(b)

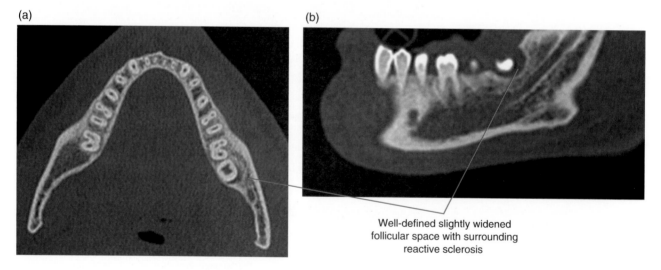

Well-defined slightly widened
follicular space with surrounding
reactive sclerosis

Figure 5.37 Chronic pericoronitis related to 38: axial (a) and corrected sagittal (b) MDCT image.

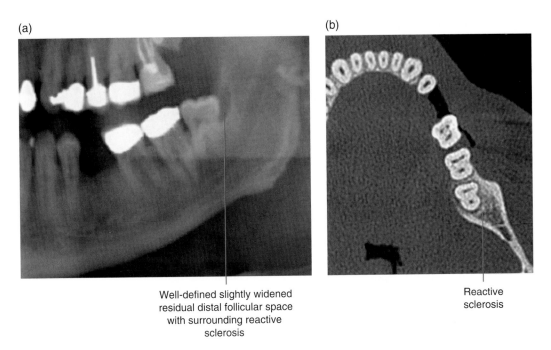

(a)

(b)

Well-defined slightly widened
residual distal follicular space
with surrounding reactive
sclerosis

Reactive
sclerosis

Figure 5.38 Chronic pericoronitis related to 38: cropped panoramic radiograph (a) and axial MDCT image (b).

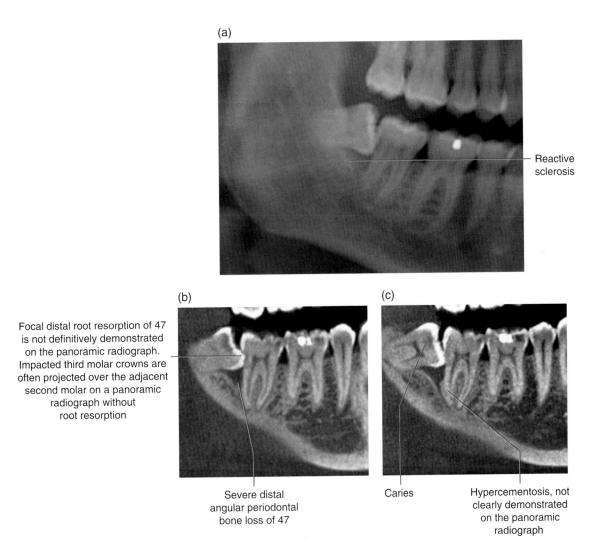

(a)

Reactive
sclerosis

(b)

(c)

Focal distal root resorption of 47
is not definitively demonstrated
on the panoramic radiograph.
Impacted third molar crowns are
often projected over the adjacent
second molar on a panoramic
radiograph without
root resorption

Severe distal
angular periodontal
bone loss of 47

Caries

Hypercementosis, not
clearly demonstrated
on the panoramic
radiograph

Figure 5.39 Chronic pericoronitis related to 48 with periodontal bone loss and resorption of 47: cropped panoramic radiograph (a) and two corrected sagittal CBCT images (b,c).

5.4 **Osteomyelitis of the jaws** (Figures 5.40–5.42)

- Infection and inflammation of the jaws with associated bone destruction.
- There are various classifications. From a radiological perspective, two broad groups can be considered:
  - Acute (suppurative, rarefying).
  - Chronic (non-suppurative, sclerosing). Often demonstrates acute phases. Osteomyelitis present for more than 4 weeks is usually considered to be chronic.
- More commonly seen in the mandible, especially posteriorly.
- Symptoms vary: can be very severe in some acute cases and mild or even essentially asymptomatic in some chronic cases. Chronic cases usually exhibit acute phases.
- Odontogenic and traumatic compound fracture microbial infections are the most common causes.
- Some cases are presumed to be seeded from distant infection (haematogenous spread).
- Occasionally, no infectious agent is identified and culture results are negative, especially in the chronic cases, where some may be related to chronic recurrent multifocal osteomyelitis (CRMO).
- Occasionally chronic osteomyelitis is related to SAPHO syndrome (synovitis, acne, pustulosis, hyperostosis and osteomyelitis).

Radiological features

- MDCT usually demonstrates more features although CBCT may be sufficient in some cases. MDCT is the imaging modality of choice if there is clinically evident or suspected soft tissue involvement, and intravenous contrast should be considered. Insufficiently examined with 2D radiography.
  - Can be focal or extensive, involving large segments of the jaw.
  - Lucent destruction of bone, with ill-defined borders in the acute cases and more well-defined borders in chronic cases. The number of lucent foci can be few, even one, or extensive and scattered.
  - Early cases may demonstrate a hypodense appearance of the trabeculae.
  - Adjacent sclerosis is seen in time. Can be extensive, related to the degree of chronicity. Chronic cases often demonstrate a segment of sclerotic bone with varying degrees of multifocal lucent bony destruction.
  - Sequestra formation is a key feature.
  - Focal destruction of cortices is often seen.
  - Periosteal response (periosteal new bone formation) is also a common feature. Can be exuberant, especially in the younger patient.
- MRI may be useful. May demonstrate the presence of active inflammation not identified on MDCT:
  - Decreased T1 signal and increased T2 and short T1 inversion recovery (STIR) signal related to marrow oedema. Gadolinium contrast enhancement of the marrow and often the adjacent soft tissues.
  - Sequestra demonstrate low T1, T2 and STIR signal.
- Nuclear medicine studies are occasionally employed.

Differential diagnosis

	Key radiological differences
Fibrous dysplasia	Can resemble chronic osteomyelitis although sequestra and periosteal response are not seen in this condition.
Malignant lesions	Differentiation can sometimes be difficult. Bony destruction by some malignant tumours may leave residual bone that resembles sequestra. Some malignancies stimulate sclerosis in the adjacent bone and others stimulate periosteal response. Secondary infection of a malignant lesion should also be considered. Malignant lesions usually demonstrate more aggressive bone destruction. Aggressive destruction of periosteal new bone formation is a malignant feature.
Paget disease	Usually involves the entire mandible. Sequestra and periosteal response are not seen.

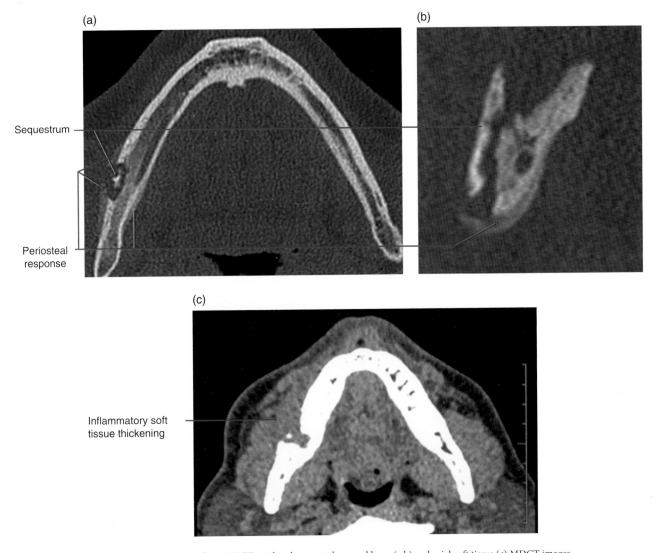

Figure 5.40 Right mandibular body osteomyelitis: MDCT axial and corrected coronal bone (a,b) and axial soft tissue (c) MDCT images.

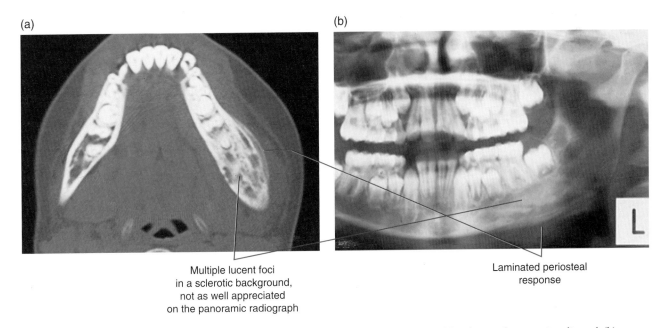

Figure 5.41 Left mandibular body chronic osteomyelitis with a few acute episodes: axial MDCT image (a) and cropped panoramic radiograph (b).

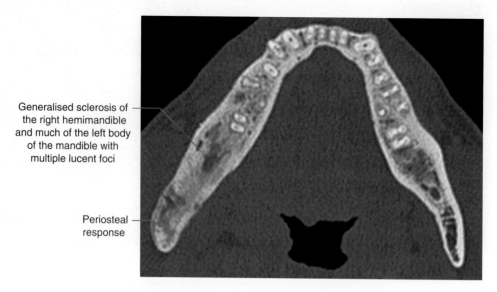

Generalised sclerosis of the right hemimandible and much of the left body of the mandible with multiple lucent foci

Periosteal response

Figure 5.42 Chronic osteomyelitis right mandible: axial MDCT image.

5.5 Dentoalveolar and jaw infections involving the adjacent soft tissues
(Figures 5.43–5.46)

- The extent of soft tissue involvement from dentoalveolar and jaw infections varies substantially. This can range from:
  - A small soft tissue inflammatory focus over the effaced cortex, where it may or may not be draining through the mucosa into the oral cavity.
  to:
  - Cellulitis and abscess collection, which may be life threatening. This may be superficial and may drain at the skin surface. It may involve various spaces, including the submandibular, sublingual, masticator, parapharyngeal and parotid spaces. Potential complications include airway compromise, cavernous sinus thrombosis, cerebral abscess, orbital infections and mediastinitis.
- For the acutely infected sick patient, the imaging should be performed as efficiently as possible and the findings reported to the appropriate clinician immediately.
- Abscess collections usually require surgical drainage.
- Obviously, paragnathic soft tissue infections may be unrelated to the teeth and jaws, for example dermal and salivary gland infections.

Radiological features

- This section is limited to describing the soft tissue involvement (from dentoalveolar infections and osteomyelitis) in the region adjacent to the jaws.
- Where there is more than minor soft tissue involvement or if there is suspicion for cellulitis or abscess collection related to a dentoalveolar infection or osteomyelitis, MDCT with intravenous contrast is the first modality of choice. CBCT is insufficient. While MRI may be useful in some cases, it is less sensitive in demonstrating the dentoalveolar and jaw changes.
- Postintravenous contrast MDCT features include:
  - Thickening of the skin and subcutaneous fat stranding or streaking (linear densities).
  - Fat planes often demonstrate increased density 'dirty' appearances representing the inflammatory infiltrate.
  - Involved muscles are swollen and enhanced.
  - Abscess collection presents as a spherical or lobulated fluid density focus with rim enhancement.
  - Naturally, if this originates from the teeth and jaws, it should also be radiologically demonstrated (refer to sections 5.1–5.4).

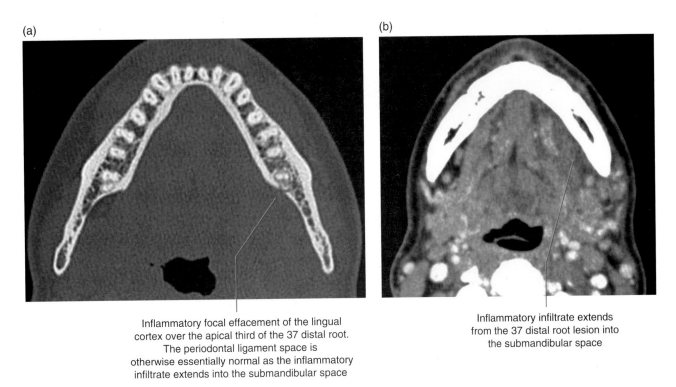

Inflammatory focal effacement of the lingual cortex over the apical third of the 37 distal root. The periodontal ligament space is otherwise essentially normal as the inflammatory infiltrate extends into the submandibular space

Inflammatory infiltrate extends from the 37 distal root lesion into the submandibular space

Figure 5.43 Submandibular space cellulitis related to an inflammatory lesion of 37 distal root: axial bone (a) and soft tissue (b) MDCT images.

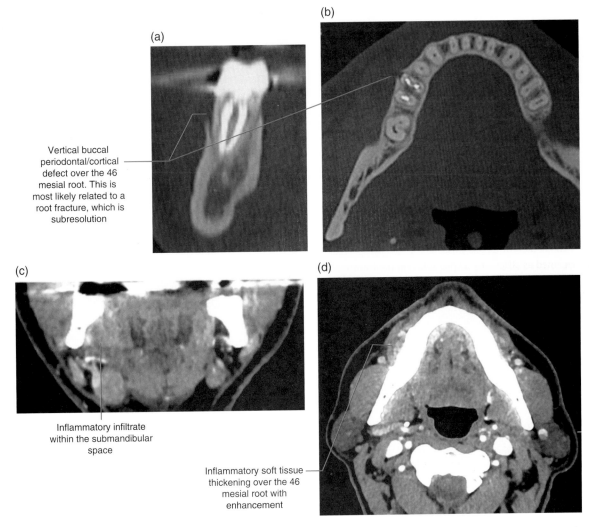

Vertical buccal periodontal/cortical defect over the 46 mesial root. This is most likely related to a root fracture, which is subresolution

Inflammatory infiltrate within the submandibular space

Inflammatory soft tissue thickening over the 46 mesial root with enhancement

Figure 5.44 Buccal inflammatory lesion of endodontically treated 46 mesial root with soft tissue involvement: postintravenous contrast corrected coronal and axial bone (a,b) and coronal and axial soft tissue (c,d) MDCT images.

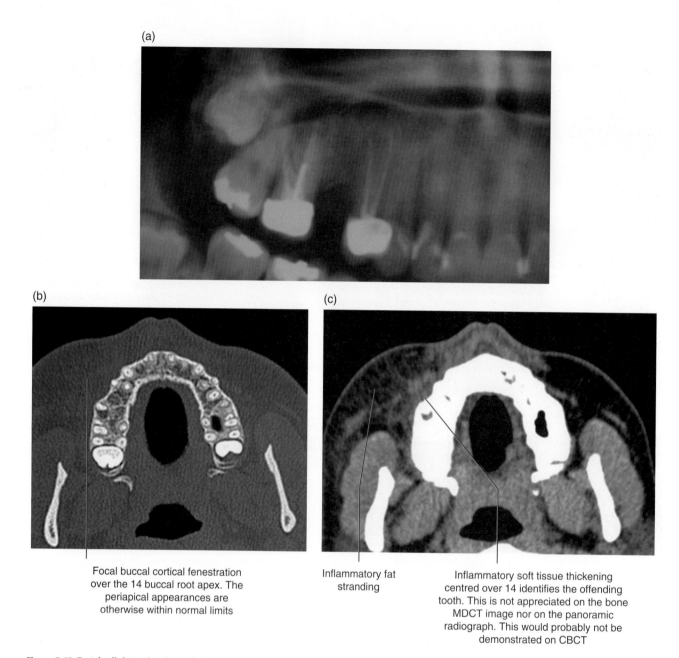

(a)

(b)

Focal buccal cortical fenestration over the 14 buccal root apex. The periapical appearances are otherwise within normal limits

(c)

Inflammatory fat stranding

Inflammatory soft tissue thickening centred over 14 identifies the offending tooth. This is not appreciated on the bone MDCT image nor on the panoramic radiograph. This would probably not be demonstrated on CBCT

Figure 5.45 Facial cellulitis related to endodontically treated 14 buccal root. The offending tooth could not be clinically identified: cropped panoramic radiograph (a) and axial bone (b) and soft tissue (c) MDCT images.

(a)

(b)

(c)

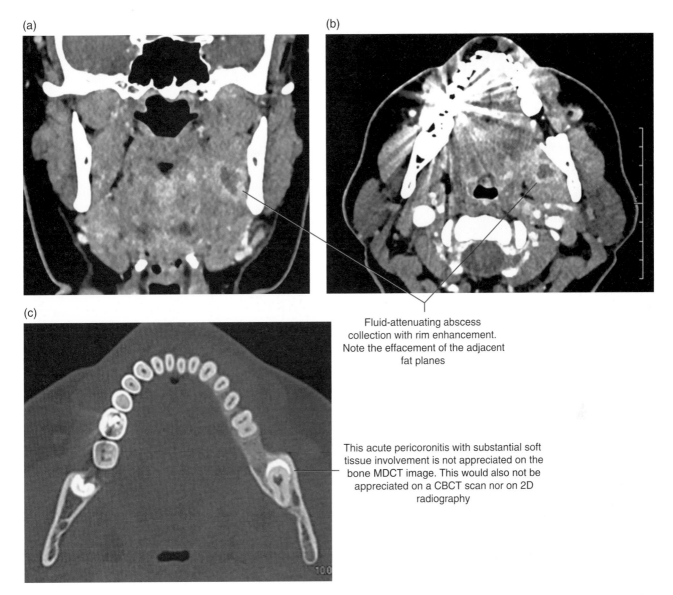

Fluid-attenuating abscess
collection with rim enhancement.
Note the effacement of the adjacent
fat planes

This acute pericoronitis with substantial soft
tissue involvement is not appreciated on the
bone MDCT image. This would also not be
appreciated on a CBCT scan nor on 2D
radiography

Figure 5.46 Left masticator space cellulitis with collection arising from acute pericoronitis related to impacted 38: postintravenous contrast coronal and axial soft tissue (a,b) and axial bone (c) MDCT images.

CHAPTER 6

Osteoradionecrosis and Osteonecrosis of the Jaws

6.1 Osteoradionecrosis of the jaws
(Figures 6.1–6.6)

- Clinically exposed bone of more than 3 months' duration is a definition. Other definitions have been described. Some include the size of the bone exposure and may require presence of the exposed bone over a longer period.
- Most commonly seen in the mandible, especially posteriorly.
- Pain is not a constant feature.
- Infection is often secondary but may also be a contributing factor.
- Contributing factors include trauma, including teeth extractions.

Radiological features
- Osteoradionecrosis (ORN) is a clinical diagnosis and can be present with minimal or negative radiological findings.
- Common postradiotherapy changes (Figure 6.6) which do not in themselves indicate the presence of ORN include:
  - Widening of periodontal ligament spaces, sometimes irregular. There may be sclerotic thickening of the lamina dura.
  - Sclerotic change. The sclerotic bone may occasionally demonstrate a slightly ground-glass architecture.
  - Not infrequently, extractions have been performed peri-radiotherapy. In these cases, delayed or non-healing tooth sockets may be demonstrated.
- Multidetector computed tomography (MDCT) may show relevant soft tissue changes but cone beam computed tomography (CBCT) may be sufficient. 2D radiography is not optimal. MDCT is recommended if there is secondary infection with soft tissue involvement.
  - The involved bone often primarily demonstrates ill-defined lucent focus/foci. Early changes may be limited to the cortices.

- The affected region is often largely sclerotic, resembling chronic osteomyelitis, with or without lucent foci. However, postradiotherapy sclerotic bone changes are often seen in the absence of ORN.
  - Sequestra may or may not be present.
  - Periosteal new bone formation is *not* a feature, usually not seen. May be present if secondarily infected.
  - Delayed or non-healing postextraction tooth sockets may be present but this is another common postradiotherapy finding.
  - Occasionally, there may be pathological fracture.
- Magnetic resonance imaging (MRI) features can be similar to osteomyelitis.
  - Decreased T1 signal and increased T2 and short T1 inversion recovery (STIR) signal related to marrow oedema. Gadolinium contrast enhancement of the marrow.
  - Sequestra demonstrate low T1, T2 and STIR signal.

Differential diagnosis

	Key radiological differences
Malignant lesions	Malignant bony destruction can resemble the lucencies seen with ORN. Differentiation of postradiotherapy irregular periodontal ligament space from that related to a malignant lesion can also be difficult. MDCT and MRI may demonstrate a soft tissue mass related to the malignancy.
Chronic osteomyelitis	Can be difficult to differentiate radiologically. Periosteal response is not usually seen with ORN unless there has been secondary infection.

Atlas of Oral and Maxillofacial Radiology, First Edition. Bernard Koong.
© 2017 John Wiley & Sons Ltd. Published 2017 by John Wiley & Sons Ltd.

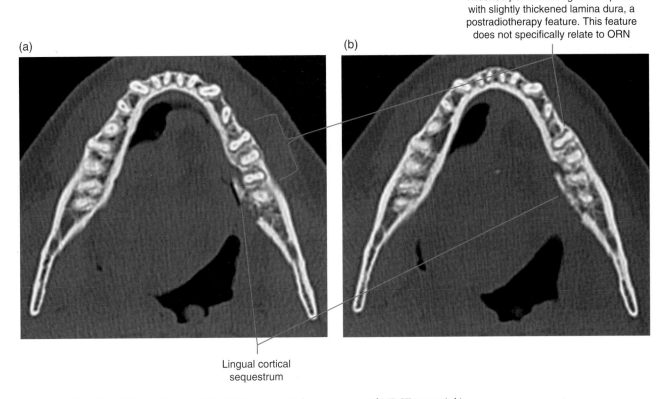

(a)

(b)

Widened periodontal ligament spaces
with slightly thickened lamina dura, a
postradiotherapy feature. This feature
does not specifically relate to ORN

Lingual cortical
sequestrum

Figure 6.1 ORN of the left body of the mandible with lingual cortical sequestrum: axial MDCT images (a,b).

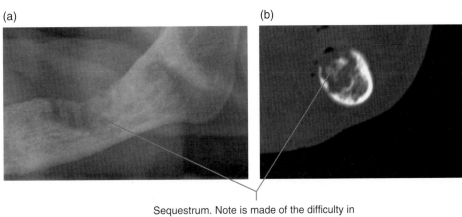

(a)

(b)

Sequestrum. Note is made of the difficulty in
definitively identifying the sequestrum on the
panoramic radiograph. Sequestra within the jaws
cannot be excluded with intraoral and panoramic
radiography

Figure 6.2 ORN with sequestrum of the left body of the mandible: cropped panoramic radiograph (a) and corrected coronal MDCT image (b).

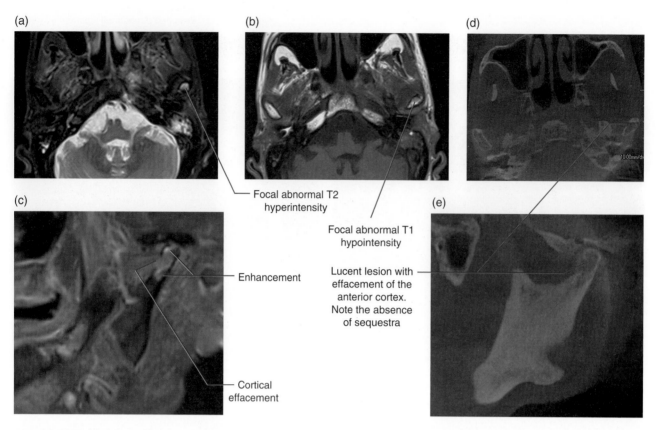

(a)

(b)

(d)

Focal abnormal T2
hyperintensity

(c)

(e)

Focal abnormal T1
hypointensity

Enhancement

Lucent lesion with
effacement of the
anterior cortex.
Note the absence
of sequestra

Cortical
effacement

Figure 6.3 ORN of the left mandibular condyle: axial T2 (a), T1 (b) and postgadolinium corrected sagittal (c) MRI images and axial (d) and corrected sagittal (e) CBCT images.

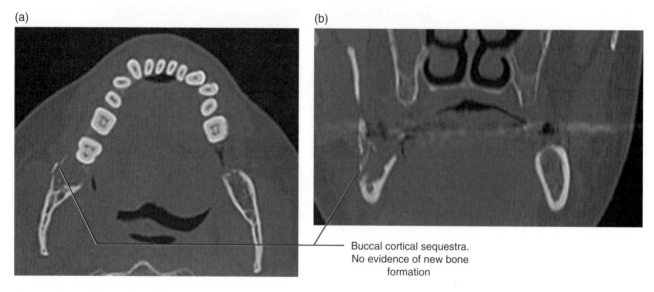

(a)

(b)

Buccal cortical sequestra.
No evidence of new bone
formation

Figure 6.4 ORN at the 48 socket with buccal cortical sequestrum: axial (a) and coronal (b) MDCT images.

(a)   (b)

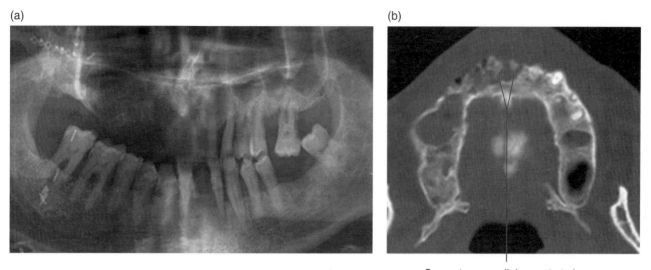

Sequestra are well demonstrated on
MDCT but not appreciated on the
panoramic radiograph. Sequestra
within jaws also cannot be excluded
with intraoral radiography

Figure 6.5 ORN with sequestra at the anterior maxilla: cropped panoramic radiograph (a) and axial MDCT image (b).

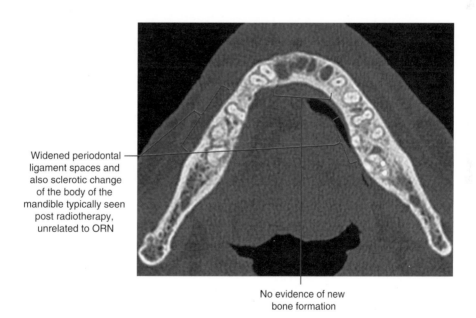

Widened periodontal
ligament spaces and
also sclerotic change
of the body of the
mandible typically seen
post radiotherapy,
unrelated to ORN

No evidence of new
bone formation

Figure 6.6 Lack of new bone formation within anterior tooth sockets several months post extraction related to radiotherapy. No clinical or radiological evidence of ORN: axial MDCT image.

6.2 Osteonecrosis of the jaws (Figure 6.7)

- *Synonyms*: ONJ, medication-related osteonecrosis of the jaws, MRONJ, bisphosphonate-related ONJ, BRONJ.
- Exposed necrotic bone. Some definitions require that this bony exposure persists for at least 8 weeks.
- Related to antiresorptive and antiangiogenic drugs. BRONJ is presently most common. Other potential causes include long-term steroid therapy.
- Trauma is a significant contributing factor, including dentoalveolar surgical procedures and irritation from dentures.
- Most commonly seen in the posterior mandible.
- May be secondarily infected.

Radiological features
- MDCT has the advantage of demonstrating relevant soft tissue changes but CBCT may be sufficient. This is insufficiently examined with 2D radiography. MDCT is recommended if there is secondary infection with soft tissue involvement.
- Osteonecrosis is a clinical diagnosis and can be present without significant radiological findings.
- Radiological appearances are similar to ORN. However, the commonly seen postradiotherapy appearance of widened periodontal ligament spaces, thickened lamina dura and sclerotic changes in the irradiated bone is usually not seen (see section 6.1).
- Air/gas may be seen in cases where there is secondary infection.

(a) (b)

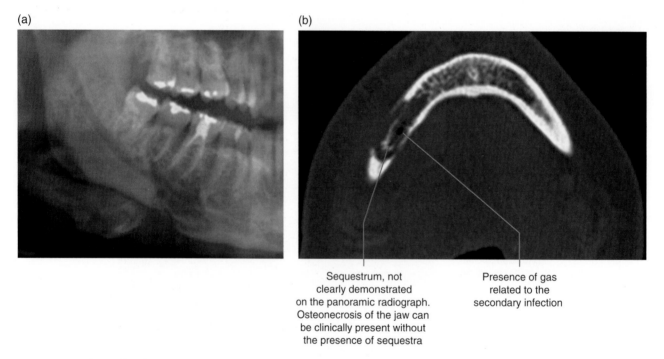

Sequestrum, not clearly demonstrated on the panoramic radiograph. Osteonecrosis of the jaw can be clinically present without the presence of sequestra

Presence of gas related to the secondary infection

Figure 6.7 Secondarily infected right mandibular osteonecrosis of the jaw related to bisphosphonate therapy, with presence of a sequestrum: panoramic radiograph (a) and axial MDCT image (b).

CHAPTER 7

Hamartomatous/Hyperplastic Bony Opacities and Prominences Involving the Jaws

7.1 Torus palatinus (Figures 7.1 and 7.2)

- Midline bony prominence at the oral aspect of the hard palate.
- Variable size and shape. Often very slow increase in size. Normal overlying mucosa, which may be traumatised.
- 20% of US population. Variable incidence in various ethnic groups.
- More common in females.
- Usually identified in the young adult or older.
- The nature of palatine torus is often clinically apparent, requiring radiological investigation only when there is clinical doubt, patient concern or alteration of the overlying mucosa, including ulcers and exposed bone.
- Usually no treatment unless the torus compromises the design/retention of a denture or there is an associated chronic ulcer.

Radiological features

- If imaging is clinically indicated, multidetector computed tomography (MDCT) or cone beam computed tomography (CBCT) is recommended.
  - Poorly depicted on a panoramic radiograph, demonstrating a blurred opaque appearance often projected over the roots of the maxillary teeth.
- Bony prominence centred at the oral surface of the palatal midline.
- Variable morphology, ranging from a small sessile appearance to one with an asymmetric lobulated surface.
- Usually internally homogeneous and isodense with cortical bone. Larger tori may demonstrate internal trabecular bone.

Appearance of large tomographically blurred opacity superimposed over the roots of the maxillary teeth bilaterally reflects one large torus palatinus

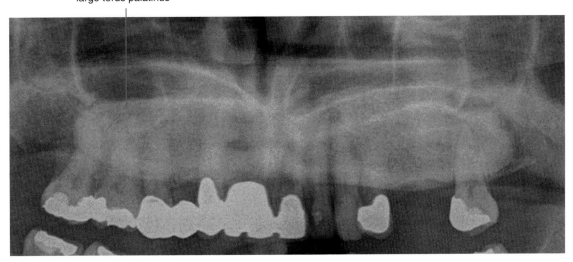

Figure 7.1 Torus palatinus: cropped panoramic radiograph.

Atlas of Oral and Maxillofacial Radiology, First Edition. Bernard Koong.
© 2017 John Wiley & Sons Ltd. Published 2017 by John Wiley & Sons Ltd.

(a)

(b)

(c)

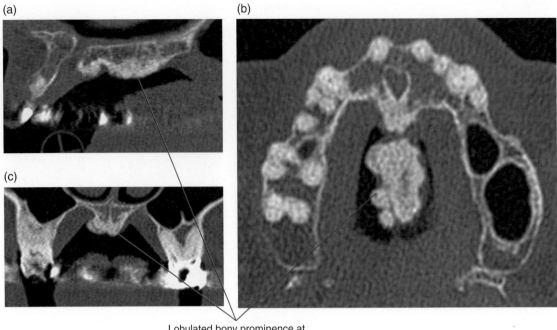

Lobulated bony prominence at
the palatal midline largely isodense
with cortical bone. It is contiguous with
the palatal cortex

Figure 7.2 Torus palatinus: sagittal (a), axial (b) and coronal (c) MDCT images.

7.2 **Torus mandibularis** (Figures 7.3 and 7.4)

- Bony prominence(s) at the lingual aspect of the body of the mandible.
- Variable in number, size and shape. Often very slow increase in size. Normal overlying mucosa, which may be traumatised. Most often seen in the premolar regions.
- Less common than the torus palatinus. Variable incidence in various ethnic groups.
- More common in females.
- Usually identified in the adult.
- The nature of these tori (torus) is often clinically apparent, requiring radiological investigation only when there is clinical doubt, patient concern or alteration of the overlying mucosa, including ulcers and exposed bone.
- Usually no treatment unless the torus compromises the design/retention of a denture or there is an associated chronic ulcer.

Radiological features

- If imaging is clinically indicated, MDCT or CBCT is recommended.
  - Poorly depicted on intraoral and panoramic radiographs, demonstrating opaque appearance(s) projected over the tooth roots at the level of the alveolar crest.
- Bony prominence(s) at the lingual surface of the mandibular alveolar process.
- Variable number, size and morphology, ranging from a small sessile unilateral prominence to multiple bilateral large shelf-like protuberances.
- Usually internally homogeneous and isodense with cortical bone. Larger tori may demonstrate internal trabecular bone.

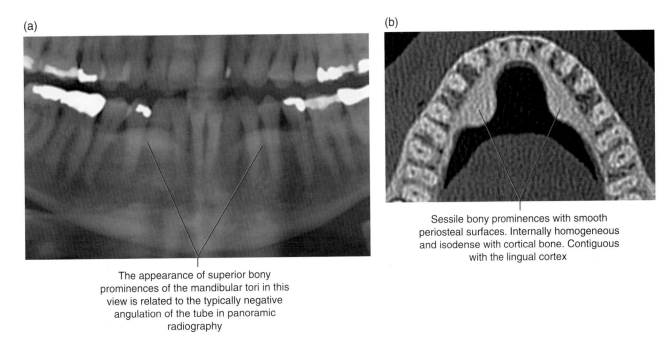

(a)

(b)

The appearance of superior bony prominences of the mandibular tori in this view is related to the typically negative angulation of the tube in panoramic radiography

Sessile bony prominences with smooth periosteal surfaces. Internally homogeneous and isodense with cortical bone. Contiguous with the lingual cortex

Figure 7.3 Bilateral torus mandibularis: panoramic radiograph (a) and axial CBCT image (b).

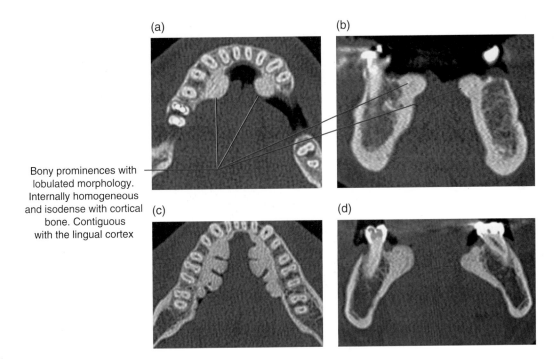

(a)

(b)

Bony prominences with lobulated morphology. Internally homogeneous and isodense with cortical bone. Contiguous with the lingual cortex

(c)

(d)

Figure 7.4 Torus mandibularis: axial (a, c) and coronal (b, d) CBCT images.

7.3 Exostoses (Figures 7.5–7.7)

- In relation to the jaws, this term usually refers to cortical bony prominences associated with the alveolar processes, occasionally with internal trabecular bone. There is no cartilaginous cap. Some consider the maxillary and mandibular tori as exostoses.
  - It should be noted that the term exostoses is sometimes used synonymously with osteochondromas, although the latter demonstrate a cartilaginous cap. Hereditary multiple exostoses is a condition characterised by the development of multiple osteochondromas.
  - In the region of the head, bony exostoses, isodense with cortical bone, may also be seen within the external auditory canals (swimmer's/surfer's ear).
- Most commonly seen at the buccal aspects of the maxillary alveolar process, sometimes palatally. Mandibular exostoses are more often seen buccally, although this may be the result of lingual prominences often being considered to be mandibular tori.

- Variable number, size and morphology. Overlying mucosa is normal unless traumatised.
- The nature of these prominence(s) is often clinically apparent, requiring radiological investigation only when there is clinical doubt, patient concern or alteration of the overlying mucosa, including ulcers and exposed bone.
- Exostoses of the alveolar processes of the jaws do not usually require treatment unless they compromise the design/retention of a denture or there is an associated chronic ulcer.

Radiological features

- If imaging is clinically indicated, MDCT or CBCT is recommended.
  - Poorly depicted on intraoral and panoramic radiographs, demonstrating opaque appearance(s) projected over the tooth roots, often approximating the alveolar crests.
- Variable number, size and morphology.
- Usually internally homogeneous and isodense with cortical bone. May demonstrate internal trabecular bone, especially larger prominences.

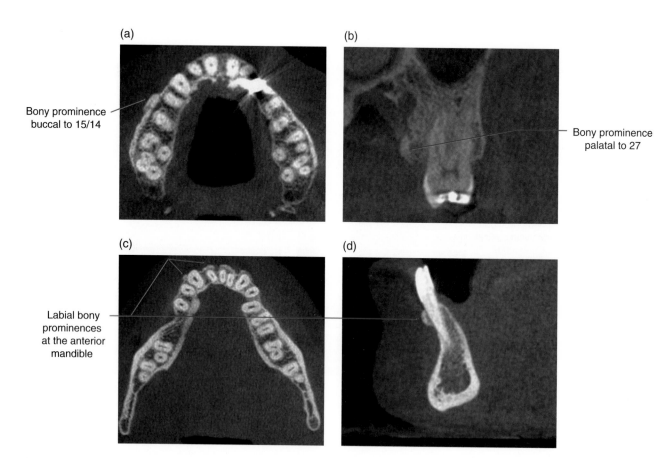

(a) Bony prominence buccal to 15/14

(b) Bony prominence palatal to 27

(c) Labial bony prominences at the anterior mandible

(d)

Figure 7.5 Maxillary and mandibular exostoses: axial (a, c), coronal (b) and sagittal (d) CBCT images.

(a)

(b)

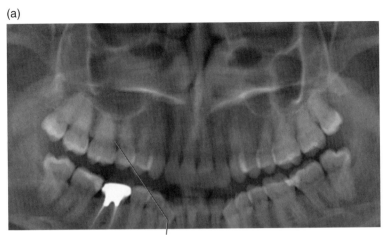
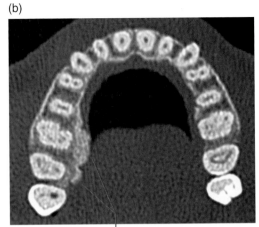

Appearance of a tomographically
blurred opacity reflects the
exostoses, which are poorly
examined in these views

Lobulated bony prominences
internally largely isodense
with cortical bone

Figure 7.6 Palatal exostoses, right maxilla: panoramic radiograph (a) and axial MDCT image (b).

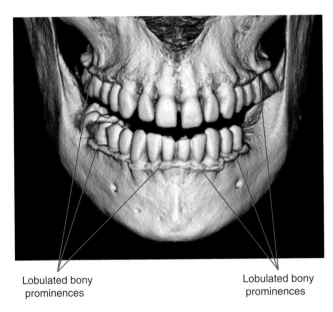

Lobulated bony
prominences

Lobulated bony
prominences

Figure 7.7 Bilateral buccal/labial exostoses, maxillary and mandibular alveolar processes: surface-rendered CBCT image.

7.4 Bone island (Figures 7.8–7.19)

- *Synonym*: enostosis (pl. enostoses).
- A focus of mature compact bone within cancellous bone. Generally considered to be hamartomas.
- Affects any bone. When seen within the jaws, it is more common in the mandible.
- Variable size.
- Asymptomatic and does not require treatment. Usually identified incidentally.
- Often diagnosed radiologically (in the absence of symptoms), not requiring biopsy.

Radiological features
- MDCT or CBCT is recommended if 2D radiographic appearances are not classical and there is doubt about the true identity of the opacity. CT is also recommended if there is suggestion of a surrounding lucent margin or if there are multiple opacities where the appearances are not typical of bone islands.
- Well-defined opacity often with an irregular border. Many borders demonstrate thorny appearances (brush-like border), where these radiating spicules blend with the adjacent normal trabecular bone.
- Internally usually homogeneously isodense with cortical bone. Some demonstrate heterogeneity with variable patterns with regions which are hypodense to cortical bone.
- In the jaws, bone islands often extend to the cortices with no expansion. When adjacent to teeth, they are usually contiguous with the lamina dura with preservation of the periodontal ligament space.
- May slowly increase in size over time.
- There may be more than one bone island; occasionally four or five may be seen in the jaws. However, if there are also opacities within other facial bones, the skull base or cervical spine in the appropriate clinical setting, malignant osteoblastic metastases should be considered. Multiple bone islands have been seen in a few cases of Gardner syndrome.
- Occasionally associated with root resorption, usually only seen with larger bone islands.
- Associated displacement of teeth or interruption of eruption is extremely rare.

Differential diagnosis

Key radiological differences

Other entities which may appear opaque, including:

Dense reactive sclerosis associated with periapical inflammatory lesions	Usually centred at the root apices. While a small inflammatory periapical lucency or subtle inflammatory widening of the apical periodontal ligament space may not be appreciated on 2D radiography, these changes are almost always demonstrated with MDCT or CBCT.
Mature periapical osseous dysplasia	There is usually a lucent margin (which can be extremely narrow) around the opacity, with adjacent surrounding sclerotic borders.
Root remnant	Surrounding periodontal ligament space and lamina dura and a root canal may be seen internally. Morphology resembles a root. Positioned at a site where a root would be expected to be normally located. Sometimes, differentiation can be difficult.
Osteoblastic metastases	Usually multiple and seen within more than one bone, e.g. jaws and/or skull base and/or cervical spine. Most often seen with prostate and breast metastatic lesions. It should be noted that these sclerotic malignant metastatic lesions do not always demonstrate bony destruction and may be quite benign in appearance.
Bony prominences	May resemble bone islands on 2D radiography. The bony prominence may be apparent clinically. A bony prominence is obviously demonstrated with MDCT and CBCT.
Sialolith (salivary calculus)	May be projected over the mandible on 2D radiography or panoramic radiograph. MDCT or CBCT clearly demonstrates that this opacity is not within bone.
Hypercementosis	Presence of periodontal ligament space and lamina dura around the opacity.
Cementoblastoma	Surrounding lucent margin is usually observed and is usually internally heterogeneous. Usually associated with pain.
Osteoid osteoma/ osteoblastoma	Variable heterogeneous internal appearance. Associated with pain.

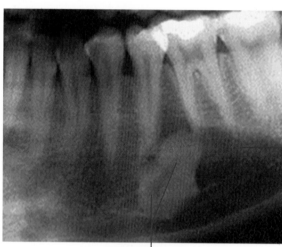

Well-defined opacity isodense with cortical bone. Note the brush-like border mesially. It is difficult to evaluate the relationship with the lamina dura of 36 and 35 in this view

Anterior loop of the mandibular canal and mental foramen

Figure 7.8 Bone island, left mandible: cropped panoramic radiograph.

(a) (b)

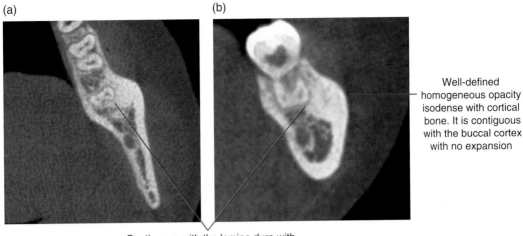

Well-defined
homogeneous opacity
isodense with cortical
bone. It is contiguous
with the buccal cortex
with no expansion

Contiguous with the lamina dura with
preservation of the periodontal ligament
spaces and no root resorption

Figure 7.9 Bone island, 37: axial (a) and cross-sectional (b) CBCT images.

(a) (b)

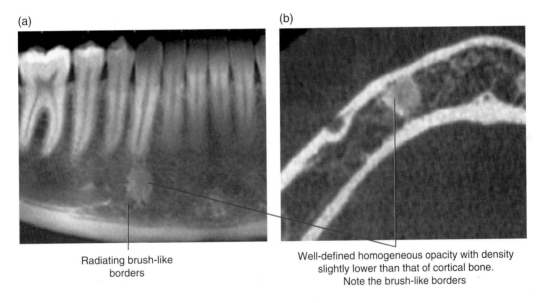

Radiating brush-like
borders

Well-defined homogeneous opacity with density
slightly lower than that of cortical bone.
Note the brush-like borders

Figure 7.10 Bone island, 43 region: panoramic radiograph (a) and axial CBCT image (b).

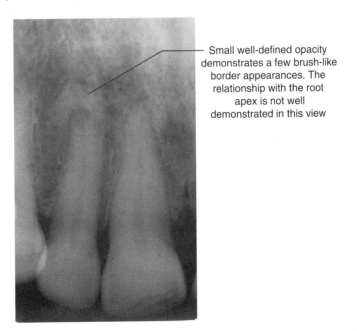

Small well-defined opacity
demonstrates a few brush-like
border appearances. The
relationship with the root
apex is not well
demonstrated in this view

Figure 7.11 Bone island, 12: periapical radiograph.

(a)

(b)

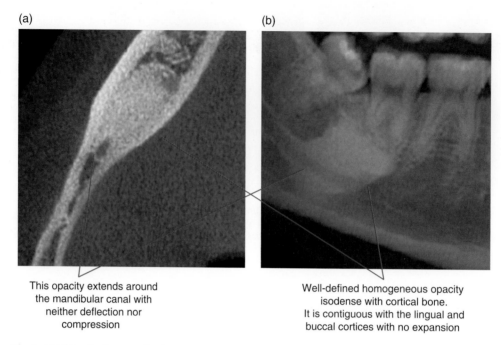

This opacity extends around
the mandibular canal with
neither deflection nor
compression

Well-defined homogeneous opacity
isodense with cortical bone.
It is contiguous with the lingual and
buccal cortices with no expansion

Figure 7.12 Bone island: axial (a) and volume-rendered panoramic (b) CBCT images.

Well-defined homogeneous
opacity isodense with cortical bone.
It is contiguous with the lingual
and buccal cortices with no expansion

(a)

(b)

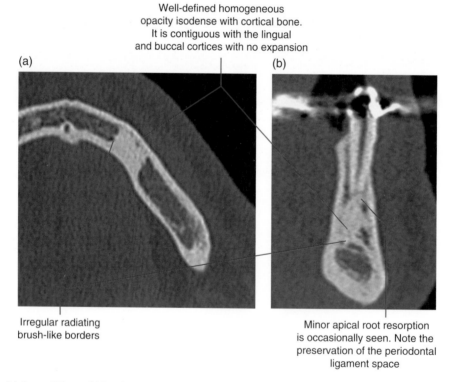

Irregular radiating
brush-like borders

Minor apical root resorption
is occasionally seen. Note the
preservation of the periodontal
ligament space

Figure 7.13 Bone island, left mandible: axial (a) and cross-sectional (b) CBCT images.

(a)

(b)

(c)

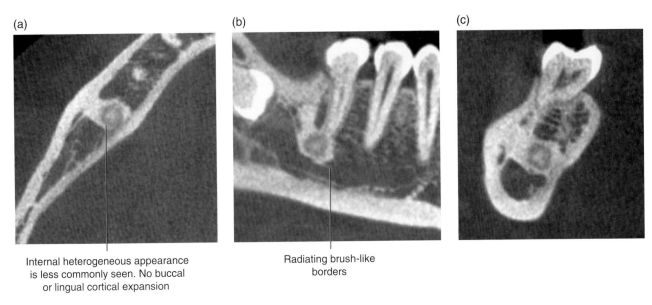

Internal heterogeneous appearance
is less commonly seen. No buccal
or lingual cortical expansion

Radiating brush-like
borders

Figure 7.14 Bone island, 46: axial (a), corrected sagittal (b) and cross-sectional (c) CBCT images.

(a)

(b)

(c)

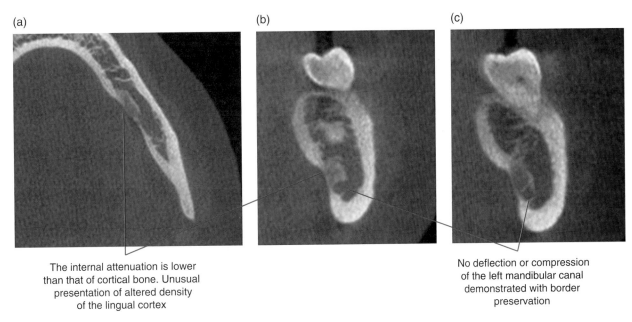

The internal attenuation is lower
than that of cortical bone. Unusual
presentation of altered density
of the lingual cortex

No deflection or compression
of the left mandibular canal
demonstrated with border
preservation

Figure 7.15 Bone island, left mandible: axial (a) and cross-sectional (b, c) CBCT images.

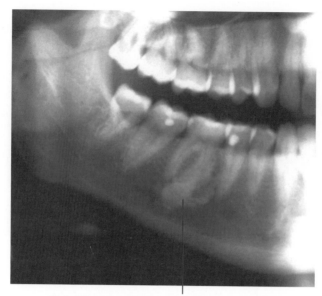

Well-defined irregular opacity isodense with cortical bone. Note the brush-like borders. The mesial root resorption is occasionally seen. The periodontal ligament space is likely preserved, not well demonstrated in this view

Figure 7.16 Bone island, 46: cropped panoramic radiograph.

(a) (b)

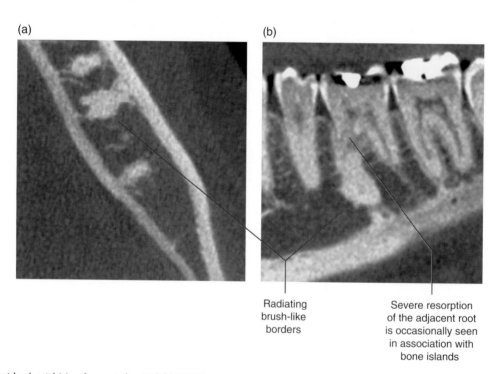

Radiating brush-like borders

Severe resorption of the adjacent root is occasionally seen in association with bone islands

Figure 7.17 Bone island: axial (a) and corrected sagittal (b) CBCT images.

(a)

(b)

Well-defined opacity isodense
with cortical bone. Note the
brush-like borders

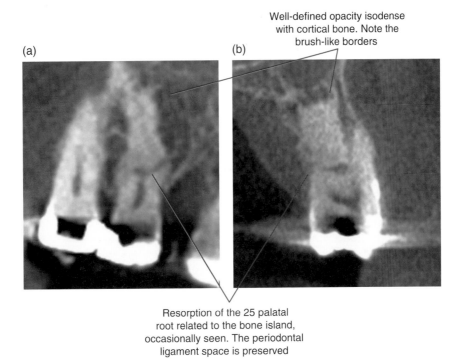

Resorption of the 25 palatal
root related to the bone island,
occasionally seen. The periodontal
ligament space is preserved

Figure 7.18 Bone island, 25: corrected sagittal (a) and cross-sectional (b) CBCT images.

Minimal expansion,
which is rarely seen

Well-defined
homogeneous
opacity isodense
with cortical bone

Contiguous with
the lamina dura with
preservation of the
periodontal ligament
space and no root
resorption

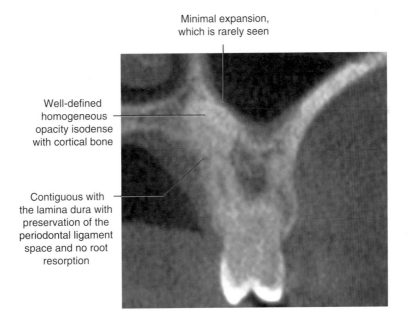

Figure 7.19 Bone island, 26 palatal root: cross-sectional CBCT image.

CHAPTER 8

Cysts and Cyst-like Lesions Involving the Jaws

ODONTOGENIC CYSTS AND CYST-LIKE LESIONS

8.1 Radicular cyst (Figures 8.1–8.10)

- *Synonym*: periapical cyst.
- A true epithelium-lined cyst related to a non-vital tooth.
- Most common jaw cyst.
- Often asymptomatic until it causes swelling or is secondarily infected.

Radiological features

- Computed tomography (CT) is more sensitive in identifying the presence of these lesions than 2D radiography. Multidetector CT (MDCT) may demonstrate more features but cone beam CT (CBCT) is likely to be sufficient for many, especially smaller lesions.
- Corticated lucent lesion centred at the apical foramen of a tooth root. Usually homogeneous fluid attenuation internally (MDCT soft tissue window).
  - Occasionally centred upon the foramen of a lateral canal at the 'side' (non-apical surface) of a tooth root.
  - Often demonstrates a periapical 'tear-drop' morphology in relation to the offending tooth root apex.
  - The border can be more sclerotic if secondarily infected. However, in acute secondary infection, there may be focal regions of absent cortical borders.
  - Longstanding lesions may demonstrate internal dystrophic calcifications.
- Demonstrates mass-type effect when sufficiently large.
  - Displacement and resorption of tooth roots.
  - Expansion with thinning of the jaw cortices.
  - Elevation of the maxillary sinus and nasal cortical floors.
  - Displacement and compression/flattening of the mandibular canal.
- Post treatment, radicular cysts often demonstrate new bone formation beginning at the periphery.

- Occasionally, this bony infill of the cystic defect may be incomplete, demonstrating a residual lucency related to fibrous healing, more commonly seen with large lesions.
- At the maxillary sinus base, bony infill may result in the appearance of an antral bony prominence centred in the apical region (Figure 8.10) (the tooth may have been extracted), similar to that seen with healed periapical inflammatory lesions (see Figure 5.15). These prominences can occasionally be quite large.
- Magnetic resonance imaging (MRI): internally homogeneous low or intermediate T1 signal, homogeneous high T2 and short T1 inversion recovery (STIR) signal. There may be thin gadolinium rim enhancement.

Differential diagnosis

	Key radiological differences
Periapical inflammatory lesion	Radicular cysts usually demonstrate a spherical 'full' appearance with corticated borders. As a rule of thumb, a maximal dimension larger than 10 mm is considered by some to be more likely a radicular cyst. However, other radiological features are more important and must be taken into account.
Keratocystic odontogenic tumour (KCOT)	Rarely centred at the root apex. However, it can be difficult to identify the site of origin with larger cysts. Relative lack of expansion is a feature of the KCOT in the body of mandible.

Atlas of Oral and Maxillofacial Radiology, First Edition. Bernard Koong.
© 2017 John Wiley & Sons Ltd. Published 2017 by John Wiley & Sons Ltd.

Lateral periodontal cyst	Can be difficult to differentiate from the radicular cyst related to the lateral canal.	Bony mass lesions at the maxillary sinus bases	A post-treatment (extraction, root canal therapy, enucleation) healing/healed radicular cyst which has expanded into the maxillary sinus may infill with bone and resemble a bony mass lesion. Antral base prominences related to a healing/healed radicular cyst may be more hypodense centrally (new bone formation begins at the periphery). There may also be evidence of postextraction new bone formation within a tooth socket or presence of an endodontically treated tooth at the base of this prominence.
Postendodontic therapy apical fibrous healing	Can be difficult to differentiate as fibrous healing often demonstrates a corticated border. However, a radicular cyst tends to demonstrate a more full spherical morphology and the border of fibrous healing is usually thick and denser, sometimes with some irregularity.		
Periapical osseous (cemental) dysplasia	Immature lesions are essentially lucent but the borders are usually sclerotic rather than corticated. These lesions are often multiple, affecting more than one tooth.		

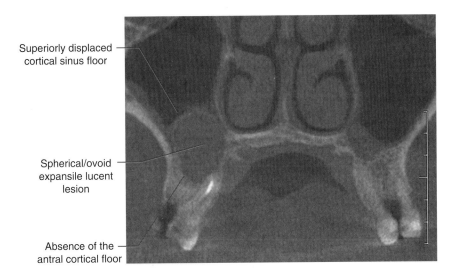

Superiorly displaced cortical sinus floor

Spherical/ovoid expansile lucent lesion

Absence of the antral cortical floor

Figure 8.1 Radicular cyst, 16: coronal CBCT image.

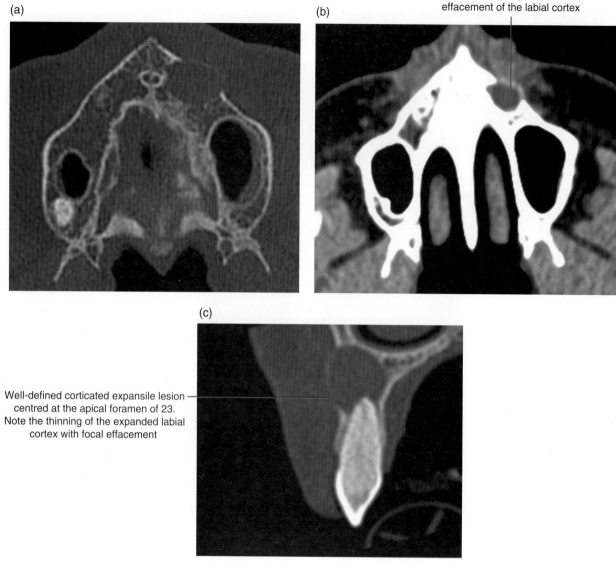

(a)

(b)

Internal homogeneous fluid density. Note that this lesion has remained well contained in spite of the focal effacement of the labial cortex

(c)

Well-defined corticated expansile lesion centred at the apical foramen of 23. Note the thinning of the expanded labial cortex with focal effacement

Figure 8.2 Radicular cyst, 23: axial bone (a), axial soft tissue (b) and corrected sagittal bone (c) MDCT images.

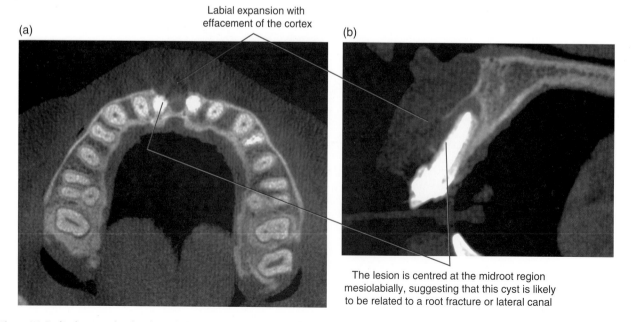

Labial expansion with effacement of the cortex

(a)

(b)

The lesion is centred at the midroot region mesiolabially, suggesting that this cyst is likely to be related to a root fracture or lateral canal

Figure 8.3 Radicular cyst related to the endodontically treated 11: axial (a) and corrected sagittal (b) CBCT images.

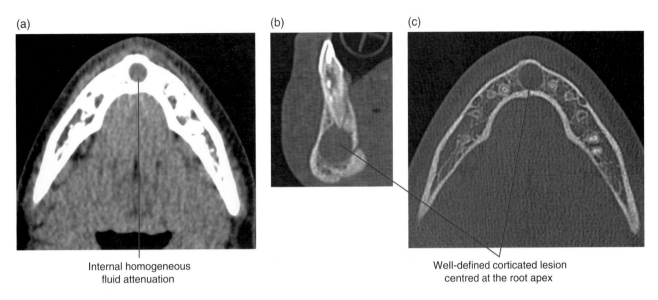

(a)

(b)

(c)

Internal homogeneous
fluid attenuation

Well-defined corticated lesion
centred at the root apex

Figure 8.4 Radicular cyst related to 31: axial soft tissue (a) and corrected sagittal (b) and axial (c) bone MDCT images.

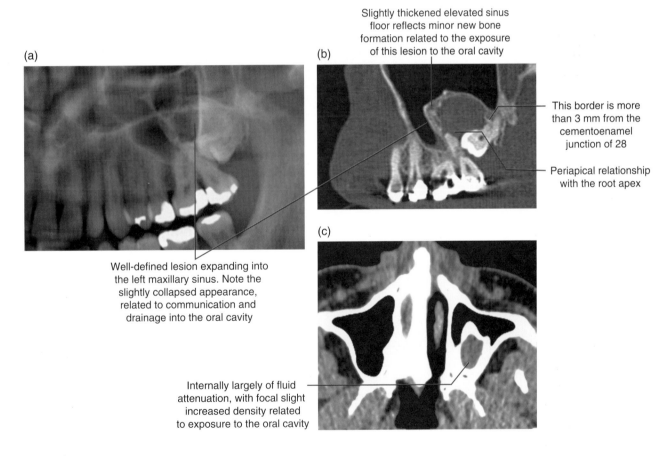

(a)

(b)

Slightly thickened elevated sinus
floor reflects minor new bone
formation related to the exposure
of this lesion to the oral cavity

This border is more
than 3 mm from the
cementoenamel
junction of 28

Periapical relationship
with the root apex

Well-defined lesion expanding into
the left maxillary sinus. Note the
slightly collapsed appearance,
related to communication and
drainage into the oral cavity

(c)

Internally largely of fluid
attenuation, with focal slight
increased density related
to exposure to the oral cavity

Figure 8.5 Radicular cyst related to 27: cropped panoramic radiograph (a), corrected sagittal bone (b) and axial soft tissue (c) MDCT images.

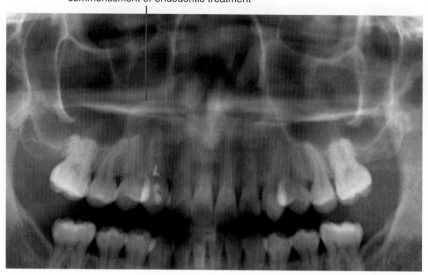

Expansile lesion centred at the apex of 13 elevating the sinus cortical floor. The slightly lobulated appearance of this dome-shaped lesion reflects some deflation related to commencement of endodontic treatment

Figure 8.6 Radicular cyst, 13: cropped panoramic radiograph.

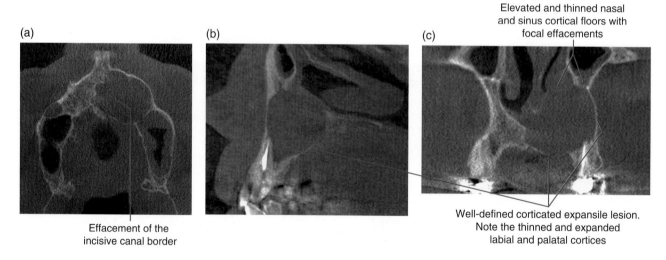

(a)

(b)

(c)

Elevated and thinned nasal and sinus cortical floors with focal effacements

Effacement of the incisive canal border

Well-defined corticated expansile lesion. Note the thinned and expanded labial and palatal cortices

Figure 8.7 Radicular cyst related to endodontically treated 23: axial (a), corrected sagittal (b) and coronal (c) CBCT images.

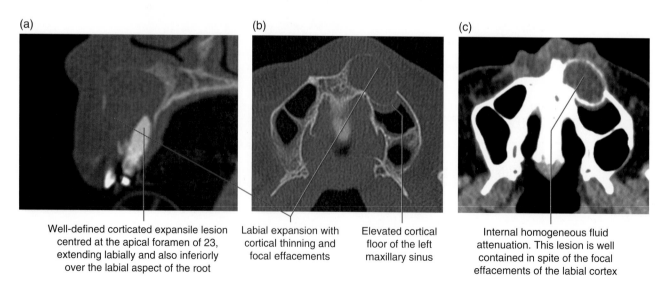

(a)

(b)

(c)

Well-defined corticated expansile lesion centred at the apical foramen of 23, extending labially and also inferiorly over the labial aspect of the root

Labial expansion with cortical thinning and focal effacements

Elevated cortical floor of the left maxillary sinus

Internal homogeneous fluid attenuation. This lesion is well contained in spite of the focal effacements of the labial cortex

Figure 8.8 Radicular cyst, 23: corrected sagittal (a) and axial bone (b) and soft tissue (c) MDCT images.

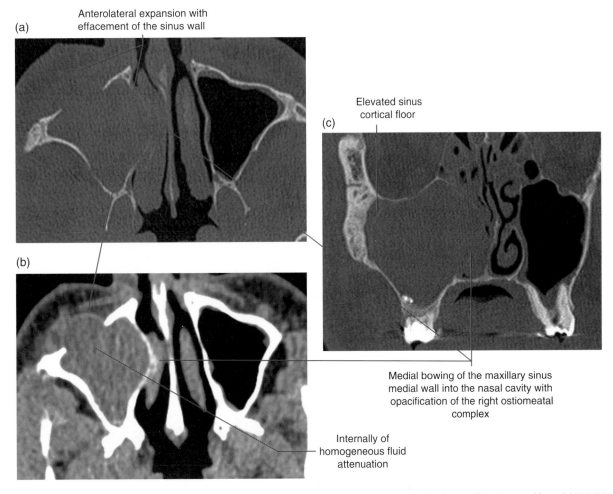

(a)

Anterolateral expansion with
effacement of the sinus wall

(c)

Elevated sinus
cortical floor

(b)

Medial bowing of the maxillary sinus
medial wall into the nasal cavity with
opacification of the right ostiomeatal
complex

Internally of
homogeneous fluid
attenuation

Figure 8.9 Radicular cyst related to 16 almost fully occupying the right maxillary sinus: axial bone (a) and soft tissue (b) and coronal bone (c) MDCT images.

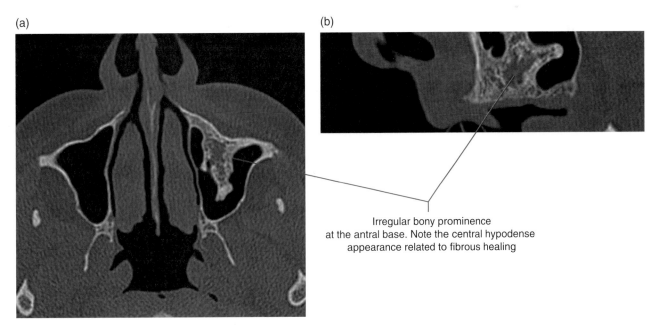

(a)

(b)

Irregular bony prominence
at the antral base. Note the central hypodense
appearance related to fibrous healing

Figure 8.10 Healed radicular cyst, left maxilla (post extraction): axial (a) and corrected sagittal (b) MDCT images.

8.2 Residual cyst (Figures 8.11 and 8.12)

- Postextraction/surgery persisting radicular cyst.
- The accepted term 'residual' for this lesion is not generic and refers only to the postextraction persisting radicular cyst. To avoid potential confusion, this author suggests consideration for the use of the term 'residual radicular cyst'.

Radiological features

- Essentially the same as the radicular cyst, but with absent tooth. The borders may appear thicker or slightly more sclerotic than those of the radicular cyst.

Differential diagnosis

- Similar to the radicular cyst, in the absence of a related tooth.

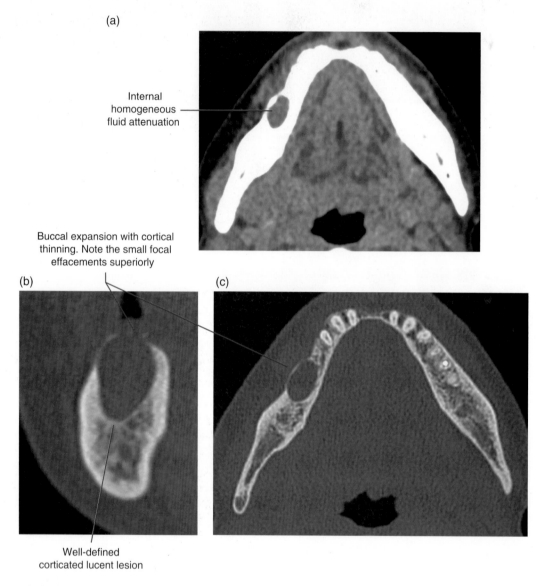

(a)

Internal homogeneous fluid attenuation

Buccal expansion with cortical thinning. Note the small focal effacements superiorly

(b)

(c)

Well-defined corticated lucent lesion

Figure 8.11 Residual radicular cyst, right mandibular body: axial soft tissue (a) and corrected coronal (b) and axial (c) bone MDCT images.

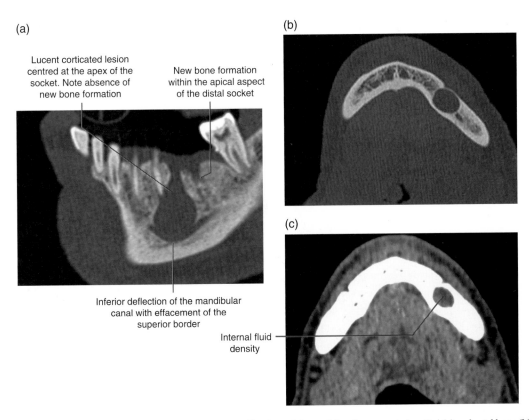

(a)

Lucent corticated lesion centred at the apex of the socket. Note absence of new bone formation

New bone formation within the apical aspect of the distal socket

(b)

(c)

Inferior deflection of the mandibular canal with effacement of the superior border

Internal fluid density

Figure 8.12 Residual radicular cyst post extraction of 36 with absence of healing of the mesial socket: corrected sagittal (a) and axial bone (b) and axial soft tissue (c) MDCT images.

8.3 Dentigerous cyst (Figures 8.13–8.23)

- *Synonym*: follicular cyst.
- A true epithelium-lined pericoronal cyst associated with an unerupted tooth.
- Second most common jaw cyst.
- Most commonly associated with the third molars.
- Often asymptomatic until it causes swelling or is secondarily infected.

Radiological features

- These lesions are better demonstrated with CT than with 2D radiography, although 2D radiography may be sufficient for small lesions which do not impinge upon critical structures. MDCT may demonstrate more features but CBCT may be sufficient for many cases.
- Presents as a corticated pericoronal lucent lesion or appearance of an enlarged follicular space of a tooth crown (5 mm or more – refer to the differential diagnosis). This pericoronal lucency may evenly surround the entire crown or may be more focal, centred at one region or limited to one side of the crown.
  - The border typically extends to the cementoenamel junction (CEJ) or at the root surface within 2–3 mm of the CEJ. With larger lesions, this border relationship with the CEJ may be difficult to appreciate (especially on 2D plain films) as the lesion may 'fold' over the root.
  - This border can be sclerotic if exposed to the oral cavity and is/was previously secondarily infected. When acutely sec-

ondarily infected, there may be focal regions of effacement of this corticated border.
- Demonstrates mass-type effect when sufficiently large.
  - Displacement of teeth. The offending tooth can be displaced substantially, depending on the size of the cyst, e.g. a maxillary third molar can be displaced to the orbital floor.
  - Resorption of adjacent tooth roots.
  - Expansion with thinning of the jaw cortices.
  - Elevation of the maxillary sinus and nasal cortical floors.
  - Displacement and compression/flattening of the mandibular canal.
- Internally, this lesion usually demonstrates homogeneous fluid attenuation (MDCT soft tissue window). Longstanding lesions may demonstrate internal dystrophic calcifications.
- Deflated dentigerous cysts (exposed and drained into the oral cavity) may not display the typical space-occupying expansile features and may also demonstrate more sclerotic borders (secondary infection). Rarely, internal opacities can be seen, which may be related to oral debris or dystrophic calcifications.
- MRI: often demonstrates internal pericoronal homogeneous low to intermediate T1 signal and homogeneous high T2 and STIR signal. These lesions may sometimes demonstrate more heterogeneous internal T1 and T2 signals, more commonly seen if the lesion is longstanding or has been exposed to the oral cavity. There may be gadolinium rim enhancement.

Differential diagnosis

Key radiological differences

Normal follicular space

Can be difficult to differentiate as an early developing dentigerous cyst appears similar. As a rule of thumb, a distance of 5 mm or more from the follicular cortex to the crown surface is considered to be more likely a cyst. Other features, such as slight displacement of the affected tooth, may be helpful.

Keratocystic odontogenic tumour

Usually non-expansile in the mandible. Likely to be attached 3 mm or more from the CEJ. Less displacement and/or resorption of tooth roots.

Unicystic ameloblastoma

Can appear very similar but this is a rare cyst and is usually substantially expansile (more than most dentigerous cysts).

Ameloblastic fibroma

Can be difficult to differentiate. Rare.

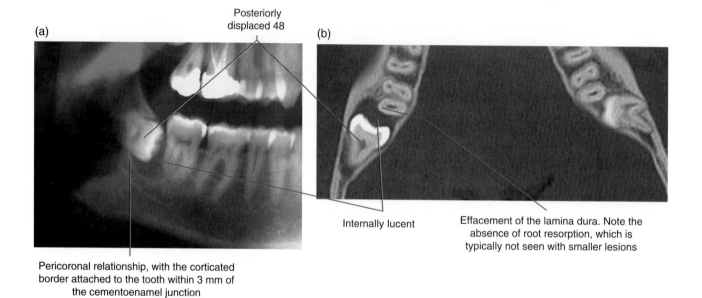

Figure 8.13 Dentigerous cyst, 48: panoramic radiograph (a) and axial MDCT image (b).

(a)

Corticated lucent lesion in a pericoronal relationship with the distally displaced 48

(b)

Corticated lucent lesion in a pericoronal relationship with the impacted 48 extending mesially and distally

(c)

Lucent lesion in a pericoronal relationship with the impacted 48, centred inferiorly. Note the sclerotic margin related to secondary infection

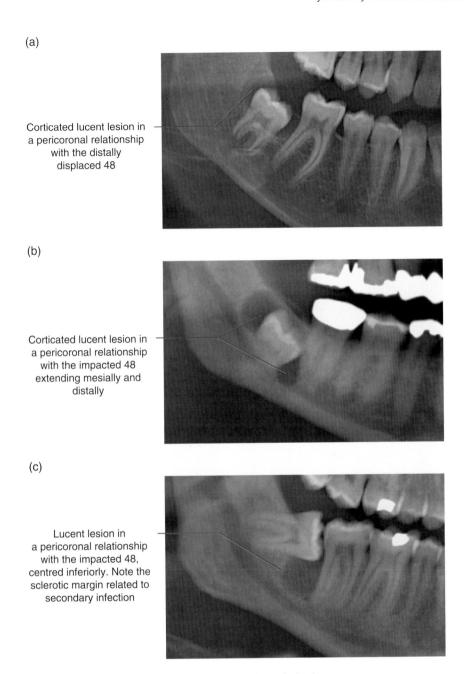

Figure 8.14 Dentigerous cysts of three different cases, 48: cropped panoramic radiographs (a–c).

(a)

(b)

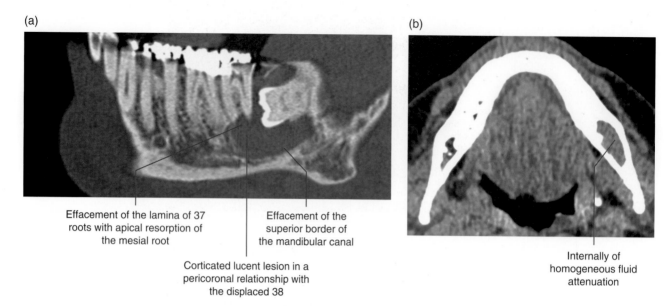

Effacement of the lamina of 37 roots with apical resorption of the mesial root

Effacement of the superior border of the mandibular canal

Corticated lucent lesion in a pericoronal relationship with the displaced 38

Internally of homogeneous fluid attenuation

Figure 8.15 Dentigerous cyst, 38: corrected sagittal bone (a) and axial soft tissue (b) MDCT images.

(a)

(b)

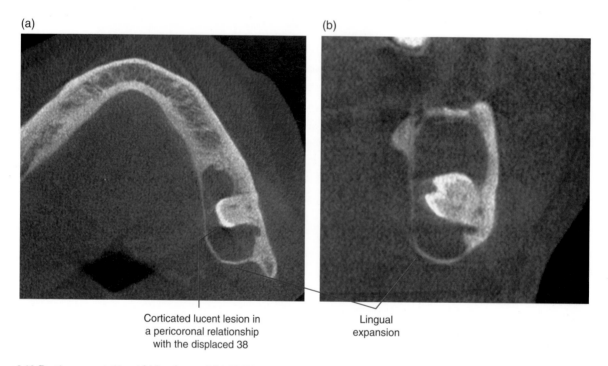

Corticated lucent lesion in a pericoronal relationship with the displaced 38

Lingual expansion

Figure 8.16 Dentigerous cyst, 38: axial (a) and coronal (b) CBCT images.

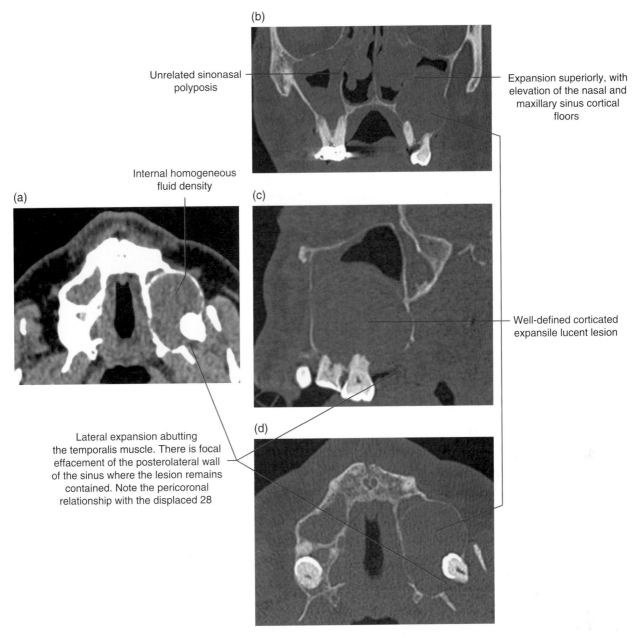

Figure 8.17 Dentigerous cyst, 28: axial soft tissue (a) and coronal (b), sagittal (c) and axial bone (d) MDCT images.

Labels in figure:
- Unrelated sinonasal polyposis
- Expansion superiorly, with elevation of the nasal and maxillary sinus cortical floors
- Internal homogeneous fluid density
- Well-defined corticated expansile lucent lesion
- Lateral expansion abutting the temporalis muscle. There is focal effacement of the posterolateral wall of the sinus where the lesion remains contained. Note the pericoronal relationship with the displaced 28

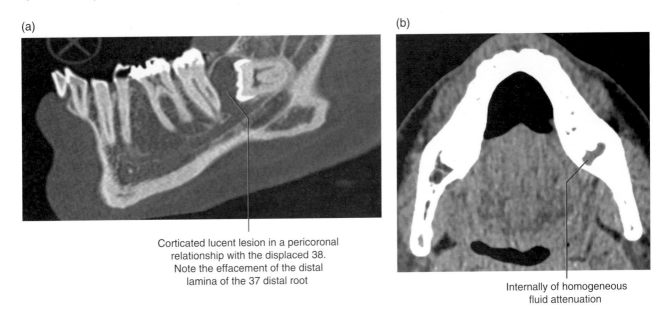

Figure 8.18 Dentigerous cyst, 38: corrected sagittal bone (a) and axial soft tissue (b) MDCT images.

Labels in figure:
- Corticated lucent lesion in a pericoronal relationship with the displaced 38. Note the effacement of the distal lamina of the 37 distal root
- Internally of homogeneous fluid attenuation

(a)

(b)

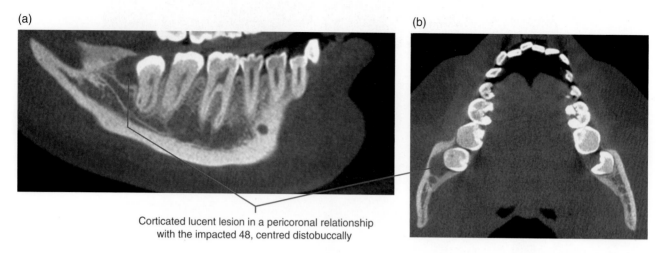

Corticated lucent lesion in a pericoronal relationship
with the impacted 48, centred distobuccally

Figure 8.19 Dentigerous cyst, 48: corrected sagittal (a) and axial (b) CBCT images.

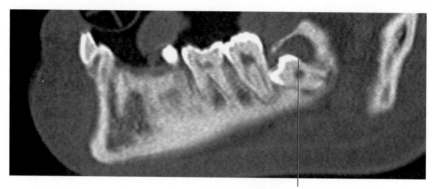

Corticated lucent lesion in
a pericoronal relationship with
the impacted 38, centred distally

Figure 8.20 Dentigerous cyst, 38: corrected sagittal CBCT image.

(a)

(b)

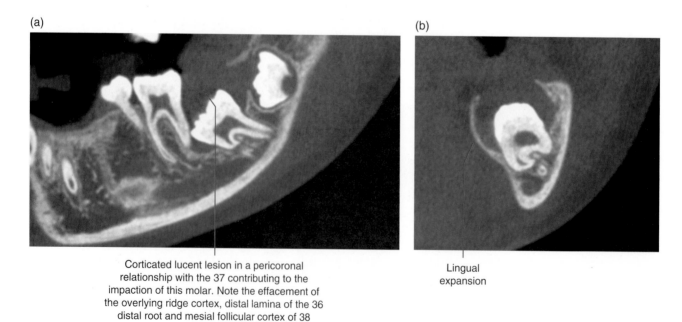

Corticated lucent lesion in a pericoronal
relationship with the 37 contributing to the
impaction of this molar. Note the effacement of
the overlying ridge cortex, distal lamina of the 36
distal root and mesial follicular cortex of 38

Lingual
expansion

Figure 8.21 Dentigerous cyst, 37: corrected sagittal (a) and coronal (b) CBCT images.

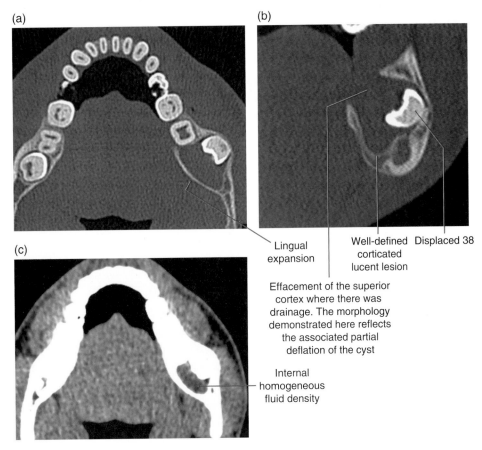

(a)

(b)

(c)

Lingual expansion

Well-defined corticated lucent lesion

Displaced 38

Effacement of the superior cortex where there was drainage. The morphology demonstrated here reflects the associated partial deflation of the cyst

Internal homogeneous fluid density

Figure 8.22 Partially deflated dentigerous cyst, 38: axial (a) and coronal bone (b) and axial soft tissue (c) MDCT images.

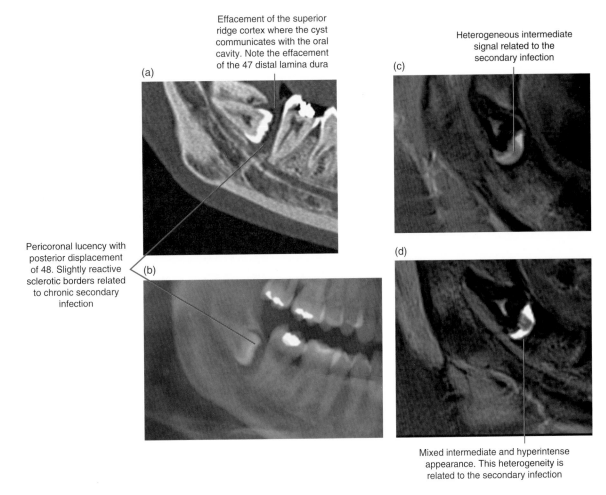

Effacement of the superior ridge cortex where the cyst communicates with the oral cavity. Note the effacement of the 47 distal lamina dura

Heterogeneous intermediate signal related to the secondary infection

(a)

(c)

Pericoronal lucency with posterior displacement of 48. Slightly reactive sclerotic borders related to chronic secondary infection

(b)

(d)

Mixed intermediate and hyperintense appearance. This heterogeneity is related to the secondary infection

Figure 8.23 Secondarily infected dentigerous cyst, 48: corrected sagittal MDCT image (a) and cropped panoramic radiograph (b). MRI images: corrected sagittal T1 image (c) and corrected sagittal STIR image (d).

8.4 Buccal bifurcation cyst (Figures 8.24–8.26)

- An epithelium-lined true cyst arising from the buccal furcation of mandibular first or second molars, most frequently the first molars.
- Similar lesions associated with the mandibular third molars are usually referred to as paradental cysts. Some consider these to be the same as the buccal bifurcation cyst.
- Can be bilateral.
- Usually seen in the younger child.
- Clinically presents with swelling and/or delayed/non-eruption of the molar.
- Can be secondarily infected.
- Postenucleation recurrence is rare and the affected tooth is usually preserved.

Radiological features
- Better examined with MDCT or CBCT than intraoral or panoramic radiography.

- A well-defined expansile corticated lucent lesion centred at the buccal furcation of a mandibular molar. There is often a tendency for this lesion to extend posteriorly from the bifurcation.
- The root is usually displaced lingually, with the occlusal surface of the tooth directed superobuccally. Root resorption is not a feature.
- If secondarily infected, periosteal new bone formation may be evident.
- MRI appearances are often those of a typical true cyst. However, this cyst can be secondarily infected, with associated alteration in signal characteristics.

Differential diagnosis

	Key radiological differences
Dentigerous cyst	The buccal bifurcation cyst is centred at the buccal furcation.

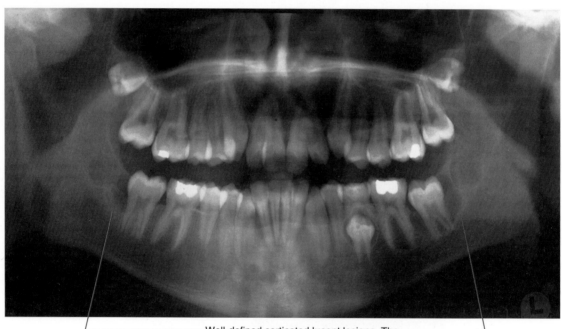

Well-defined corticated lucent lesions. The appearance of a distal relationship to 47 reflects the tendency for these lesions to extend distally from the bifurcation, which is sometimes exaggerated by the typically oblique projection of these tomograms

Figure 8.24 Bilateral buccal bifurcation cysts, 37 and 47: panoramic radiograph.

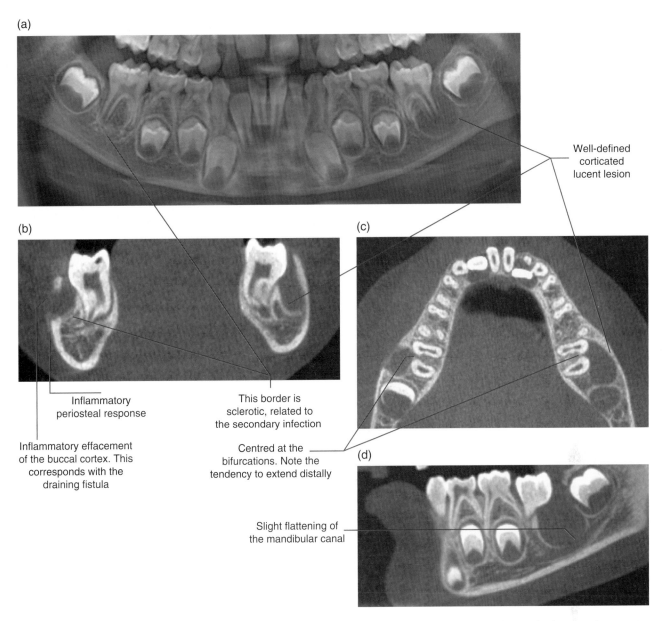

(a)

(b)

(c)

(d)

Well-defined
corticated
lucent lesion

Inflammatory
periosteal response

This border is
sclerotic, related to
the secondary infection

Inflammatory effacement
of the buccal cortex. This
corresponds with the
draining fistula

Centred at the
bifurcations. Note the
tendency to extend distally

Slight flattening of
the mandibular canal

Figure 8.25 Bilateral buccal bifurcation cysts, 36 and 46. The lesion associated with 46 is secondarily infected, with a draining fistula: cropped panoramic radiograph (a), coronal (b), axial (c) and left mandibular corrected sagittal (d) CBCT images.

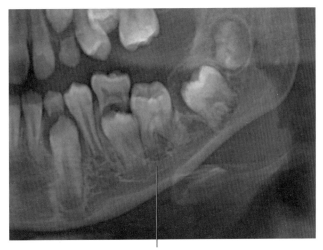

Well-defined corticated lucent lesion centred at the
buccal bifurcation of 36. Note the tilt of this tooth,
related to lingual displacement of the roots

Figure 8.26 Buccal bifurcation cyst, 36: cropped panoramic radiograph.

8.5 Keratocystic odontogenic tumour
(Figures 8.27–8.31)

- *Synonyms*: KOT, KCOT, odontogenic keratocyst, OKC.
- While considered an odontogenic tumour, this lesion demonstrates cyst-like radiological features and is therefore discussed in this section.
- Histologically, the parakeratinised epithelial lining demonstrates tumour-like infiltrative behaviour. This lesion contains viscid keratinaceous material.
- Most commonly seen in the posterior mandible.
- Multiple KCOTs may be related to basal cell naevus (Gorlin–Goltz) syndrome.
- High post-treatment recurrence rate. Requires radiological review.
- Surgical management often includes peripheral ostectomy and/or chemical treatment of the bony cyst wall. Occasionally, marsupialisation is considered for large lesions.
- Usually asymptomatic unless large or secondarily infected.

Radiological features
- A suspected KCOT requires evaluation with CT: MDCT may demonstrate features which are not seen on CBCT. MRI may be useful.
- Well-defined corticated border which may demonstrate a scalloped appearance.
- Most often unicystic and internally completely lucent on plain 2D radiographs and CBCT. With multislice CT (soft tissue algorithm) internal appearances may demonstrate slight heterogeneity, with regions of fluid density and regions of increased density related to the presence of keratinaceous material. However, the internal appearance of homogeneous fluid attenuation does not exclude the KCOT.
- Larger lesions may demonstrate internal septa, usually one or a few, which are quite prominent.
- Within the body of the mandible, it classically demonstrates little or no expansion, relative to the size of the lesion. It is usually expansile elsewhere within the mandible and in the maxilla. It can occupy much of the maxillary sinus.
- There is often variable thinning of the jaw cortices, where there may be regions of cortical effacement.
- While this lesion may displace teeth and contribute to root resorption, this occurs to a lesser degree than that usually seen with dentigerous cysts.
- May displace or compress the mandibular canal.
- When involving the posterior maxilla, evaluation of the integrity of the posterior wall of the sinus and possible extension of the lesion into the pterygopalatine fossa is important.

- MRI: variable. May demonstrate regions of increased T1 signal (keratinaceous material) and regions of increased T2/STIR signal (fluid) internally. May also demonstrate intermediate T1 and T2 homogeneous signal internally. Usually demonstrates diffusion restriction (diffusion-weighted imaging (DWI)). There may be variable gadolinium rim enhancement.

Differential diagnosis

	Key radiological differences
Dentigerous cyst	A pericoronal cystic lesion with borders which are not at the CEJ or within 2–3 mm of the CEJ is more likely a KCOT than a dentigerous cyst. Dentigerous cysts are expansile, unless deflated, usually related to exposure to the oral cavity. KCOTs are more likely to demonstrate scalloped borders.
Simple bone cyst (SBC)	SBCs usually demonstrate a much thinner and delicate corticated border than KCOTs. May also be scalloped. Effacement of lamina dura and root resorption is less often seen with SBCs. SBCs essentially do not directly displace teeth.
Odontogenic myxoma	Can appear similar in the posterior body of the mandible, as both are often not expansile and KCOTs occasionally demonstrate internal septa.
Radicular cyst	The borders of a radicular cyst demonstrate a more acute angle to the root surface of the offending tooth, usually a 'tear-drop' appearance. KCOT borders are usually at right angles or demonstrate obtuse angles in relation to the root surfaces of the apical aspect of involved roots. Radicular cysts are expansile and KCOTs are usually not expansile or minimally expansile within the body of mandible.
Ameloblastoma	The scalloped margins of KCOTs, when present, can be mistaken for a multilocular lesion on plain 2D radiography. Ameloblastomas are expansile lesions, unless quite small.

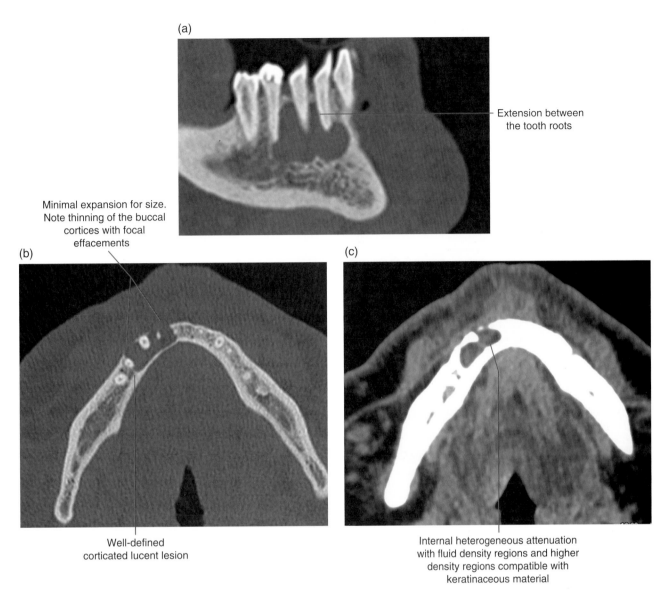

Figure 8.27 Keratocystic odontogenic tumour within the right body of the mandible: corrected sagittal (a) and axial bone (b) and axial soft tissue (c) MDCT images.

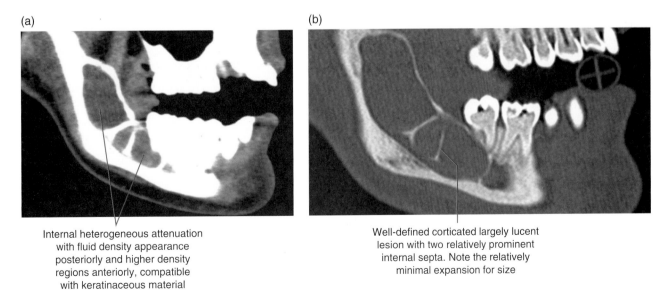

Figure 8.28 Keratocystic odontogenic tumour within the right body of the mandible: corrected sagittal soft tissue (a) and bone (b) MDCT images.

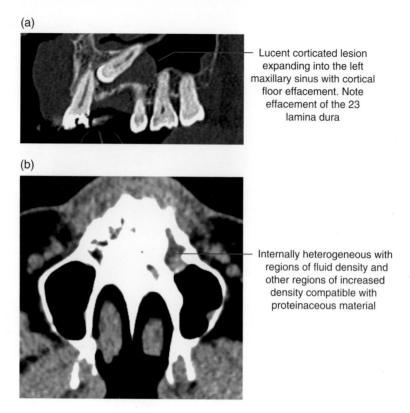

(a)

Lucent corticated lesion expanding into the left maxillary sinus with cortical floor effacement. Note effacement of the 23 lamina dura

(b)

Internally heterogeneous with regions of fluid density and other regions of increased density compatible with proteinaceous material

Figure 8.29 Keratocystic odontogenic tumour within the left posterior maxilla related to 23: corrected sagittal bone (a) and axial soft tissue (b) MDCT images.

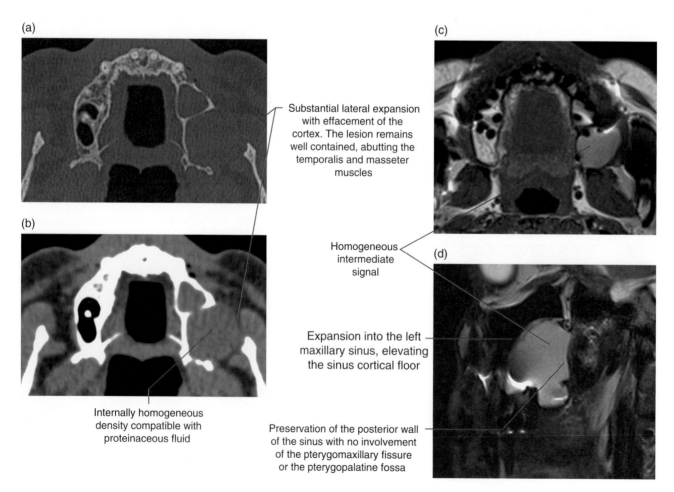

(a)

(c)

Substantial lateral expansion with effacement of the cortex. The lesion remains well contained, abutting the temporalis and masseter muscles

Homogeneous intermediate signal

(d)

(b)

Expansion into the left maxillary sinus, elevating the sinus cortical floor

Internally homogeneous density compatible with proteinaceous fluid

Preservation of the posterior wall of the sinus with no involvement of the pterygomaxillary fissure or the pterygopalatine fossa

Figure 8.30 Keratocystic odontogenic tumour within the left posterior maxilla: axial bone (a) and soft tissue (b) MDCT images. MRI images: axial T1 (c) and sagittal T2 fat-saturated (d).

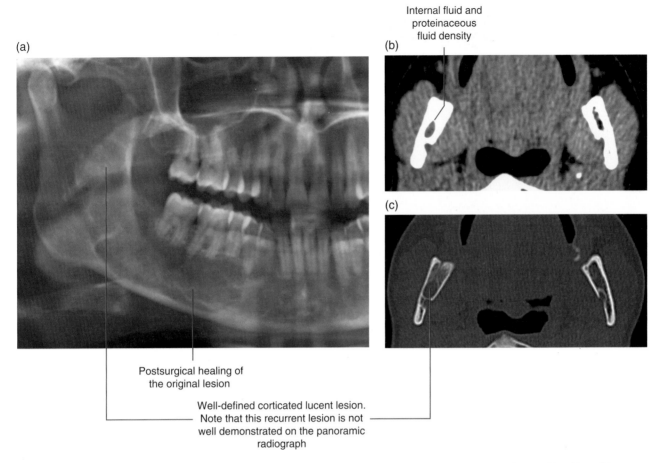

(a)

(b)

Internal fluid and
proteinaceous
fluid density

(c)

Postsurgical healing of
the original lesion

Well-defined corticated lucent lesion.
Note that this recurrent lesion is not
well demonstrated on the panoramic
radiograph

Figure 8.31 Recurrent keratocystic odontogenic tumour, right mandibular ramus: panoramic radiograph (a) and axial soft tissue (b) and bone (c) MDCT images.

8.6 Basal cell naevus syndrome (Figure 8.32)

- *Synonyms*: naevoid basal cell carcinoma syndrome (NBCCS), Gorlin–Goltz syndrome.
- An inherited syndrome demonstrating abnormalities which include multiple skin naevoid basal cell carcinomas, skeletal, central nervous system and eye abnormalities as well as multiple KCOTs of the jaws.

Radiological features
- Multiple KCOTs: refer to preceding section.
- Early calcification of the falx cerebri.

Differential diagnosis

	Key radiological differences
Buccal bifurcation cysts	Often present bilaterally in a relatively symmetric pattern, unlike the basal cell naevus syndrome.
Other cysts	Examples include radicular, residual, dentigerous cysts. More than one of these cysts may be seen. These cysts demonstrate different radiological features.

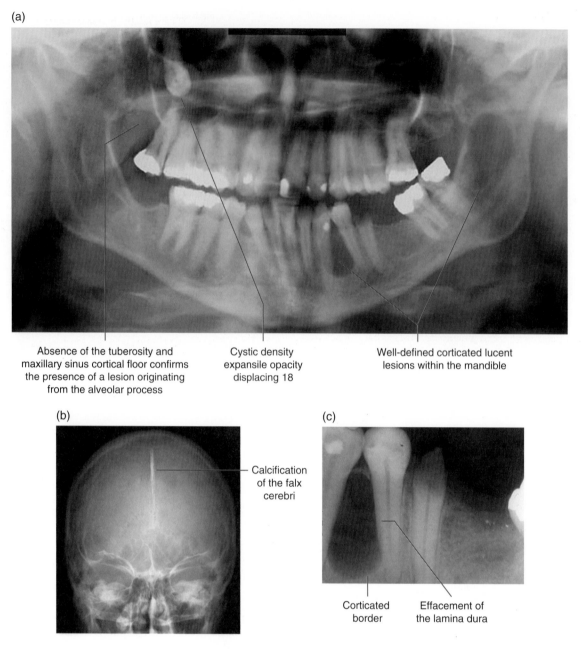

(a)

Absence of the tuberosity and
maxillary sinus cortical floor confirms
the presence of a lesion originating
from the alveolar process

Cystic density
expansile opacity
displacing 18

Well-defined corticated lucent
lesions within the mandible

(b)

Calcification
of the falx
cerebri

(c)

Corticated
border

Effacement of
the lamina dura

Figure 8.32 Multiple keratocystic odontogenic tumours and early falx cerebri calcification related to basal cell naevus syndrome: panoramic (a), posteroanterior skull (b) and periapical (33/34) (c) radiographs.

8.7 Lateral periodontal cyst (Figures 8.33 and 8.34)

- Cyst arising from the odontogenic epithelium of the lateral surface(not at the apex) of the root, unrelated to the pulp status/vitality of the tooth.
- Most often involving mandibular premolars, canines and lateral incisors. Also seen in the anterior maxilla, especially the canines and lateral incisors.

Radiological features
- MDCT may demonstrate more features but CBCT may be sufficient for most cases.

- Well-defined corticated unicystic lucent lesion centred upon the lateral (not at the apex) surface of a root surface. A multicystic variety (botyroid odontogenic cyst) has been described, but is thought to be extremely rare.
- Internally of homogeneous fluid density (MDCT soft tissue window).
- Effacement of the lamina dura of involved teeth is common. Large lesions demonstrate expansion and displacement of teeth.

Differential diagnosis

Key radiological differences

Radicular cyst | Radicular cysts related to lateral canals can appear similar. However, there is often evidence to suggest a compromised/non-vital pulp and there may be periapical inflammatory disease.

Keratocystic odontogenic tumour | KCOTs are relatively non-expansile.

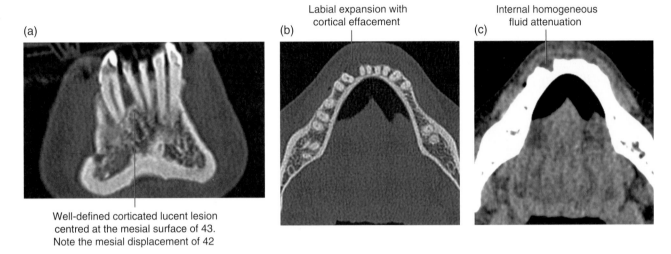

(a)

Well-defined corticated lucent lesion centred at the mesial surface of 43. Note the mesial displacement of 42

(b) Labial expansion with cortical effacement

(c) Internal homogeneous fluid attenuation

Figure 8.33 Lateral periodontal cyst, 43: coronal (a) and axial bone (b) and axial soft tissue (c) MDCT images.

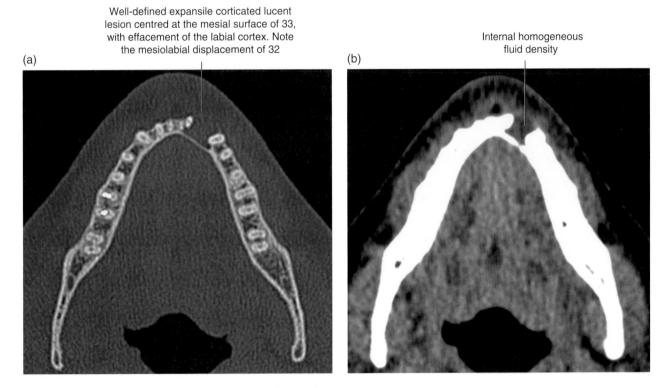

(a) Well-defined expansile corticated lucent lesion centred at the mesial surface of 33, with effacement of the labial cortex. Note the mesiolabial displacement of 32

(b) Internal homogeneous fluid density

Figure 8.34 Lateral periodontal cyst, 33: axial bone (a) and soft tissue (b) MDCT images.

8.8 Glandular odontogenic cyst (Figure 8.35)

- *Synonym*: sialo-odontogenic cyst.
- Odontogenic cyst demonstrating salivary gland-type histological features.
- Rare.
- Tendency for postsurgical recurrence.

Radiological features

- Unilocular or multilocular well-defined lesion with corticated borders.
- Expansile, with effacement of maxillary/mandibular cortices.
- Displaces teeth.

Differential diagnosis

	Key radiological differences
Other multilocular lesions	Can be difficult to differentiate, e.g. ameloblastoma and central mucoepidermoid carcinoma.
Keratocystic odontogenic tumour	Small lesions can appear similar.

NON-ODONTOGENIC CYSTS AND CYST-LIKE LESIONS

8.9 Simple bone cyst (Figures 8.36–8.45)

- *Synonyms*: unicameral bone cyst, traumatic bone cyst, haemorrhagic bone cyst, haemorrhagic cyst, solitary bone cyst, SBC, idiopathic bone cavity.
- A pseudocystic cavity in bone with connective tissue lining. There is no epithelial lining and this is not a true cyst. Usually contains serosanguinous straw-coloured fluid.
- Common. Usually in those less than 20 years old. Almost all occur within the mandible.
- Unknown aetiology.
- Most are asymptomatic, and are often incidentally identified radiologically.
- May be associated with cemento-osseous dysplasias (Figure 8.44).
- May spontaneously heal without intervention (Figure 8.45).
- Usually managed with conservative surgical exploration to exclude other cyst-like conditions. Low recurrence.

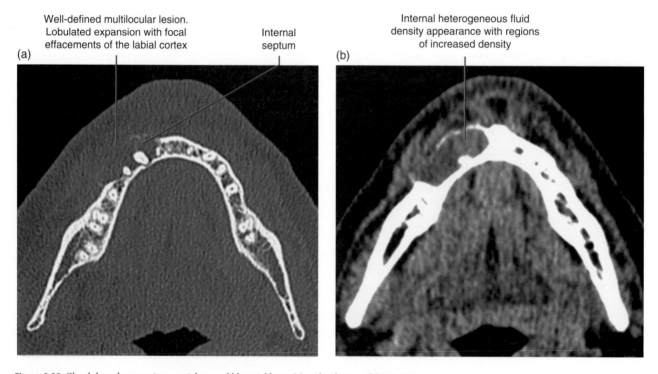

(a) Well-defined multilocular lesion. Lobulated expansion with focal effacements of the labial cortex — Internal septum

(b) Internal heterogeneous fluid density appearance with regions of increased density

Figure 8.35 Glandular odontogenic cyst, right mandible: axial bone (a) and soft tissue (b) MDCT images.

Radiological features

- When suspected, CT should be considered. MDCT demonstrates more features but CBCT may be sufficient for many cases, especially the smaller lesions. MRI may be useful.
- Unilocular well-defined corticated lucency. This corticated border is often delicate in appearance. Some regions may not demonstrate the presence of a cortex but remain well defined. The borders may be scalloped. Usually no expansion, although larger lesions may demonstrate minimal expansion.
- On 2D radiography, the margins may appear ill-defined in some regions, usually where the periphery of the lesion does not occupy the entire thickness of the jaw or where there is less trabecular bone between the cortices (e.g. inferior mandible with prominent submandibular fossae).
- In lesions where the borders scallop the buccal or lingual cortices, 2D radiography may give the impression of a multilocular lesion.
- While this lesion often scallops between the roots of teeth, most of the lamina dura is usually preserved. Tooth displacement and root resorption is rare.

- Internally, it is usually of homogeneous fluid attenuation (MCDT soft tissue window).
- MRI: homogeneous intermediate T1 signal. Homogeneous high T2 and STIR signal. May demonstrate minimal gadolinium rim enhancement.

Differential diagnosis

	Key radiological differences
Keratocystic odontogenic tumour	KCOTs usually demonstrate more corticated margins and are more likely to cause root resorption and tooth displacement than SBCs. MRI DWI usually demonstrates diffusion restriction in KCOTs.
Radicular cyst	Apical lamina dura is effaced. Usually demonstrates a tear-drop morphology of at the root apex. SBC borders often scallop between the roots. The radicular cyst, unless small or deflated, is expansile.

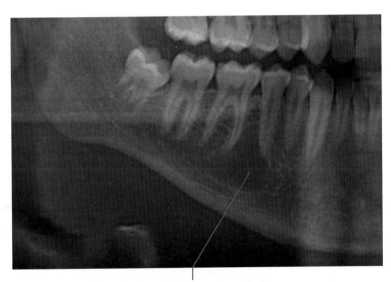

Well-defined corticated lucent lesion extending superiorly between the 45 and 46 roots. Most of the radicular lamina dura is preserved. No root resorption or tooth displacement

Figure 8.36 Simple bone cyst, right posterior body of mandible: cropped panoramic radiograph.

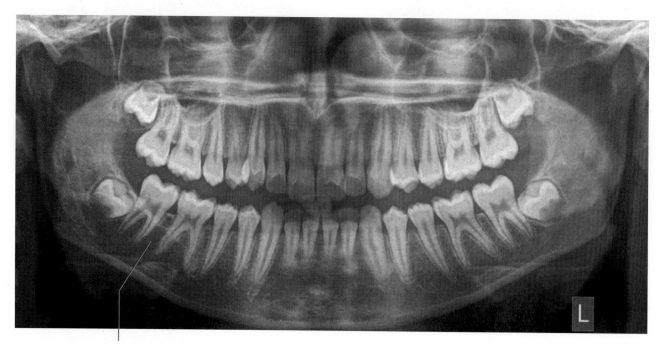

Well-defined corticated lucent lesion extending superiorly between the 48, 47 and 46 roots. Most of the radicular lamina dura is preserved. No root resorption or tooth displacement

Figure 8.37 Simple bone cyst, right posterior body of mandible: panoramic radiograph.

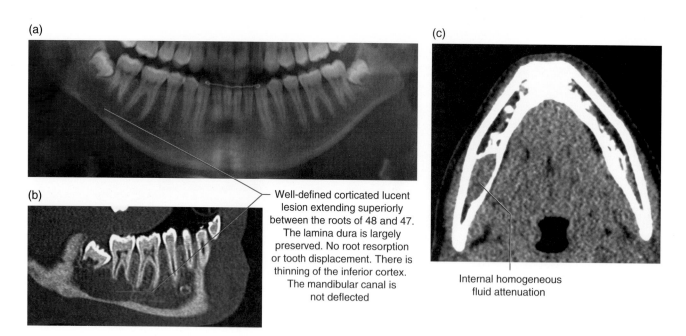

(a)

(b)

(c)

Well-defined corticated lucent lesion extending superiorly between the roots of 48 and 47. The lamina dura is largely preserved. No root resorption or tooth displacement. There is thinning of the inferior cortex. The mandibular canal is not deflected

Internal homogeneous fluid attenuation

Figure 8.38 Simple bone cyst, right posterior body of mandible: cropped panoramic radiograph (a), corrected sagittal bone (b) and axial soft tissue (c) MDCT images.

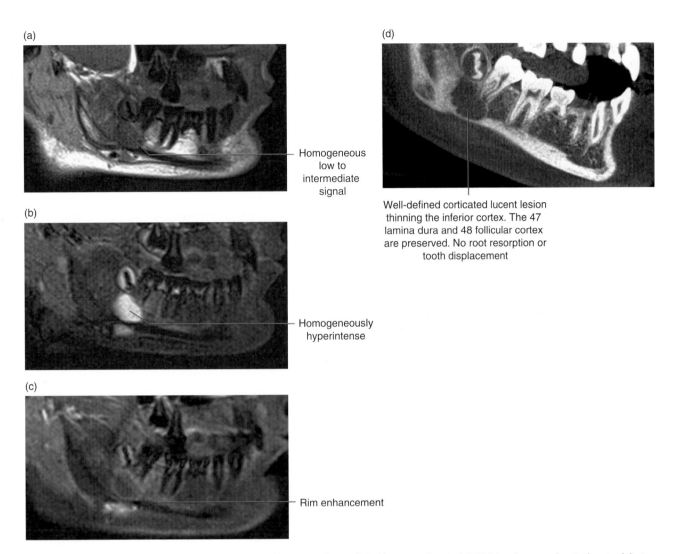

(a)

Homogeneous low to intermediate signal

(b)

Homogeneously hyperintense

(c)

Rim enhancement

(d)

Well-defined corticated lucent lesion thinning the inferior cortex. The 47 lamina dura and 48 follicular cortex are preserved. No root resorption or tooth displacement

Figure 8.39 Simple bone cyst, right posterior body of mandible: corrected sagittal T1 (a), corrected sagittal STIR (b) and corrected sagittal postgadolinium fat-saturated (c) MRI images and corrected sagittal MDCT image (d).

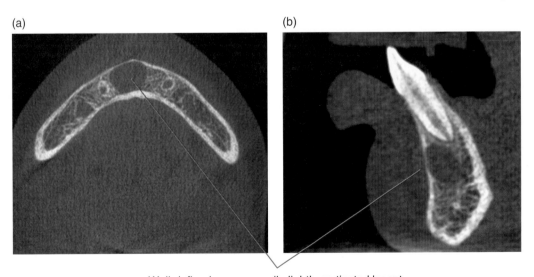

(a)

(b)

Well-defined non-expansile lightly corticated lucent lesion with slight thinning of the labial cortex, which remains preserved. Note preservation of the incisor lamina dura

Figure 8.40 Simple bone cyst, right anterior mandible: axial (a) and sagittal (b) CBCT images.

(a)

(b)

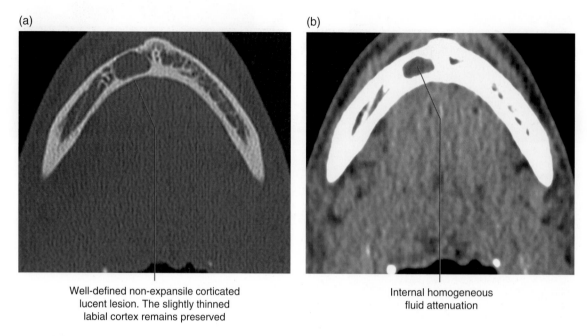

Well-defined non-expansile corticated
lucent lesion. The slightly thinned
labial cortex remains preserved

Internal homogeneous
fluid attenuation

Figure 8.41 Simple bone cyst, right mandibular parasymphysis: axial bone (a) and soft tissue (b) MDCT images.

(a)

(b)

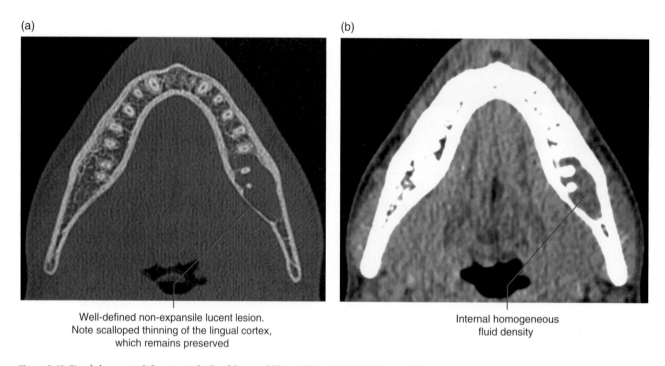

Well-defined non-expansile lucent lesion.
Note scalloped thinning of the lingual cortex,
which remains preserved

Internal homogeneous
fluid density

Figure 8.42 Simple bone cyst, left posterior body of the mandible: axial bone (a) and soft tissue (b) MDCT images.

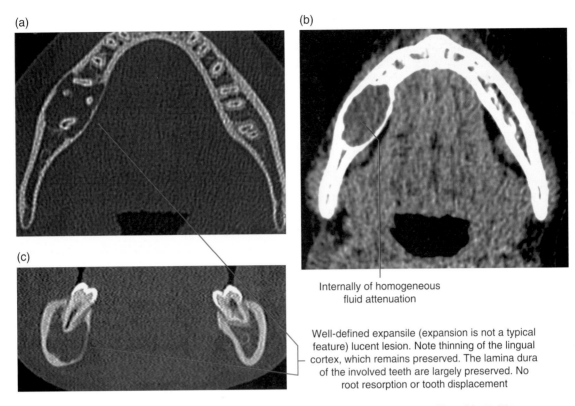

(a)

(b)

(c)

Internally of homogeneous
fluid attenuation

Well-defined expansile (expansion is not a typical
feature) lucent lesion. Note thinning of the lingual
cortex, which remains preserved. The lamina dura
of the involved teeth are largely preserved. No
root resorption or tooth displacement

Figure 8.43 Simple bone cyst, right posterior body of the mandible: axial bone (a) and soft tissue (b) and coronal bone (c) MDCT images.

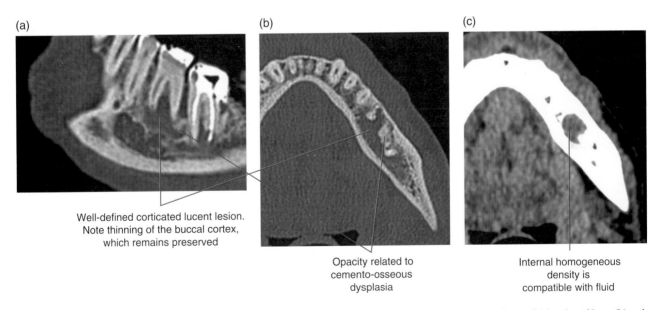

(a)

(b)

(c)

Well-defined corticated lucent lesion.
Note thinning of the buccal cortex,
which remains preserved

Opacity related to
cemento-osseous
dysplasia

Internal homogeneous
density is
compatible with fluid

Figure 8.44 Simple bone cyst associated with cemento-osseous dysplasia, left posterior body of the mandible: corrected sagittal (a) and axial bone (b) and axial soft tissue (c) MDCT images.

(a)   (b)

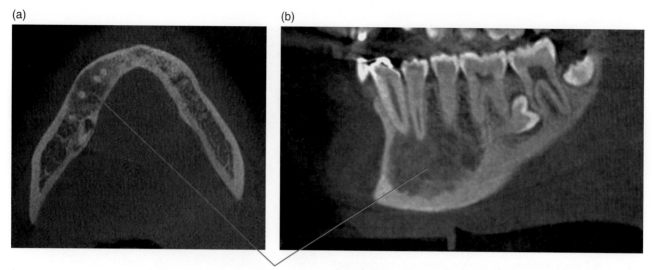

New bone formation with some remodelling related
to spontaneous healing of a simple bone cyst.
Note the minimal expansion and the thinned
preserved cortices

Figure 8.45 Spontaneously healed simple bone cyst, right mandibular body: axial (a) and corrected sagittal (b) CBCT images.

8.10 Nasopalatine duct cyst (Figures 8.46–8.48)

- *Synonyms*: nasopalatine cyst, incisive canal cyst, median palatal cyst.
- Arises from the epithelial remnants of the nasopalatine duct.
- Usually asymptomatic until large, when swelling is the most common first clinical feature. This swelling is classically fluctuant.
- Most often enucleated. Recurrence is low.

Radiological features

- MDCT may demonstrate more features but CBCT is likely to be sufficient, especially with smaller lesions.
- Well-defined, lucent, corticated lesion centred at the incisive canal.
- Often asymmetric.
- Expansile when sufficiently large. This can be seen labially and palatally. It may also expand into the nasal cavity and maxillary sinus, elevating the cortical floors.
- The expanded maxillary cortices are often thinned with focal regions of effacement.
- Displaces teeth and resorbs roots when sufficiently large.
- Internally, it is usually of homogeneous fluid attenuation (MDCT soft tissue algorithm).

- MRI: homogeneous intermediate to slightly hyperintense T1 signal. Homogeneous high T2 signal.

Differential diagnosis

Key radiological differences

Large incisive canal	Can be difficult to differentiate as the normal incisive canal is not infrequently asymmetric, with focal region(s) of asymmetric corticated prominence(s). Symmetric focal corticated widened appearance can also reflect a normal variant. Some consider that a maximal transverse dimension of the canal/foramen of more than 6 mm is more likely to reflect a cyst. However, the normal incisive canal presents with a large variation in morphology and size. Evidence of expansion, tooth displacement or resorption favours the presence of a nasopalatine duct cyst.
Radicular cyst	The radicular cyst is centred upon a root, usually apically. This is more likely to be mistaken for a nasopalatine duct cyst on 2D radiography. If a nasopalatine duct cyst is suspected, pretreatment MDCT or CBCT should be considered.

(a)

Effacement of the 21 and 22
lamina dura with no resorption.
Note that root resorption is usually
eventually seen with larger lesions

(b)

(c)

Well-defined corticated lucent focal
widening of the incisive canal

Accessory neurovascular canal
and foramen, a normal variant

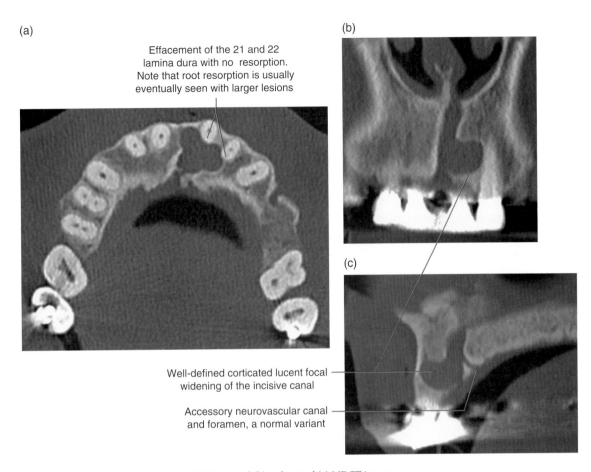

Figure 8.46 Nasopalatine duct cyst, premaxilla: axial (a), coronal (b) and sagittal (c) MDCT images.

(a)

(b)

(c)

Focal well-defined corticated
lucent widening of the incisive
canal and foramen

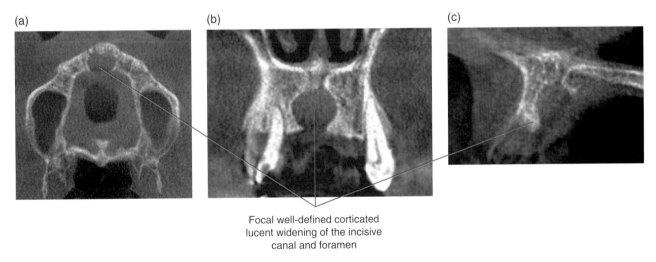

Figure 8.47 Nasopalatine duct cyst, premaxilla: axial (a), coronal (b) and sagittal (c) CBCT images.

(a)

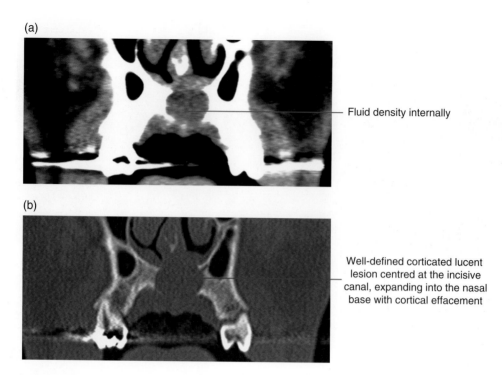

Fluid density internally

(b)

Well-defined corticated lucent lesion centred at the incisive canal, expanding into the nasal base with cortical effacement

Figure 8.48 Nasopalatine duct cyst, premaxilla: coronal soft tissue (a) and bone (b) MDCT images.

8.11 Nasolabial cyst (Figure 8.49)

- *Synonym*: nasoalveolar cyst.
- Non-odontogenic developmental cyst occurring in the naso-alar region.
- Rare.
- Low tendency for postsurgical recurrence.

Radiological features

- Not well demonstrated on 2D radiography. CBCT may be sufficient for the evaluation of bony involvement but MDCT usually demonstrates more features. Ultrasound or MRI could be considered.
- Well-defined spherical or ovoid lesion centred in the soft tissues of the nasoalar region, over the base of the premaxillary alveolar process. Most are unilateral but may be bilateral.
- Internally, it is usually isodense with proteinaceous fluid (MDCT soft tissue algorithm).
- Larger lesions may remodel the labial aspect of the alveolar process, resulting in a focal concave depression of the anterior surface usually at the level of the incisor root apices. This depression usually remains corticated. Where the depression extends to the tooth roots, there is usually associated root resorption.
- MRI: variable T1 signal. High T2 signal. There may be focal regions of intermediate signal related to proteinaceous material.

Differential diagnosis

	Key radiological differences
Periapical lesion	The focal depression at the labial surface of the maxillary alveolar process may present as a lucent appearance at the anterior root apices on 2D radiography. MDCT or CBCT usually clarifies.
Minor salivary gland lesions	Mucous retention/extravasation or cystic tumours related to minor salivary glands can appear similar.

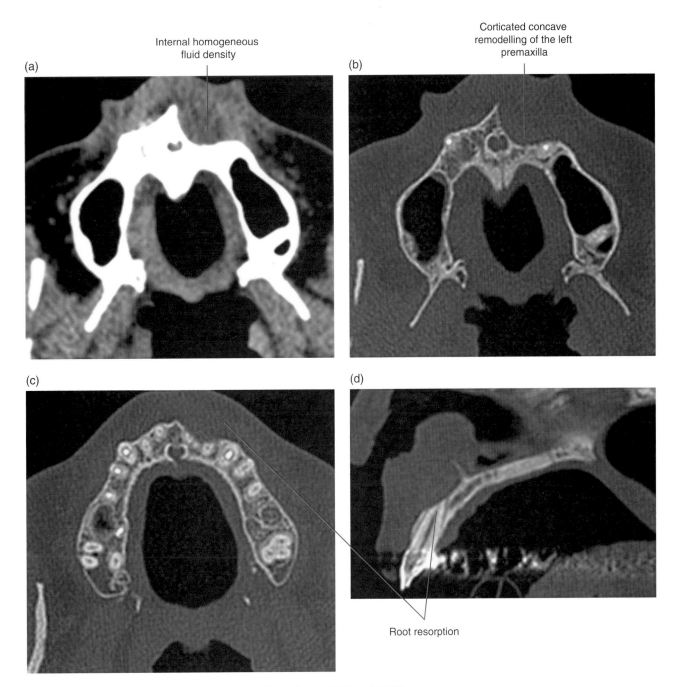

Figure 8.49 Nasolabial cyst: axial soft tissue (a) and axial (b,c) and sagittal (d) bone MDCT images.

CHAPTER 9
Fibro-osseous Lesions of the Jaws

9.1 Fibrous dysplasia (Figures 9.1–9.10; also see Figure 20.17)

- Benign genetically based sporadic condition of bone where there is abnormal remodelling with presence of dysplastic fibrous tissue and varying amounts of immature bone.
- Most common benign bone disorder.
- Can be:
  - Monostotic (one location) – majority of cases.
  - Polyostotic (multiple locations) – usually identified in young children. Can be associated with McCune–Albright syndrome.
- Growth of lesion usually ceases at the end of skeletal growth.
- May present with painless facial swelling and asymmetry. Larger lesions may impinge on nerves.
- Clinical and radiological diagnosis is often sufficient, without biopsy. Histological appearances can be 'fibro-osseous but otherwise non-specific'.
- Surgical interventions resulting in exuberant growth in the younger patient have been reported.
- Sarcomatous changes have been reported but generally considered to be rare.

Radiological features
- Best examined with multidetector computed tomography (MDCT) or cone beam computed tomography (CBCT).
- Solitary lesions are almost always limited to one bone.
- Borders are often described as ill-defined, but this is usually a plain film appearance. These lesions often demonstrate relatively well-defined borders on MDCT, CBCT and magnetic resonance imaging (MRI).
- Often hyperdense to normal bone but some may present with focal regions of increased density as well as focal regions which are hypodense and lucent compared with normal bone.
- Classical 'ground-glass' internal appearance is most frequently seen, at least in some regions of the lesion. However, other internal patterns, including cotton wool, orange peel, cyst-like and 'multilocular' appearances, are also seen.

- Expansion is an important feature, unless the lesion is extremely small. The expanded bone tends to resemble the original anatomy. That is, while expanded and slightly distorted, the general morphology of the structure is preserved. For example, expansion at the maxillary sinus base will elevate this floor, but the concave shape of this floor is maintained.
- There is often thinning and alteration of the cortical architecture, sometimes with focal regions where the cortex is absent.
- The architecture of the lamina dura of the teeth is often altered and may be indistinct. Teeth are often displaced. Root resorption is rare.
- Lesions inferior to the mandibular canal will classically deflect the canal superiorly.
- Variable MRI signal pattern is related to the amount and pattern of bone and fibrous tissue, presence of spindle cells and haemorrhage. Usually T1 and T2 hypointense. Variable gadolinium enhancement.

Differential diagnosis

Differential diagnosis	Key radiological differences
Chronic osteomyelitis	Demonstrates periosteal response and sequestra.
Ossifying fibroma	More tumour-like growth and expansion where the normal morphology is not preserved. There may be surrounding lucent margin.
Osteogenic sarcoma	More aggressive bone growth, usually with spiculation.
Paget disease	Usually older age group and usually bilateral.

Atlas of Oral and Maxillofacial Radiology, First Edition. Bernard Koong.
© 2017 John Wiley & Sons Ltd. Published 2017 by John Wiley & Sons Ltd.

(a)

(b)

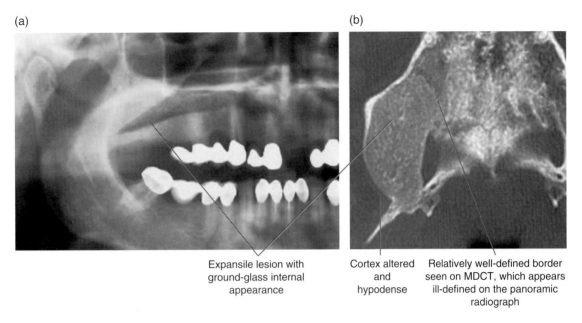

Expansile lesion with
ground-glass internal
appearance

Cortex altered
and
hypodense

Relatively well-defined border
seen on MDCT, which appears
ill-defined on the panoramic
radiograph

Figure 9.1 Fibrous dysplasia: panoramic radiograph (a) and axial MDCT image (b).

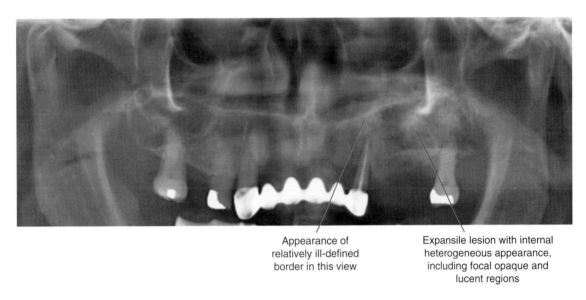

Appearance of
relatively ill-defined
border in this view

Expansile lesion with internal
heterogeneous appearance,
including focal opaque and
lucent regions

Figure 9.2 Fibrous dysplasia: cropped panoramic radiograph.

The sinus floor has been elevated and not visualised

Expansile lesion with internal homogeneous ground-glass appearance

Several cortical structures are altered and no longer visualised in this view, including the infraorbital canal and foramen

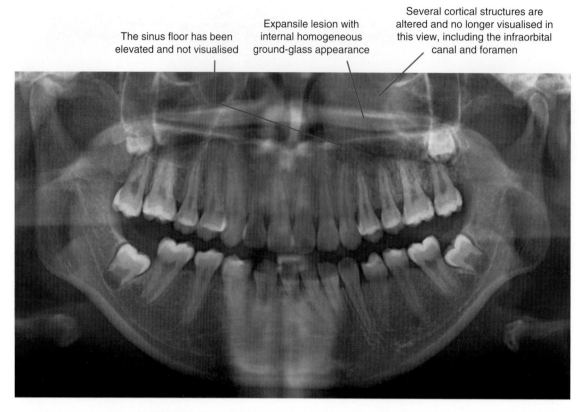

Figure 9.3 Fibrous dysplasia: panoramic radiograph.

Well-defined border

Expansile with focal cortical thinning and decreased density

Internal ground-glass appearance, with slight heterogeneity further posteriorly

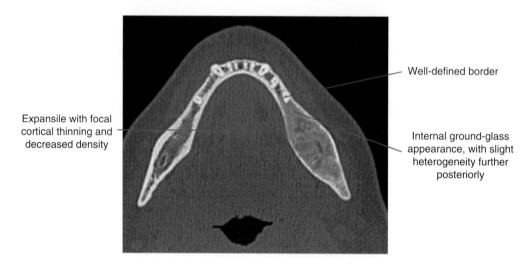

Figure 9.4 Fibrous dysplasia: axial MDCT image.

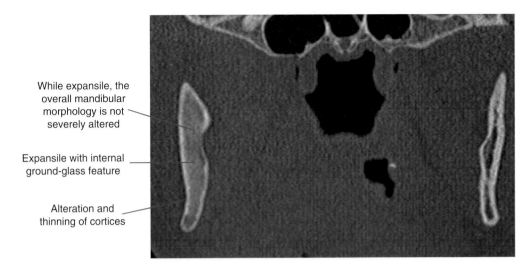

While expansile, the overall mandibular morphology is not severely altered

Expansile with internal ground-glass feature

Alteration and thinning of cortices

Figure 9.5 Fibrous dysplasia: coronal MDCT image.

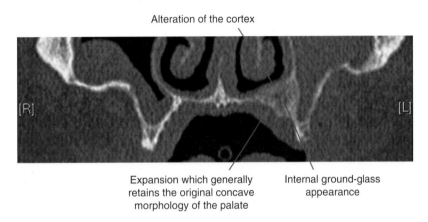

Alteration of the cortex

[R]   [L]

Expansion which generally retains the original concave morphology of the palate

Internal ground-glass appearance

Figure 9.6 Fibrous dysplasia: coronal CBCT image.

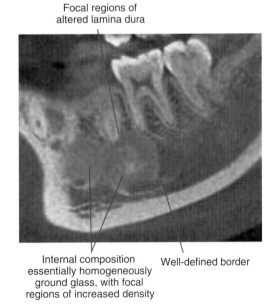

Focal regions of altered lamina dura

Internal composition essentially homogeneously ground glass, with focal regions of increased density

Well-defined border

Figure 9.7 Fibrous dysplasia: corrected sagittal CBCT image.

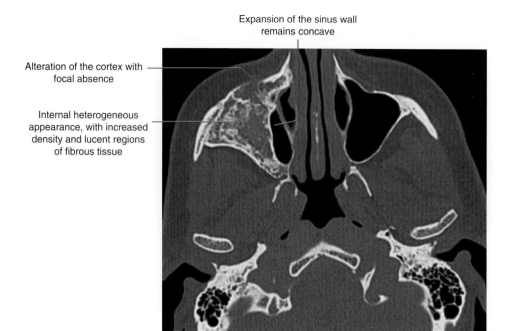

Expansion of the sinus wall remains concave

Alteration of the cortex with focal absence

Internal heterogeneous appearance, with increased density and lucent regions of fibrous tissue

Figure 9.8 Fibrous dysplasia: axial MDCT image. (Courtesy of Koong B. Diagnostic imaging of the periodontal and implant patient. In: Lindhe J, Lang NP, editors. Clinical Periodontology and Implant Dentistry. 6th ed. Wiley Blackwell; 2015. Reproduced with permission from Wiley.)

Internal heterogeneous appearance with hyper- and hypodense regions

Focal regions of altered and absent sinus cortical floor

While expansile, the overall maxillary morphology is not severely altered. That is, the concave maxillary morphology laterally, palatally, and at the nasal and maxillary antral bases is essentially maintained

Figure 9.9 Fibrous dysplasia: coronal MDCT image.

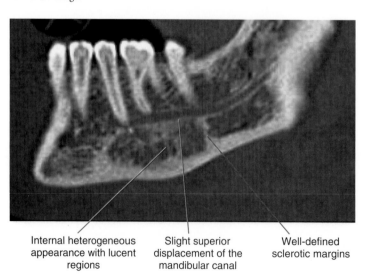

Internal heterogeneous appearance with lucent regions

Slight superior displacement of the mandibular canal

Well-defined sclerotic margins

Figure 9.10 Fibrous dysplasia: corrected sagittal CBCT image.

9.2 Cemento-osseous dysplasia

(Figures 9.11–9.21)

- Benign focal change of normal bone to fibrous tissue and metaplastic bone and/or cementum-like material.
- More common in Black and some Asian subjects and also in females.
- Most often identified in the 40 year age group.
- Three subtypes have been described:
  1 Periapical osseous dysplasia (periapical cemental dysplasia): most frequently seen type. Often multiple and involving mandibular anterior teeth. The term periapical cementoma is now rarely used.
  2 Florid osseous dysplasia: often widespread involving the alveolar processes and body of mandible. More often found in Black patients. Note that another widespread form referred to as familial gigantiform cementoma has been described, thought to be much less common than florid osseous dysplasia.
  3 Focal cemento-osseous dysplasia: has been considered to be more common in White people.
- Diagnosis is often clinical and radiological. Histological appearance is not infrequently 'fibro-osseous but otherwise non-specific'.
- Does not require treatment. Potential misdiagnosis for periapical inflammatory disease and unnecessary endodontic treatment or extraction.
- Potential secondary infection. Examples include:
  ○ Exposure to oral cavity via residual ridge atrophy at an edentulous site.
  ○ Inflammatory periodontal bone loss.

Radiological features
- MDCT or CBCT should be considered unless the appearances are definitive on 2D radiography.
- Immature lesions are usually lucent, with sclerotic margins.
- In time, internal focal opacity(s) appears and increases in size as the lesion matures over years. These opacities are usually homogeneous.
- Mature lesions present as opaque lesions demonstrating a surrounding lucent margin (band) with sclerotic borders. Occasionally, they can appear essentially opaque, where the surrounding lucent margin is essentially absent.
- Occasionally, these lesions can be internally homogeneous, demonstrating a ground-glass appearance.
- Rarely, simple bone cysts are associated with these lesions (Figure 9.18; also see Figure 8.44). However, residual opaque bone/cementum deposits usually remain present.
- The lamina dura of the involved teeth is usually absent or altered but the periodontal space is often preserved. Root resorption is rare.
- Expansion is often seen with larger lesions, where the thinned cortices are often largely preserved, although focal cortical absence is not uncommon.
- Larger lesions may displace the mandibular canal.

Differential diagnosis

	Key radiological differences
Early/immature lesions	
Chronic periapical inflammatory lesion	When there are no internal opacities, these lesions can be radiologically almost identical but cemento-osseous dysplasia is usually multiple. MDCT or CBCT may demonstrate small or low-density internal opacities of cemento-osseous dysplasia, which are not demonstrated on 2D radiography.
Mature lesions	
Bone island	No surrounding lucent margin and adjacent trabeculae run into the opacity.
Odontoma	Internal odontoid structures. Often pericoronal.
Cementoblastoma	Irregular root resorption. Usually painful.
Ossifying fibroma	Rarely, these lesions can appear very similar, especially with larger cemento-osseous dysplasia lesions. The ossifying fibroma has more of a mass effect, especially on the affected dentition. Cemento-osseous dysplasia is often multiple; ossifying fibroma is a solitary lesion.

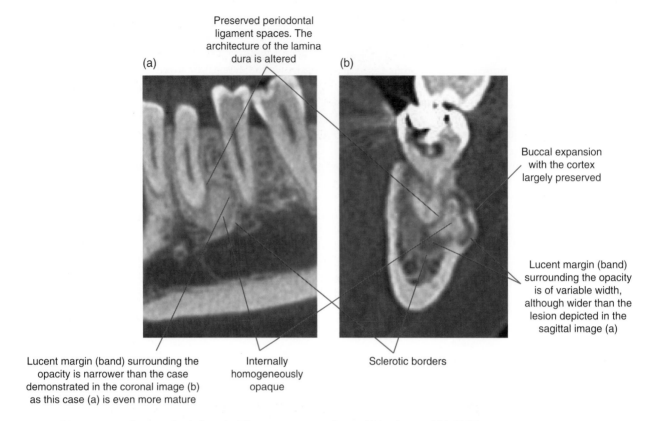

(a)   (b)

Preserved periodontal ligament spaces. The architecture of the lamina dura is altered

Buccal expansion with the cortex largely preserved

Lucent margin (band) surrounding the opacity is of variable width, although wider than the lesion depicted in the sagittal image (a)

Lucent margin (band) surrounding the opacity is narrower than the case demonstrated in the coronal image (b) as this case (a) is even more mature

Internally homogeneously opaque

Sclerotic borders

Figure 9.11 Mature periapical osseous dysplasia – two different cases: corrected sagittal (a) and coronal (b) CBCT images.

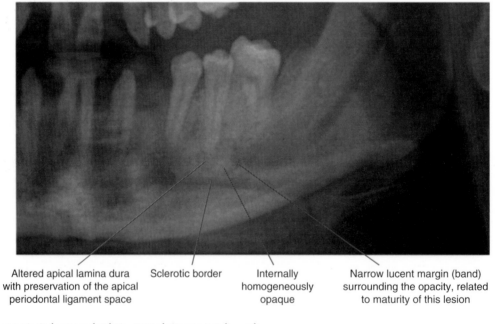

Altered apical lamina dura with preservation of the apical periodontal ligament space

Sclerotic border

Internally homogeneously opaque

Narrow lucent margin (band) surrounding the opacity, related to maturity of this lesion

Figure 9.12 Mature periapical osseous dysplasia: cropped panoramic radiograph.

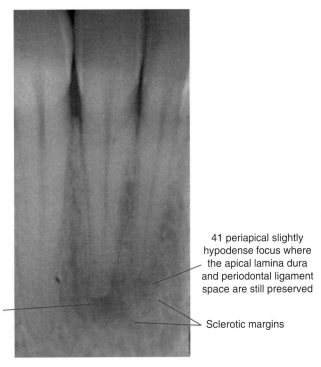

42 periapical hypodense focus. The apical lamina dura is not appreciated. No internal opacities demonstrated

41 periapical slightly hypodense focus where the apical lamina dura and periodontal ligament space are still preserved

Sclerotic margins

Figure 9.13 Early periapical osseous dysplasia, 42 and 41: cropped periapical radiograph. Note: The 42 apical appearances are similar to chronic periapical inflammatory lesions. However, MDCT or CBCT would probably demonstrate preservation of the apical periodontal ligament space and the altered architecture of the lamina dura. These techniques may also demonstrate internal calcifications not appreciated on intraoral radiographs.

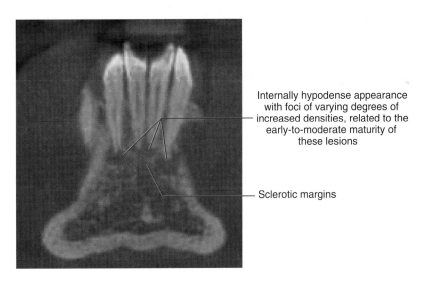

Internally hypodense appearance with foci of varying degrees of increased densities, related to the early-to-moderate maturity of these lesions

Sclerotic margins

Figure 9.14 Periapical osseous dysplasia: coronal CBCT image.

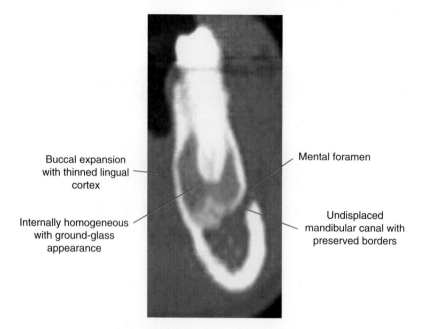

Buccal expansion with thinned lingual cortex

Internally homogeneous with ground-glass appearance

Mental foramen

Undisplaced mandibular canal with preserved borders

Figure 9.15 Periapical osseous dysplasia: corrected coronal CBCT image.

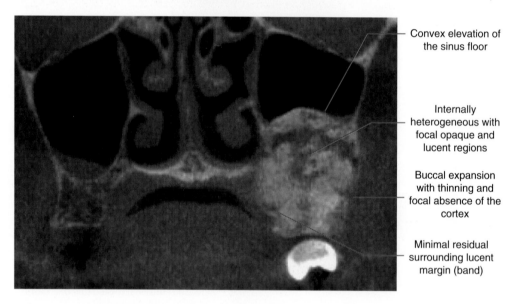

Convex elevation of the sinus floor

Internally heterogeneous with focal opaque and lucent regions

Buccal expansion with thinning and focal absence of the cortex

Minimal residual surrounding lucent margin (band)

Figure 9.16 Mature focal cemento-osseous dysplasia: coronal CBCT image.

Buccal expansion with a focal hypodense appearance of the cortex

Small focal absence of the labial cortex

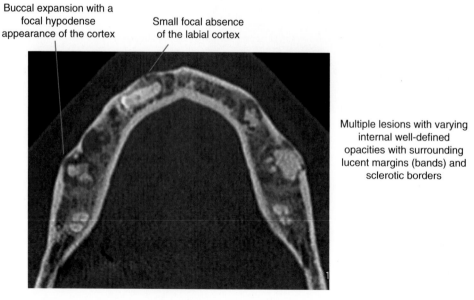

Multiple lesions with varying internal well-defined opacities with surrounding lucent margins (bands) and sclerotic borders

Figure 9.17 Florid osseous dysplasia: axial CBCT image.

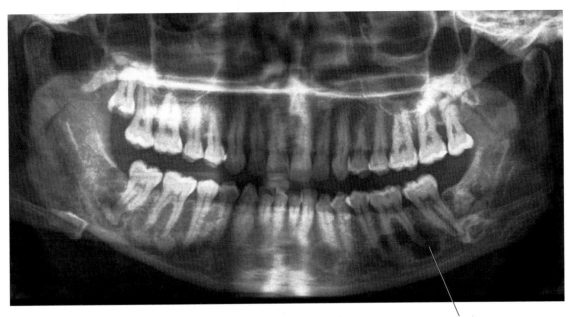

Simple bone cyst associated with this
lesion. Note the opacity centred at
the 36 mesial root apex

Figure 9.18 Florid osseous dysplasia: panoramic radiograph. There are multiple lesions associated with most of the mandibular teeth and the maxillary second and third molars, with varying well-defined internal opacities. Note the variable residual surrounding lucencies and the sclerotic margins.

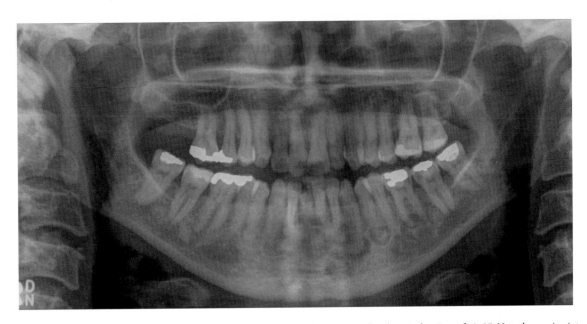

Figure 9.19 Florid osseous dysplasia: panoramic radiograph. There are multiple lesions centred at the apical regions of 48–37. Note the varying internal opacities which reflect the different stages of maturity of these lesions. Sclerotic margins are demonstrated.

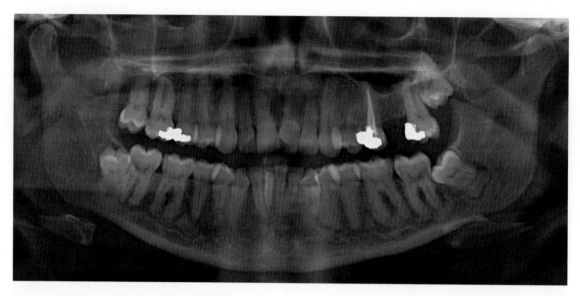

Figure 9.20 Florid osseous dysplasia: panoramic radiograph. There are multiple lesions centred at the apices of most of the mandibular teeth. Note the internal homogeneous opacities with relatively narrow surrounding residual lucent margin (band), related to the degree of maturity of these lesions. The margins are sclerotic.

(a)   (b)   (c)

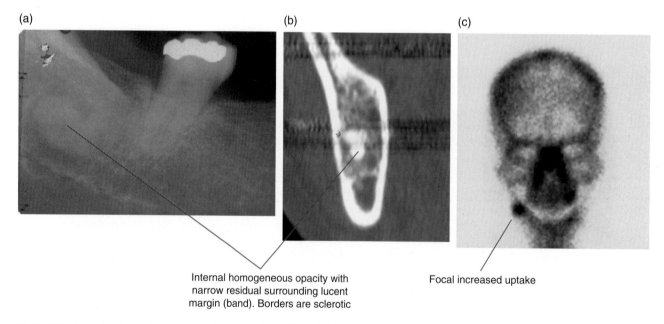

Internal homogeneous opacity with narrow residual surrounding lucent margin (band). Borders are sclerotic

Focal increased uptake

Figure 9.21 Mature focal cemento-osseous dysplasia: periapical radiograph (a), coronal MDCT (b) and technetium bone scan (c) images.

9.3 Ossifying fibroma (Figures 9.22 and 9.23)

- *Synonyms*: cemento-ossifying fibroma, cementifying fibroma, juvenile ossifying fibroma.
- Classified, behaves and managed as a benign tumour but often discussed in relation to fibro-osseous lesions.
- Composed of fibrocellular tissue with varying amounts of mineralised bone/cementum-like material.
- Internal histological appearances can resemble fibrous dysplasia and cemento-osseous dysplasia.

- Can be aggressive or indolent, tending to be more aggressive in the younger patient.
- More often seen in females.
- Much less common than cemento-osseous dysplasia and fibrous dysplasia.
- In the jaws, it is considered to be most common within the posterior body of the mandible, although it also presents elsewhere.
- Often presents as a painless swelling, sometimes with displacement of teeth.
- Usually surgically enucleated. Recurrence is not likely.

Radiological features

- MDCT may demonstrate soft tissue changes, although CBCT is likely to be sufficient for many cases.
- Tumour-like mixed-density expansile lesion.
- Well-defined borders, which may be corticated. A surrounding lucent margin (band) may be present, possibly only at one or a few aspects of these lesions.
- Internal density varies substantially, depending on the amount of mineralised material. It can be essentially lucent. The pattern of the mineralised material also varies, from ground-glass appearances (similar to fibrous dysplasia) to homogeneous opacities (similar to cemento-osseous dysplasia).
- Variable T1- and T2-weighted MRI signal patterns, related to the varying amounts of fibrous/mineralised tissue and the pattern of the mineralised tissue. Gadolinium enhancement is also variable, from homogeneous enhancement to focal regions of enhancement.
- Usually demonstrates tumour-like mass effect:
  - Displaces anatomic structures such as the mandibular canal, paranasal sinuses and nasal cavity.
  - Displaces teeth with effacement of the lamina dura. May cause root resorption.
  - Expanded jaw cortices are often thinned and altered. The expanded cortices are classically largely preserved, although focal regions of cortical absence may be seen.
- Adjacent bone can be sclerotic.

Differential diagnosis

Key radiological differences

Fibrous dysplasia	Borders are less well defined and there is no surrounding lucent margin. Expansion is not tumour like, resembling the original anatomy. Root resorption is rare.
Cemento-osseous dysplasia	Periapical osseous dysplasia and florid osseous dysplasia are usually multifocal. Less tumour-like growth, especially in relation to teeth.
Multilocular lesions including giant cell lesions	Presence of internal septa.
Lesions with internal calcifications, including calcifying cystic odontogenic tumour, adenomatoid odontogenic tumour and the rare calcifying epithelial odontogenic tumour (Pindborg tumour)	The internal calcifications of these lesions are usually small.

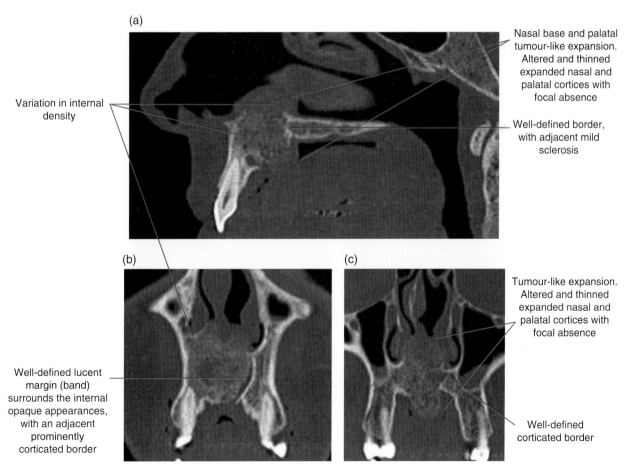

(a)

Variation in internal density

Nasal base and palatal tumour-like expansion. Altered and thinned expanded nasal and palatal cortices with focal absence

Well-defined border, with adjacent mild sclerosis

(b)

(c)

Well-defined lucent margin (band) surrounds the internal opaque appearances, with an adjacent prominently corticated border

Tumour-like expansion. Altered and thinned expanded nasal and palatal cortices with focal absence

Well-defined corticated border

Figure 9.22 Ossifying fibroma: sagittal (a) and coronal (b,c) MDCT images.

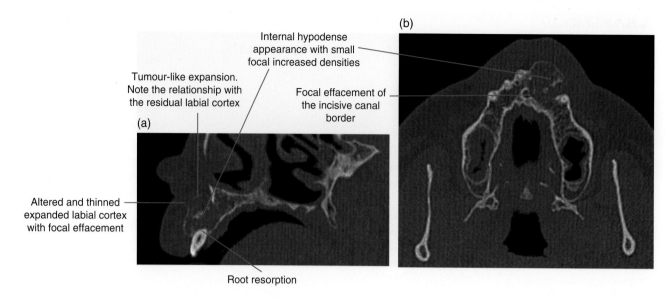

Figure 9.23 Ossifying fibroma: corrected sagittal (a) and axial (b) MDCT images.

CHAPTER 10
Benign Tumours Involving the Jaws

ODONTOGENIC BENIGN TUMOURS

10.1 Ameloblastoma (Figures 10.1–10.9)

- *Synonym*: adamantinoma.
- Benign, slow-growing but locally aggressive tumour of odontogenic epithelium.
- Three subtypes: solid/multicystic (by far the most common subtype), unicystic and desmoplastic.
  - Malignant forms or transformation are very rare:
    - malignant ameloblastoma (histologically benign but with metastases)
    - ameloblastic carcinoma (ameloblastoma with histological malignant features).
- Any age group but more common in the third to sixth decades.
- Most commonly seen in the posterior mandible. Maxillary lesions most commonly occur posteriorly.
- Usually asymptomatic until it causes painless swelling.
- Large lesions may involve adjacent structures, including the upper airway passages, orbit and skull base. Posterior maxillary lesions are of particular concern in this regard.
- Surgical excision beyond radiologically identified margins. May involve resections.
- High recurrence rate, especially the more solid/multicystic subtype. Requires radiological review over an extended period.

Radiological features
- Multidetector computed tomography (MDCT) usually demonstrates more features but cone beam computed tomography (CBCT) may be sufficient. 2D radiography is insufficient. Magnetic resonance imaging (MRI) may be useful in some cases. MDCT is best for surgical planning as MRI (with gadolinium) may overestimate the extent of the lesion.
- Most commonly presents as a multilocular lesion (solid/multicystic) with well-defined corticated or sclerotic borders.
  - The internal septa are classically thick and curved. Some may demonstrate the classic 'soap bubble' appearance.
  - The cystic locules vary in size and one or a few may be substantially larger than others.

- The unicystic ameloblastoma is unilocular (lucent internally) and often demonstrates extreme expansion for its size. Most are associated with the unerupted mandibular third molars.
- The desmoplastic subtype may demonstrate more internal septa, which are more irregular and sclerotic in appearance.
- Unless small, the jaw cortices are usually expanded and thinned, with regions of effacements.
- When involving a tooth root, there is often substantial root resorption. Tooth displacement is often seen when the lesion abuts the crown.
- MDCT – soft tissue algorithm: solid/multicystic lesions demonstrate variably heterogeneous overall soft tissue density attenuation between the septa. Sometimes, the hypodense cystic locules are demonstrated within. Occasionally, one or a few of the locules are particular large, usually of internal fluid density. Larger lesions tend to demonstrate heterogeneous contrast enhancement, with non-enhancing hypodense foci.
- MRI: solid/multicystic lesions components demonstrate heterogeneous T1 low to intermediate signal and T2 intermediate to bright signal. Larger cystic locules demonstrate homogeneous T1 low to intermediate signal and T2/short T1 inversion recovery (STIR) hyperintensity. Solid portions and septations usually enhance. Larger cystic locules usually demonstrate rim enhancement.

Differential diagnosis

Other lesions which may appear multilocular including:	Key radiological differences
Giant cell granuloma	Internal septa are usually much finer than the ameloblastoma. Also usually seen in the younger population (unless brown tumour related to hyperparathyroidism).
Odontogenic myxoma	Presence of one or a few straight septa is a feature. Typically demonstrates mild expansion for size.

Atlas of Oral and Maxillofacial Radiology, First Edition. Bernard Koong.
© 2017 John Wiley & Sons Ltd. Published 2017 by John Wiley & Sons Ltd.

Aneurysmal bone cyst	Fine internal septa and typically extremely expansile.	Vascular malformation/ haemangioma	Often demonstrates serpiginous appearance. Prebiopsy evaluation with MRI should be considered if this suspected.
Ossifying fibroma	When this lesion demonstrates appearance of internal septa, they tend to be larger and less distinct. Internal septa are uncommon and mandibular lesions demonstrate mild expansion for size.	Dentigerous cyst	May not be able to radiologically differentiate from the unicystic ameloblastoma in a pericoronal relationship with an unerupted tooth.
Keratocystic odontogenic tumour			

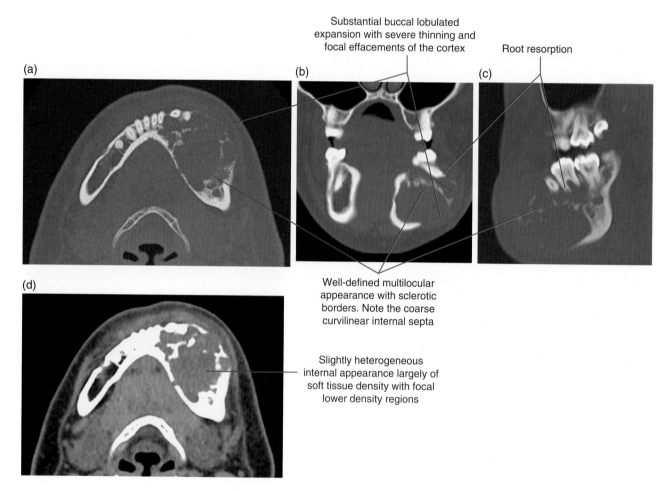

Substantial buccal lobulated expansion with severe thinning and focal effacements of the cortex

Root resorption

(a) (b) (c)

(d)

Well-defined multilocular appearance with sclerotic borders. Note the coarse curvilinear internal septa

Slightly heterogeneous internal appearance largely of soft tissue density with focal lower density regions

Figure 10.1 Ameloblastoma of the left mandible: axial (a), coronal (b) and corrected sagittal (c) bone and axial soft tissue (d) MDCT images.

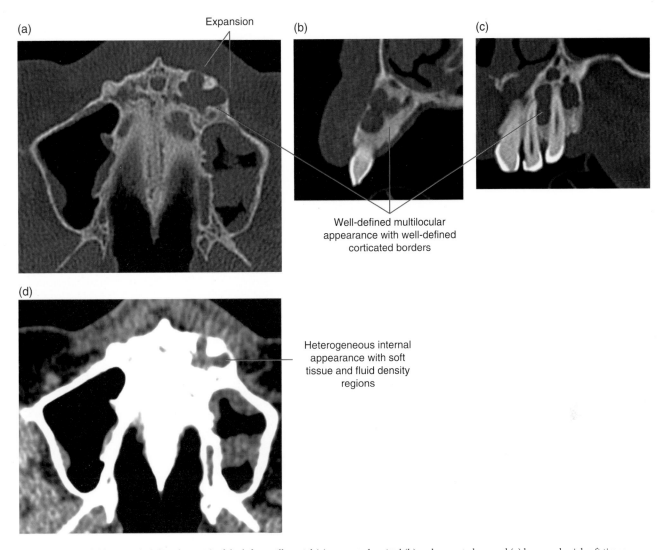

(a)

Expansion

(b)

(c)

Well-defined multilocular
appearance with well-defined
corticated borders

(d)

Heterogeneous internal
appearance with soft
tissue and fluid density
regions

Figure 10.2 Ameloblastoma (solid/multicystic) of the left maxilla: axial (a), corrected sagittal (b) and corrected coronal (c) bone and axial soft tissue (d) MDCT images.

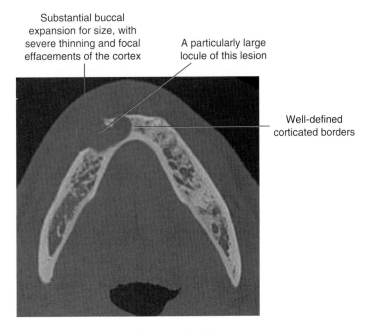

Substantial buccal
expansion for size, with
severe thinning and focal
effacements of the cortex

A particularly large
locule of this lesion

Well-defined
corticated borders

Figure 10.3 Ameloblastoma (solid/multicystic) of the right mandible: axial MDCT image.

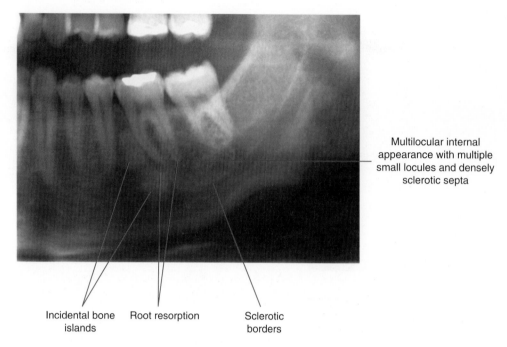

Multilocular internal
appearance with multiple
small locules and densely
sclerotic septa

Incidental bone
islands

Root resorption

Sclerotic
borders

Figure 10.4 Ameloblastoma (solid/multicystic) of the left posterior body of the mandible: cropped panoramic radiograph.

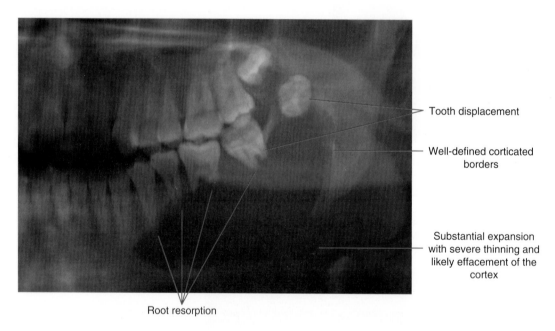

Tooth displacement

Well-defined corticated
borders

Substantial expansion
with severe thinning and
likely effacement of the
cortex

Root resorption

Figure 10.5 Unicystic ameloblastoma of the left posterior mandible: cropped panoramic radiograph.

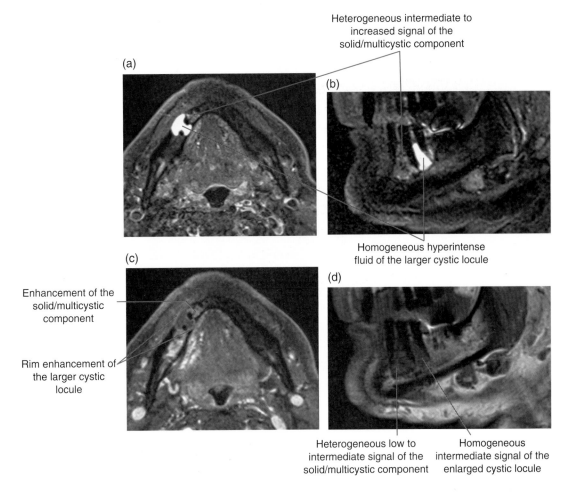

Figure 10.6 Ameloblastoma (solid/multicystic) of the right body of mandible (also refer to MDCT of this case in Figure 10.7): MRI; axial STIR (a), corrected sagittal STIR (b), axial T1 postgadolinium fat-saturated (c) and corrected sagittal T1 (d) images.

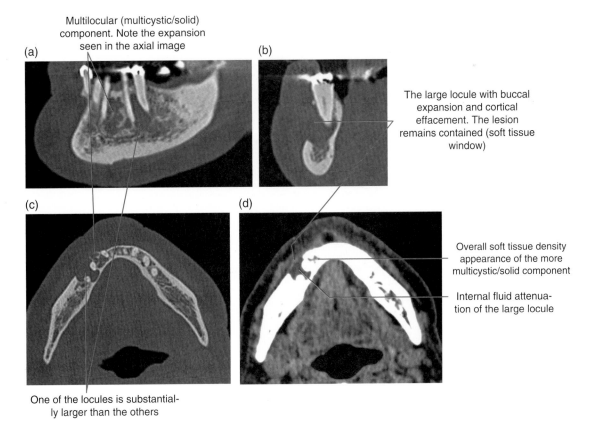

Figure 10.7 Ameloblastoma (solid/multicystic) of the right body of the mandible (also refer to MRI of this case in Figure 10.6): MDCT; corrected sagittal (a), corrected coronal (b) and axial (c) bone and axial soft tissue (d) images.

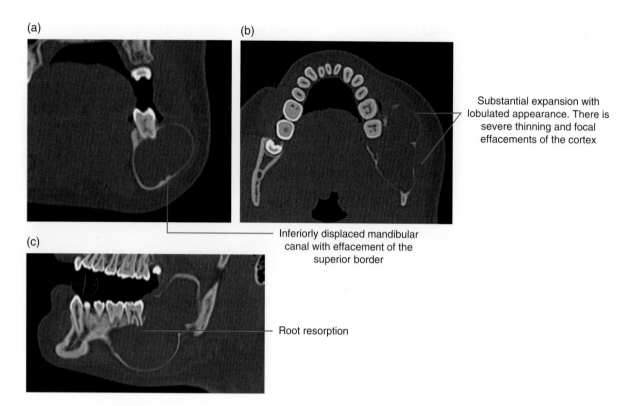

(a)

(b)

Substantial expansion with
lobulated appearance. There is
severe thinning and focal
effacements of the cortex

(c)

Inferiorly displaced mandibular
canal with effacement of the
superior border

Root resorption

Figure 10.8 Unicystic ameloblastoma of the left posterior mandible: coronal (a), axial (b) and corrected sagittal (c) MDCT images.

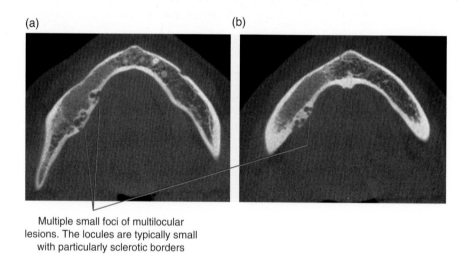

(a)

(b)

Multiple small foci of multilocular
lesions. The locules are typically small
with particularly sclerotic borders

Figure 10.9 Recurrent ameloblastoma of a right mandibular fibular graft: axial MDCT images (a,b).

10.2 Calcifying epithelial odontogenic tumour (Figure 10.10)

- *Synonyms*: Pindborg tumour, CEOT.
- Rare locally invasive epithelial odontogenic tumour with amyloid-like material where there may be calcific foci.
- Asymptomatic until expansion is noted.
- More commonly seen in the posterior mandible, many associated with unerupted teeth.
- Surgical excision. This lesion is considered less aggressive than the ameloblastoma but postsurgical radiological review over an extended period is recommended.

Radiological features
- MDCT demonstrates more features than CBCT.
- Variable presentation:
  - may be unilocular or multilocular
  - may demonstrate substantially variable internal calcifications
  - borders are also variable, ranging from well-defined cortex to poorly defined destructive margins.
- May displace teeth.

Differential diagnosis

May resemble unilocular lucent lesions such as cystic lesions, multilocular lesions or lesions which demonstrate internal calcifications

Key radiological differences

The more common location of the calcifying epithelial odontogenic tumour (CEOT) in the posterior mandible, associated with an unerupted tooth, may be a useful feature.

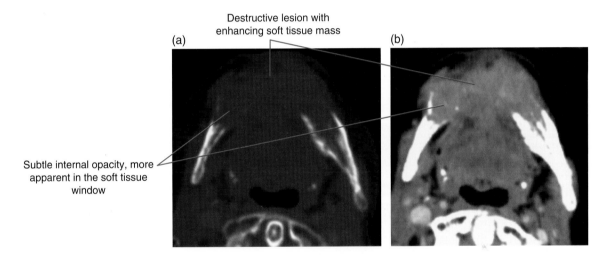

Destructive lesion with enhancing soft tissue mass

(a)   (b)

Subtle internal opacity, more apparent in the soft tissue window

Figure 10.10 Calcifying epithelial odontogenic tumour: axial bone (a) and postcontrast soft tissue (b) MDCT images.

10.3 Odontoma (Figures 10.11–10.14)

- *Synonyms*: compound/complex odontoma, compound/complex composite odontoma, odontome.
- Considered to be a hamartoma of odontogenic tissues, with the presence of variable combinations of enamel, dentin, cementum and pulp. Not a true tumour.
- Variable morphological appearances, ranging from those containing tooth-like structures (compound) to a more amorphous mix of calcified dental tissues (complex).
- Usually identified in the second decade.
- Complex odontomas are more commonly seen in the posterior mandible.
- Compound odontomas occur more commonly in the anterior maxilla.
- Many are associated with unerupted teeth. Often contributes to altered eruption or impaction of adjacent teeth. May contribute to the malformation of the adjacent teeth.
- Otherwise asymptomatic.
- Surgical excision. Does not recur. Occasionally left in situ if small and not affecting the dentition, especially those discovered later in life.

Radiological features
- MDCT or CBCT should be considered.
- Opacity of variable internal appearance with surrounding lucent margin (lucent band/zone) and a corticated border.
- Internal density is variable, depending on the proportion of the various dental tissues. Tooth-like structures are seen in the compound variety. The complex odontoma demonstrates a more homogeneous internal appearance with densities varying from dentin/cementum to enamel.
- Often affects the position, development and eruption of the adjacent teeth, which are occasionally malformed.

Differential diagnosis

	Key radiological differences
Cemento-osseous dysplasia (COD)	Mature lesions may resemble the complex odontoma. CODs are often multiple and the borders are usually sclerotic.
Ossifying fibroma	Odontomas are usually denser, with variable presence of enamel.

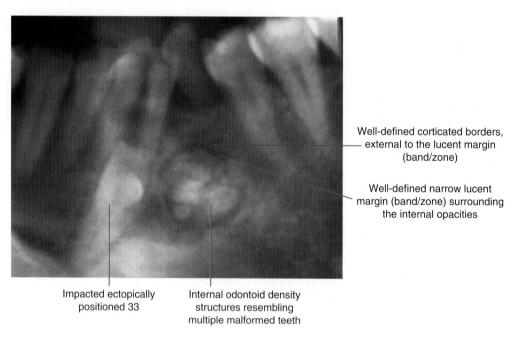

Well-defined corticated borders, external to the lucent margin (band/zone)

Well-defined narrow lucent margin (band/zone) surrounding the internal opacities

Impacted ectopically positioned 33

Internal odontoid density structures resembling multiple malformed teeth

Figure 10.11 Compound odontoma centred at the 33 region: cropped panoramic radiograph.

Well-defined lucent margin (band/zone) surrounding the internal opacities

Well-defined corticated borders, external to the lucent margin (band/zone)

(a)

(b)

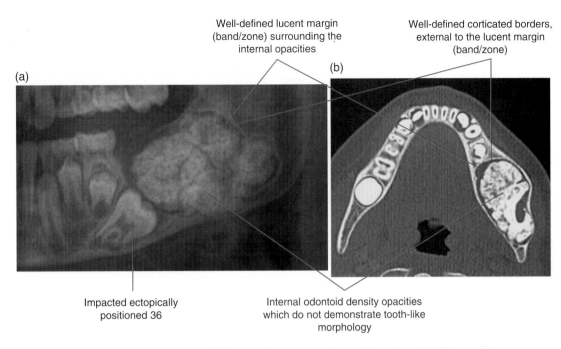

Impacted ectopically positioned 36

Internal odontoid density opacities which do not demonstrate tooth-like morphology

Figure 10.12 Complex odontoma of the left posterior mandible: cropped panoramic radiograph (a) and axial MDCT image (b).

Internal odontoid density structures resembling multiple malformed teeth

Impacted 21

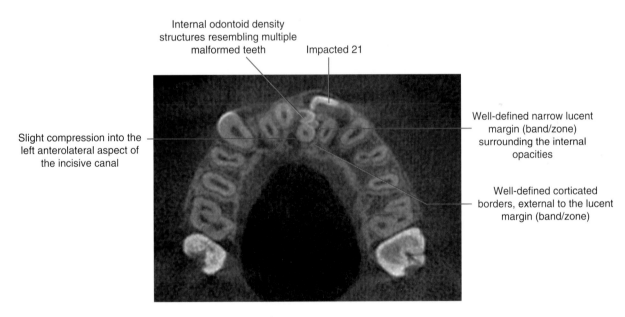

Slight compression into the left anterolateral aspect of the incisive canal

Well-defined narrow lucent margin (band/zone) surrounding the internal opacities

Well-defined corticated borders, external to the lucent margin (band/zone)

Figure 10.13 Compound odontoma centred at the 21 region: axial CBCT image.

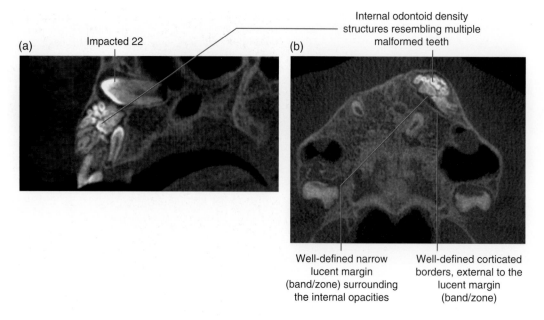

Figure 10.14 Compound odontoma of the left anterior maxilla: corrected sagittal (a) and axial (b) CBCT images.

10.4 Ameloblastic fibroma (Figure 10.15)

- A benign mixed odontogenic tumour arising from ectomesenchymal tissues without formation of the calcified dental tissues.
- Rare. Most occur in the first and second decades of life.
- Asymptomatic unless large enough to cause expansion or interfere with tooth development/eruption.
- Most are seen within the posterior mandibular alveolar process.
- Conservative excision/enucleation. Low rate of recurrence.

Radiological features
- MDCT or CBCT should be considered, rather than 2D radiography.
- Well-defined, usually corticated lesion.
- Usually unilocular. May be multilocular, usually when larger.
- Larger lesions cause expansion with cortical thinning.
- May interrupt tooth development/eruption or displace teeth.

Differential diagnosis

Key radiological differences

Dentigerous cyst	May be very difficult to differentiate from a pericoronal ameloblastic fibroma. Less likely to be a dentigerous cyst if the margins are not at the cementoenamel junction (CEJ) or at the root surface within 2–3 mm of the CEJ.
Keratocystic odontogenic tumour (KCOT)	Within the mandibular body, the KCOT demonstrates limited expansion for size. It is usually lucent internally and usually only demonstrates one or a few septa when large.
Ameloblastoma	Demonstrates coarser septa than ameloblastic fibroma. Substantial root resorption is a feature.
Giant cell granuloma	Demonstrates fine internal septa. Larger giant cell granulomas typically demonstrate lobulated expansion with a tendency for substantial tooth root resorption.
Aneurysmal bone cyst	Often extremely expansile, unless small. MRI may demonstrate fluid–fluid levels.
Odontogenic myxoma	Usually demonstrates a few straight septa internally and limited expansion for size.

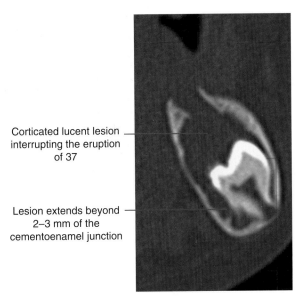

Corticated lucent lesion interrupting the eruption of 37

Lesion extends beyond 2–3 mm of the cementoenamel junction

Figure 10.15 Ameloblastic fibroma, 37: corrected coronal CBCT image.

10.5 Ameloblastic fibro-odontoma
(Figures 10.16–10.18)

- *Synonym*: AFO.
- A benign mixed odontogenic tumour involving ectomesenchymal tissues with the presence of enamel and dentin. Demonstrates histological features of the ameloblastic fibroma and complex odontoma.
- Usually identified in the first and second decades of life.
- Most are identified within the alveolar process of the posterior mandible, often approximating the alveolar crest.
- Often interrupts tooth eruption.
- Slow growing and expansile when large.
- Conservative excision/enucleation. Recurrence rate is considered to be low.

Radiological features
- MDCT is likely to demonstrate more features but CBCT may be sufficient.
- Well-defined, usually corticated lesion.

- Small lesions are often internally lucent, although some demonstrate one or a few opacities. Larger lesions usually present with more internal calcifications, with some of odontoid densities. Substantially large lesions may present with substantial internal odontoid calcifications.

Differential diagnosis

Key radiological differences

Ameloblastic fibroma	Difficult to differentiate unless there are internal calcifications.
Odontoma	An early developing odontoma appears very similar to an ameloblastic fibro-odontoma (AFO) with internal calcifications. AFO calcifications tend to be smaller and more diffused.
	Large AFOs demonstrate substantial internal odontoid calcifications similar in appearance to those of an odontoma. However, there are large lucent regions within the lesion in AFOs, usually not seen in odontomas.

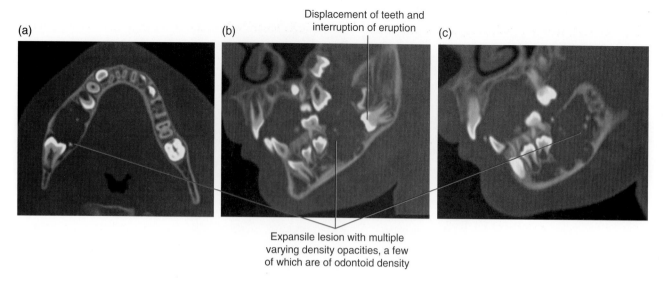

(a)

(b)

Displacement of teeth and interruption of eruption

(c)

Expansile lesion with multiple varying density opacities, a few of which are of odontoid density

Figure 10.16 Ameloblastic fibro-odontoma of the right body of the mandible: axial (a) and corrected sagittal (b,c) MDCT images.

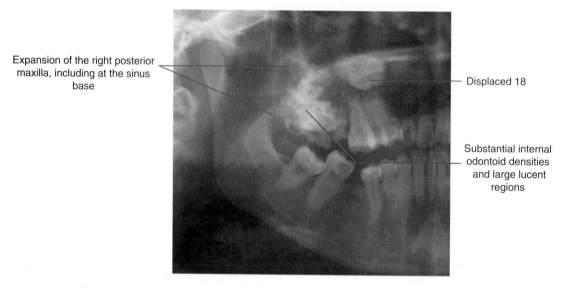

Expansion of the right posterior maxilla, including at the sinus base

Displaced 18

Substantial internal odontoid densities and large lucent regions

Figure 10.17 Ameloblastic fibro-odontoma of the right posterior maxilla: cropped panoramic radiograph.

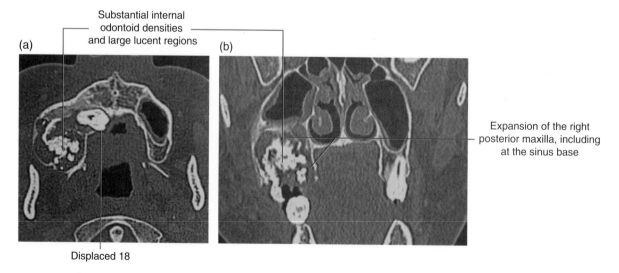

Substantial internal odontoid densities and large lucent regions

(a)

(b)

Expansion of the right posterior maxilla, including at the sinus base

Displaced 18

Figure 10.18 Ameloblastic fibro-odontoma of the right posterior maxilla: axial (a) and coronal (b) MDCT images.

10.6 Adenomatoid odontogenic tumour
(Figure 10.19)

- *Synonym*: AOT.
- A benign mixed odontogenic tumour with epithelium arranged in a variety of patterns within a mature connective tissue stroma. This lesion has been considered to be a hamartoma.
- Rare. Most occur in the second decade of life. More common in females.
- Within bone (central), the follicular type (pericoronal relationship to an unerupted tooth) is more common than the extrafollicular variant. Can occur in soft tissues (peripheral).
- Most are seen in the maxillary canine region.
- Conservative excision. Rare recurrence.

Radiological features
- MDCT would demonstrate more features although CBCT may suffice.
- Well-defined corticated lesion.
- Some may be lucent but most demonstrate variable internal calcifications. Subtle calcifications are more likely to be identified on MDCT, especially in the soft tissue window.
- Larger lesions will often displace teeth and may expand and thin the jaw cortices.

Differential diagnosis

	Key radiological differences
Calcifying cystic odontogenic tumour	Difficult to differentiate as this lesion also tends to occur anteriorly.
Ameloblastic fibro-odontoma	Most commonly seen in the posterior mandible.
Calcifying epithelial odontogenic tumour	Most commonly seen in the posterior mandible.
Dentigerous cyst	Less likely to be a dentigerous cyst if the margins are not at the CEJ or at the root surface within 2–3 mm of the CEJ. Dentigerous cysts are almost always completely lucent – occasionally, long-standing dentigerous cysts or those exposed to the oral cavity may demonstrate internal calcifications.
Keratocystic odontogenic tumour	Can appear similar to the adenomatoid odontogenic tumour (AOT) which is internally lucent.

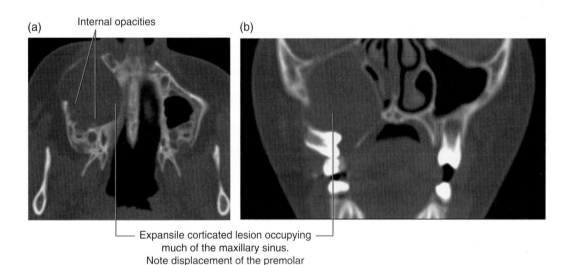

(a) Internal opacities

(b)

Expansile corticated lesion occupying much of the maxillary sinus. Note displacement of the premolar

Figure 10.19 Adenomatoid odontogenic tumour of the right maxilla: axial (a) and coronal (b) MDCT images.

10.7 Calcifying cystic odontogenic tumour
(Figure 10.20)

- *Synonyms*: CCOT, calcifying odontogenic cyst (COC), Gorlin cyst.
- Rare odontogenic tumour with spectrum of presentations, ranging from solid to cystic varieties and, extremely rarely, a more aggressive variant. Some authors consider this entity as a cystic tumour with calcifying potential, since most present as such.
- Most commonly seen in the anterior segments of the jaw, especially the maxilla.
- May be associated with an impacted tooth.
- Sometimes associated with odontomas. Association with other odontogenic tumours is extremely rare.
- Surgical enucleation. Recurrence is rare.

Radiological features
- MDCT would demonstrate more features although CBCT may suffice.
- Unilocular expansile lesion.
- Borders range from being corticated to ill defined.

- Usually largely lucent with variable internal calcifications. Some cases may not demonstrate internal calcifications. Subtle calcifications are more likely to be identified on MDCT, especially in the soft tissue window.
- Displaces teeth and resorbs roots.

Differential diagnosis

	Key radiological differences
Dentigerous cyst	Usually does not demonstrate internal calcifications. However, calcifying cystic odontogenic tumours may not demonstrate internal calcifications. Also, long-standing dentigerous cysts or those exposed to the oral cavity may occasionally demonstrate internal calcifications.
Other cyst-like lesions which demonstrate internal calcifications, such as AFO, AOT and CEOT	Can be difficult to differentiate, especially the AOT, which tends to occur anteriorly. AFOs and CEOTs usually present posteriorly.

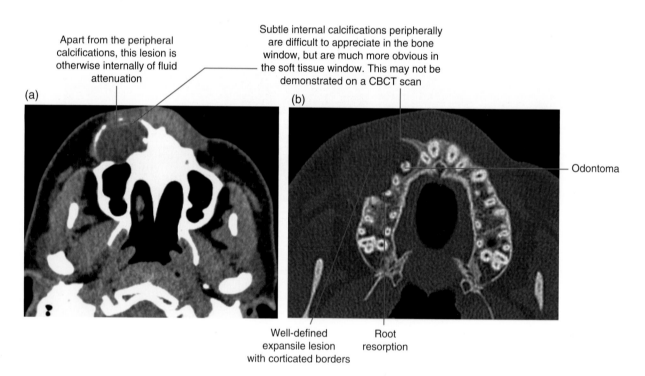

(a) Apart from the peripheral calcifications, this lesion is otherwise internally of fluid attenuation

(b) Subtle internal calcifications peripherally are difficult to appreciate in the bone window, but are much more obvious in the soft tissue window. This may not be demonstrated on a CBCT scan

Odontoma

Well-defined expansile lesion with corticated borders

Root resorption

Figure 10.20 Calcifying cystic odontogenic tumour with odontoma of the right maxilla: axial soft tissue (a) and bone (b) MDCT images.

10.8 Odontogenic myxoma (Figures 10.21 and 10.22)

- *Synonyms*: myxoma, myxofibroma.
- A benign odontogenic tumour characterised by the presence of stellate and spindle-shaped cells and collagen fibres in an abundant myxoid/mucoid matrix.
- Usually asymptomatic until larger, when there may some expansion and/or discomfort.
- More commonly seen within the body of the mandible, most common in the posterior segment.
- Surgical excision/resection beyond radiologically identified margins.
- Relatively high recurrence rate. This is related to the gelatinous nature of this lesion, which extends into the adjacent marrow spaces. Postsurgical radiological review is recommended.

Radiological features

- MDCT demonstrates more features and is the preferred technique but CBCT may be sufficient for some cases. Further characterisation with MRI may be useful, considered by some to be an important modality, in combination with MDCT.
- Usually presents as a well-defined, corticated, multilocular lesion where one or a few of the septa are flat/straight rather than curved. Subtle septa are more likely to be identified on MDCT, especially in the soft tissue window.
- Small lesions, especially those occurring pericoronally, may appear as unilocular lucent lesions.
- Usually demonstrates relatively limited expansion relative to size.
- May displace teeth, although root resorption is usually not a feature.
- MRI: homogeneous intermediate T1 signal; homogeneous high T2/STIR signal. Usually demonstrates gadolinium enhancement peripherally and little or no enhancement centrally.

Differential diagnosis

Other lesions with multilocular appearance, including ameloblastoma, giant cell granulomas, aneurysmal bone cysts, keratocystic odontogenic tumour and vascular malformations

Key radiological differences

The presence of one or a few flat/straight septa among others is a feature of the odontogenic myxoma. Relatively limited expansion for size is typical but the keratocystic odontogenic tumour also demonstrates this feature. If there is suspicion for a vascular lesion, postcontrast MDCT and MRI must be considered in further evaluation.

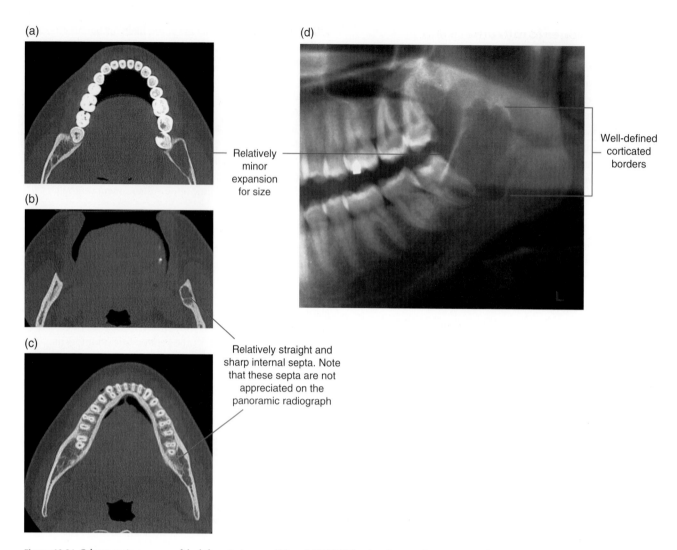

Figure 10.21 Odontogenic myxoma of the left posterior mandible: axial MDCT (a–c) and cropped panoramic radiograph (d) images.

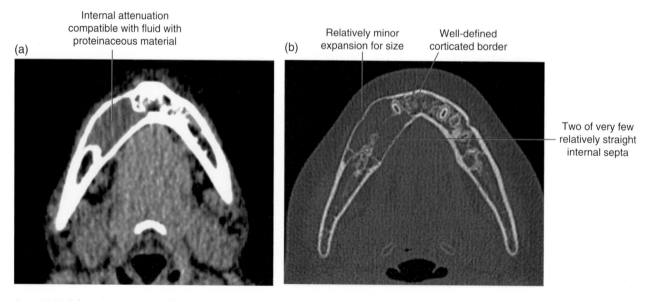

Figure 10.22 Odontogenic myxoma of the right mandible: axial soft tissue (a) and bone (b) MDCT images.

10.9 Cementoblastoma (Figure 10.23)

- *Synonym*: benign cementoblastoma.
- A benign odontogenic tumour largely composed of cementum-like tissue related to a tooth root. Histological features resemble the osteoblastoma. Some consider that the cementoblastoma is essentially an osteoblastoma occurring at the tooth root apex.
- Occurs more commonly in males, most often younger than 25 years old.
- Most commonly seen at the mandibular first molar region, centred apically.
- Pain is commonly reported. The pulp status of the involved tooth is usually normal.
- Surgical excision. When the lesion is completely excised, recurrence is not considered to be common. However, post-surgical radiological review should be considered.

Radiological features

- Should be examined with MDCT or CBCT.
- Well-defined, largely opaque lesion with a surrounding lucent margin (band) and a corticated/slightly sclerotic border, centred at the apical aspect of a tooth root.
- Internal opaque architecture varies from being unstructured to a sunburst/'spokes of a wheel' appearance.
- Root resorption is commonly seen.
- Expansile when sufficiently large.

Differential diagnosis

Key radiological differences

Mature periapical osseous dysplasia	The lucent margin (band) around the internal opacity is usually less defined and the surrounding opaque border is wider, often more sclerotic in appearance. In addition, root resorption is not commonly seen with periapical osseous dysplasia and these lesions are more likely to be multiple, and are asymptomatic.
Bone island	No surrounding lucent margin with corticated border. Usually internally homogeneous and root resorption is only occasionally seen.
Severe hypercementosis	Surrounding periodontal ligament space is usually much narrower and well defined. Usually internally homogeneous and contiguous with the root, with no resorption.
Reactive sclerosis related to a periapical inflammatory lesion	Usually ill defined with no surrounding lucency. MDCT or CBCT will almost always demonstrate a periapical hypodense/lucent appearance or widening of the apical periodontal ligament space.

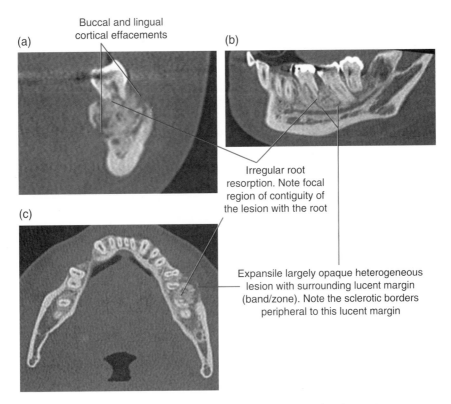

(a) Buccal and lingual cortical effacements

(b)

Irregular root resorption. Note focal region of contiguity of the lesion with the root

(c)

Expansile largely opaque heterogeneous lesion with surrounding lucent margin (band/zone). Note the sclerotic borders peripheral to this lucent margin

Figure 10.23 Cementoblastoma at the 36–37 region: corrected coronal (a), corrected sagittal (b) and axial MDCT images.

NON-ODONTOGENIC BENIGN TUMOURS INVOLVING THE JAWS

10.10 Osteoma (Figures 10.24–10.29)

- A benign, slow-growing, mature bony prominence at the periosteal surface. It remains uncertain if this is a hamartoma or a true benign tumour.
- Three types can be seen, consisting of:
  - compact bone (ivory osteoma)
  - cancellous bone
  - combination of compact and cancellous.
- Almost exclusively involving membranous bones of the skull and face, most commonly occurring within the paranasal sinuses (especially the frontal sinus and ethmoidal air cells – refer to Chapter 19), skull vault and mandible.
- When involving the mandible, they most commonly occur at the posterior mandible, often the medial aspect of the ramus or inferior border of the posterior body. They may also be seen at the condyle and coronoid processes.
- May be solitary or multiple. Gardner syndrome should be considered when there are multiple osteomas.
- Usually asymptomatic, often incidentally identified, unless large with a mass effect or causing clinically detectable asymmetry.

- Only require surgical excision if there is a mass effect or there is a cosmetic issue.

Radiological features
- MDCT or CBCT.
- Well-defined, focal, opaque prominence of variable bony appearance, often with a smooth convex or lobulated surface. Usually sessile in morphology although sometimes peduculated.
- Internally varies from being homogeneous and isodense with cortical bone (ivory osteoma) to those with variable internal cancellous bone appearance and varying thickness of the overlying cortical bone.
- Larger osteomas displace the adjacent soft tissues. Those occurring within the paranasal sinuses potentially distort the sinuses and may contribute to occlusion or narrowing of drainage pathways.

Differential diagnosis

	Key radiological differences
Osteochondroma of the mandibular condyle and coronoid process	Osteochondromas demonstrate more irregular morphology with more heterogeneous, sometimes sclerotic, internal appearances.

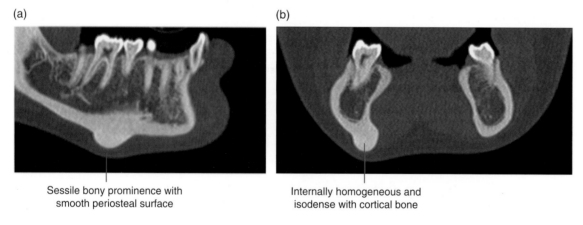

(a)

(b)

Sessile bony prominence with smooth periosteal surface

Internally homogeneous and isodense with cortical bone

Figure 10.24 Osteoma at the inferior body of the right mandible: corrected sagittal (a) and coronal (b) MDCT images.

(a)

(b)

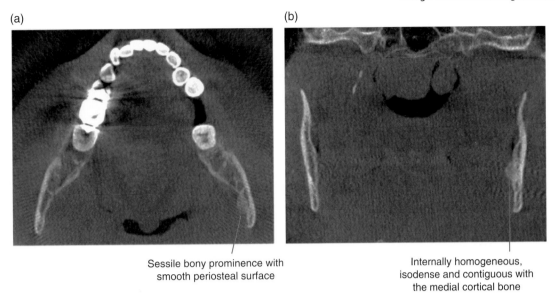

Sessile bony prominence with
smooth periosteal surface

Internally homogeneous,
isodense and contiguous with
the medial cortical bone

Figure 10.25 Osteoma at the medial aspect of the left mandibular ramus: axial (a) and coronal (b) CBCT images.

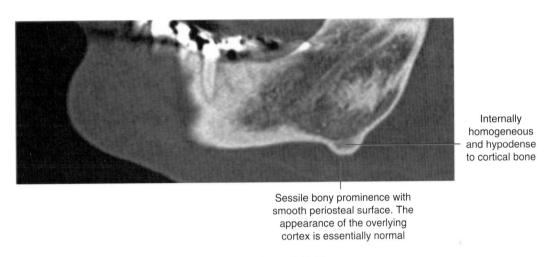

Internally
homogeneous
and hypodense
to cortical bone

Sessile bony prominence with
smooth periosteal surface. The
appearance of the overlying
cortex is essentially normal

Figure 10.26 Osteoma at the inferior left angle of the mandible: corrected sagittal CBCT image.

(a)

(b)

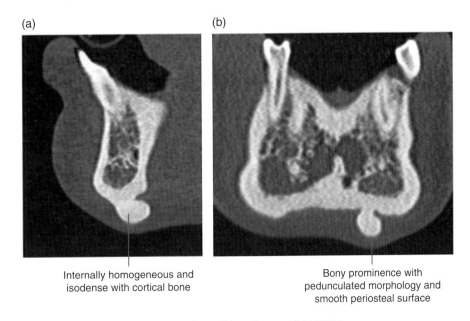

Internally homogeneous and
isodense with cortical bone

Bony prominence with
pedunculated morphology and
smooth periosteal surface

Figure 10.27 Osteoma at the inferior anterior mandible: corrected sagittal (a) and coronal (b) MDCT images.

(a)

(c)

(b)

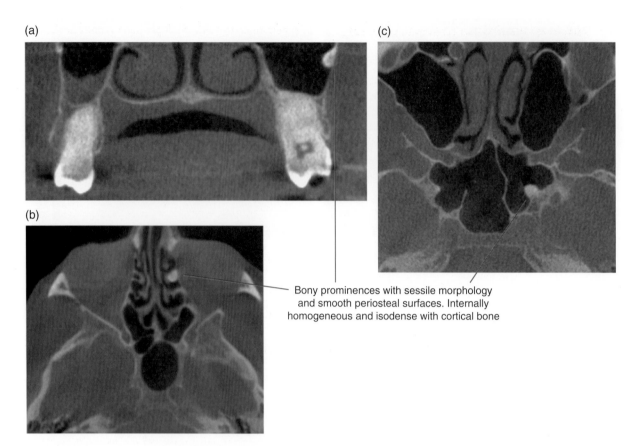

Bony prominences with sessile morphology and smooth periosteal surfaces. Internally homogeneous and isodense with cortical bone

Figure 10.28 Maxillary, ethmoidal and sphenoidal osteomas: CBCT images of three different cases. Maxillary osteoma – coronal image (a). Ethmoid osteoma – axial image (b). Sphenoid osteoma – axial image (c).

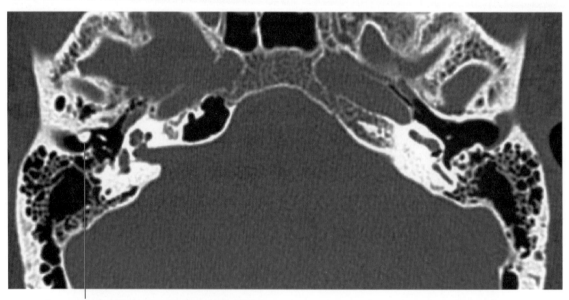

Bony prominence with sessile morphology and smooth periosteal surface. Internally homogeneous and isodense with cortical bone

Figure 10.29 Osteoma of the right external auditory canal: axial MDCT image.

10.11 Gardner syndrome (Figures 10.30–10.32)

- *Synonym*: familial colorectal polyposis.
- A rare autosomal dominant syndrome characterised by multiple intestinal polyps. Other features include osteomas of the skull and facial bones, epidermoid cysts, fibromas, desmoid tumours and a number of other tumours.
- High propensity for the intestinal polyps to undergo malignant change at an early age.
- With the jaws, there may be multiple osteomas and dental anomalies, including multiple unerupted teeth and supernumerary teeth. Multiple bone islands have also been seen. Multiple odontomas have also been described.
- Osteomas may develop earlier than the colonic polyps. The jaw features may contribute to early diagnosis.

Radiological features within the jaws

- There may be multiple osteomas and dental anomalies. Multiple bone islands have also been seen. There may be multiple odontomas. Note that these entities may be present and unrelated to Gardner syndrome.

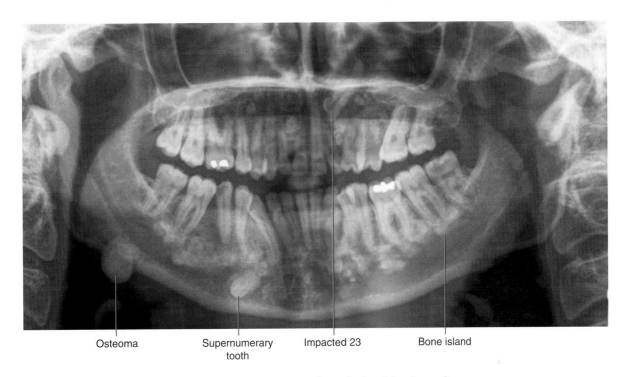

Osteoma   Supernumerary tooth   Impacted 23   Bone island

Figure 10.30 Gardner syndrome: panoramic radiograph. Multiple osteomas, bone islands and dental anomalies.

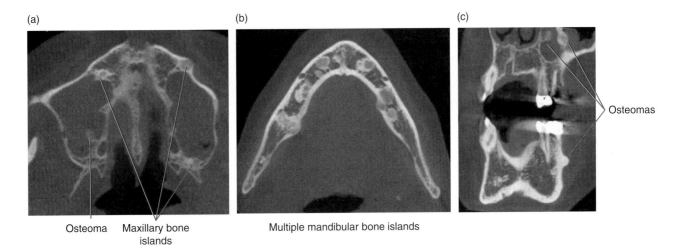

(a)   (b)   (c)

Osteoma   Maxillary bone islands   Multiple mandibular bone islands   Osteomas

Figure 10.31 Gardner syndrome: axial (a,b) and corrected coronal (c) MDCT images.

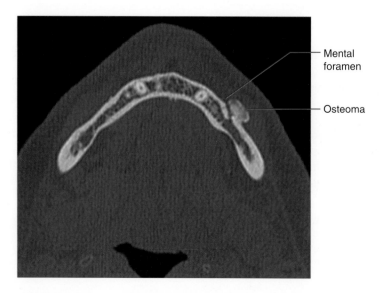

Figure 10.32 Gardner syndrome: axial MDCT image.

10.12 Osteochrondroma

- Refer to Chapter 18

10.13 Schwannoma (within the jaws)
(Figure 10.33)

- *Synonym*: neurilemmoma.
- A benign tumour of the Schwann cell, usually well encapsulated. Belongs to the group of nerve sheath tumours (refer to Chapter 20).
- May arise from any peripheral nerve with Schwann cells, including the cranial nerves. When it affects the trigeminal nerve, it is most commonly seen at the skull base. May also occur in patients with neurofibromatosis type 2.
- Within the jaws, it most commonly affects the mandibular division of the trigeminal nerve.
- Asymptomatic until large enough to affect nerve function, when there may be pain or other sensory changes.

Radiological features (when seen within the jaws)
- Expansile, corticated lucent lesion with mass effect, including displacement of teeth, root resorption and cortical effacements.
- In the mandible, smaller lesions demonstrate focal corticated expansion of the mandibular canal and/or mental/mandibular foramina. Classically, it demonstrates a fusiform morphology, although this is not always seen.
- MRI should be considered when a schwannoma is suspected: typically T1 isointense with brain; high T2 signal; homogeneous gadolinium enhancement.

Differential diagnosis (for lesions within the jaws)

	Key radiological differences
Vascular malformations/ haemangiomas	Usually demonstrates serpiginous or multilocular appearances.
Malignant lesions within the mandibular canal	Usually demonstrates destruction of the canal borders and the widening of the canal is usually more irregular.

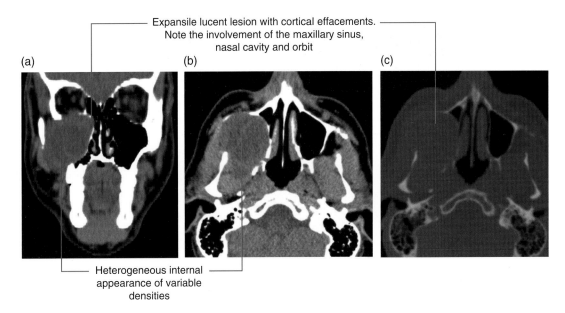

Expansile lucent lesion with cortical effacements. Note the involvement of the maxillary sinus, nasal cavity and orbit

(a) (b) (c)

Heterogeneous internal appearance of variable densities

Figure 10.33 Schwannoma of the right maxilla: coronal (a) and axial (b) soft tissue and axial bone (c) MDCT images.

10.14 Osteoblastoma

- A rare benign bone tumour which produces osteoid tissue and primitive woven bone.
  - Very similar to the osteoid osteoma. Many consider that the osteoblastoma represents a larger osteoid osteoma.
  - Some consider the cementoblastoma as an osteoblastoma centred at a tooth root apex.
- Histological differentiation from the low-grade osteogenic sarcoma can be challenging.
- Rarely seen in the jaws, more commonly in the mandible than the maxilla. Most commonly occurs in the spine and long bones. Also in flat bones.
- More common in males. Most commonly presents in the second to third decades of life.
- Most present with dull pain which is usually not worse at night. Not usually relieved with nonsteroidal anti-inflammatory drugs. Swelling is noted when sufficiently large.
- Surgical excision, usually with a wide margin. May recur.
- Postsurgical radiological review is recommended. The possibility of incorrect histological diagnosis (osteosarcoma) should be considered.

Radiological features

- MDCT is recommended. CBCT may be insufficient. MRI may be useful although it often overestimates the lesion.

- Variable radiological presentation: ranges from lytic lesions to variable internal opaque appearances.
- Internal opacities demonstrate a variety of patterns, ranging from coarse septum-like architecture to more amorphous appearances. There is often a lucent margin (band/zone) surrounding the internal opaque structure(s).
- Borders can be ill defined or well demarcated, even corticated.
- Expansile and displaces teeth when sufficiently large.
- May be associated with a soft tissue mass.

Differential diagnosis

	Key radiological differences
Osteoid osteoma	Smaller but otherwise very similar in appearance.
Cemento-osseous dysplasia	Can be similar in appearance. Osteoblastoma demonstrates more tumour features.
Osteogenic sarcoma	More aggressive malignant features, including destruction of cortical boundaries and invasion of the adjacent structures. This malignancy is often associated with a more prominent soft tissue mass.

10.15 Osteoid osteoma (Figure 10.34)

- A rare benign bone tumour which is considered by many to be a smaller variant of the osteoblastoma.
- More common in males.
- Usually seen in children and younger adults.
- Usually presents with nocturnal pain. Usually relieved with nonsteroidal anti-inflammatory drugs. There may be associated soft tissue swelling.
- Very rarely seen in the jaws. Most commonly seen in the long bones of the limbs, especially the femur.

Radiological features
- MDCT is recommended. CBCT may be insufficient.
- Usually presents as a well-defined lesion with sclerotic margins centred at the jaw cortex.
- Internally, these lesions may be lucent or may demonstrate central opacity.

Differential diagnosis

	Key radiological differences
Cemento-osseous dysplasia	Often centred apically (periapical osseous dysplasia).
Cementoblastoma	Often centred apically.

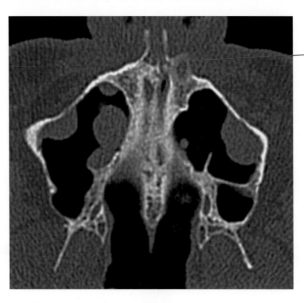

Lesion centred at the cortex, with sclerotic borders. Note the central opacity with surrounding lucency

Figure 10.34 Osteoid osteoma of the left premaxilla. History of nocturnal unexplained pain: axial MDCT image.

10.16 Desmoplastic fibroma (Figure 10.35)

- Extremely rare benign fibrous bone tumour which is locally destructive. Metastases have not been reported.
- Demonstrates slim fibroblasts within an abundant collagen fibre matrix. Often histologically difficult to differentiate from other fibrous-type lesions. Of particular concern is differentiating these lesions from low-grade fibrosarcomas. Some consider these lesions as the bony equivalent of the soft tissue desmoid tumours.
- Most commonly seen in the jaws, pelvis and femur. In the jaws, it most commonly occurs within the posterior mandible.
- Usually presents with swelling and associated dysfunction. Sometimes with pain.
- Aggressive surgical excision/resection. High recurrence rate. Postsurgical radiological review is recommended.

Radiological features

- MDCT is the technique of choice over CBCT. MRI may be useful in further characterisation.
- Ill-defined lesion with aggressive borders, not typical of most benign tumours. Some lesions may be largely well defined but there are usually one or a few regions where the borders are more aggressive and ill defined in appearances.
- Internally, small lesions may be lucent but larger lesions usually demonstrate a multilocular appearance with coarse and irregular septa. One or a few of these septa may demonstrate an angular configuration.
- There is often destruction of the jaw cortex with extension into the soft tissues.
- MRI: low T1 signal; foci of high T2 signal with surrounding intermediate signal; heterogeneous gadolinium enhancement.

Differential diagnosis

	Key radiological differences
Fibrosarcoma	The difficulty is often associated with the aggressive appearance of the borders of the desmoplastic fibroma. The appearance of coarse internal septa, especially if there are one or a few which demonstrate an angular appearance, favours the desmoplastic fibroma.
Other multilocular lesions	The aggressive features of the desmoplastic fibroma borders are not seen in other benign lesions with multilocular appearances. Coarse internal septa of the desmoplastic fibroma, especially the presence of one or a few which demonstrate an angular appearance, may be helpful.

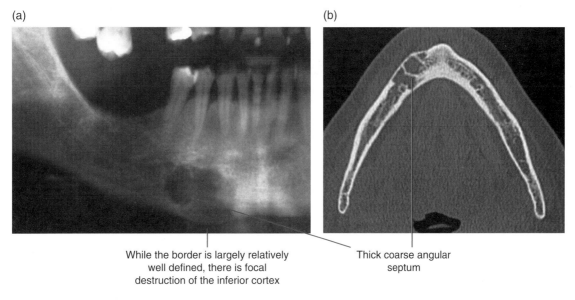

(a)   (b)

While the border is largely relatively well defined, there is focal destruction of the inferior cortex

Thick coarse angular septum

Figure 10.35 Desmoplastic fibroma of the inferior body of the right mandible: cropped panoramic radiograph (a) and axial MDCT image (b).

CHAPTER 11

Malignant Tumours Involving the Jaws

11.1 Imaging of malignancies involving the jaws

- Multidetector computed tomography (MDCT) is often the imaging modality of choice (at least initially) in the evaluation of malignancies involving the jaws, often with intravenous contrast. Magnetic resonance imaging (MRI) is also essential. Single-photon emission computed tomography and positron emission tomography/computed tomography may be required.
- Radiological malignant features can be identified on intraoral radiographs, panoramic radiographs and cone beam computed tomography (CBCT), which are commonly applied techniques in dentistry. The presence of a malignancy may well be first discovered by one of these techniques. However, if there is clinical suspicion for a malignancy in the maxillary or mandibular regions, 2D radiography is inadequate. CBCT is also insufficient as the adjacent soft tissues are poorly demonstrated, which may be important.
- Malignant lesions in the jaws share common features. Section 11.2 describes these while section 11.3 highlights some of the specific features of malignancies which more commonly involve the jaws.

11.2 Radiological features of malignancies involving the jaws (Figures 11.1–11.18)

- Borders.
  - Most demonstrate poorly defined invasive borders, which may demonstrate irregular lucent extensions into the adjacent marrow spaces. Occasionally, several small, ill-defined lucencies may be seen not far from the main lesion.
  - Occasionally, multiple 'punched out' lucencies with slightly more defined borders may be seen. Most commonly associated with multiple myeloma.
  - Some malignancies may sometimes not demonstrate aggressive borders, e.g. mucoepidermoid carcinoma and prostate and breast metastases.

- Internal appearances.
  - Usually lucent. There may occasionally be residual bone remnants within.
  - Osteoblastic metastatic lesions are usually sclerotic.
    - Breast and prostate metastatic lesions are typically sclerotic. There may be associated aggressive-appearing lucencies or destruction of adjacent cortices. However, these sclerotic lesions may be relatively benign in appearance.
    - Multiple sclerotic foci involving several visualised bones of the head and neck should raise the suspicion for metastatic disease. However, similar appearances may be seen in patients who have been or are on related drug therapies.
  - Osteogenic sarcomas variably produce tumour bone.
  - Mucoepidermoid carcinoma involving bone often presents as a multilocular lesion.
- Maxillary or mandibular cortices.
  - When a malignant lesion extends to or is centred at a bony boundary, there is usually cortical destruction, often with irregular edges.
  - Periosteal response at the involved cortex.
    - Most do not demonstrate a periosteal response, unless there is secondary infection. However:
      - sometimes the edges of the destroyed cortex may be slightly raised; this is considered a type of periosteal response associated with aggressive lesions (Codman triangle)
      - occasionally there is a lamina periosteal response adjacent to the cortical lesion; the periosteal response over the destroyed cortex is usually also destroyed
      - occasionally spiculation (sunburst appearance) is seen, i.e. multiple linear opacities extending outwardly from the site of cortical involvement; this is a form of periosteal response classically described in association with the osteosarcoma; prostate metastases may also demonstrate this feature.

Atlas of Oral and Maxillofacial Radiology, First Edition. Bernard Koong.
© 2017 John Wiley & Sons Ltd. Published 2017 by John Wiley & Sons Ltd.

- There is usually variable soft tissue mass over the region of involved/destroyed cortex (demonstrated on MDCT or MRI).
- Dentoalveolar structures.
  - Irregular widening of the periodontal ligament spaces of the teeth. There may be focal regions of widening of the periodontal ligament spaces with relatively normal appearances between.
  - Destruction of the lamina dura of tooth roots. This is often seen with the irregular widening of the periodontal ligament spaces. There may be focal destruction of the lamina dura interspersed with regions of relatively normal-appearing lamina dura.
  - This malignant widening of the periodontal ligament spaces and destruction of the lamina dura may involve any surface of any tooth root.
  - Destruction of follicular cortices of unerupted teeth. There may be displacement of the calcified dental structures within the follicle.
  - Tooth displacement and root resorption are not typically seen. However:
    - root resorption is occasionally seen
    - teeth may occasionally appear to be in a displaced position if a significant amount of surrounding bone is destroyed; this is usually related to a lack of alveolar bone support rather than displacement by the malignant lesion.

- Sometimes, all or most of the alveolar bone around the teeth is destroyed, giving the classically described appearance of 'teeth floating in space'.
- Mandibular canal.
  - Where a malignant lesion extends to this canal, the borders are usually destroyed.
  - A malignant lesion may traverse along, largely/partly within, the mandibular canal. There is usually lobulated or irregular widening with focal regions of canal border destruction.

11.3 Features of some malignancies which more commonly involve the jaws

- Squamous cell carcinoma (SCCa) (Figures 11.1 and 11.2).
  - When it involves the jaws, SCCa usually presents as a lytic destructive lesion with invasive borders (refer to section 11.2). Teeth are not usually affected and may appear to be 'floating in space'. Early bony involvement may appear as a focal erosion of the cortex.
  - Within the oral cavity, it most commonly occurs at the lateral border of the tongue. It also occurs on the lip, floor of the mouth and over the alveolar processes. SCCa can very rarely arise from odontogenic epithelium within bone, including odontogenic cysts.

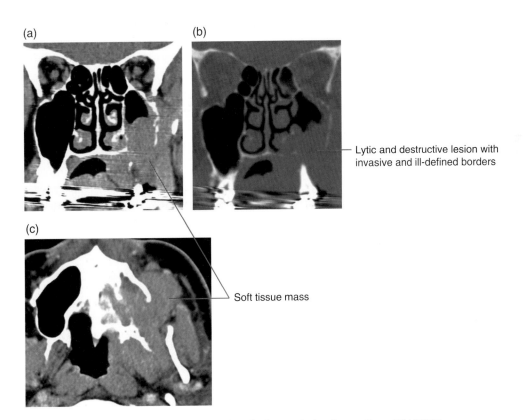

(a) (b) (c)

— Lytic and destructive lesion with invasive and ill-defined borders

— Soft tissue mass

Figure 11.1 Squamous cell carcinoma of the left maxilla: coronal and axial soft tissue (a,c) and coronal bone (b) MDCT images.

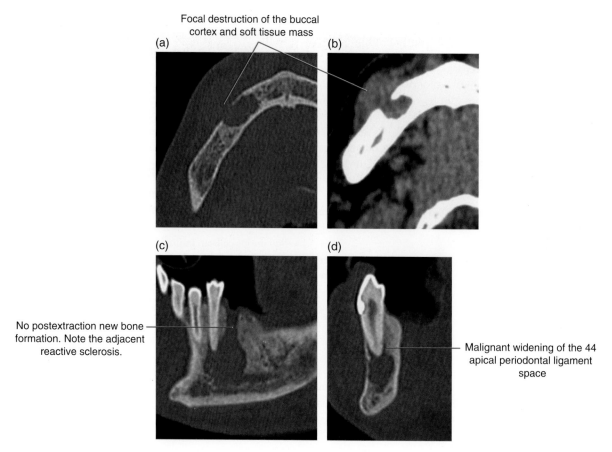

Figure 11.2 Squamous cell carcinoma; secondarily infected, 45 region: axial, corrected sagittal and corrected coronal bone (a,c,d) and axial soft tissue (b) MDCT images.

- Metastatic lesions (Figures 11.3 and 11.4).
  - More often in the older age group.
  - Occasionally, a metastatic lesion involving the jaws is the first identified evidence of the presence of malignant disease.
  - Usually present as lytic lesions with aggressive features (refer to section 11.2).
  - Osteoblastic metastatic lesions (e.g. breast and prostate) are often sclerotic in appearance. Prostate metastases may demonstrate a spiculated periosteal response.
- Lymphomas and leukaemias (Figures 11.5–11.10).
  - Malignancies involving white blood cells.
    - Leukaemia usually arises from within bone marrow. Four main types.
    - Lymphoma arises from lymphoid tissue. Two main types.
  - When these malignancies involve the jaws, there are similar radiological features.

- Lytic destructive or infiltrative lesions with ill-defined borders which demonstrate invasive features.
- In some cases the marrow spaces may be replaced with tumour tissue while the trabecular and cortical bone remains intact (as demonstrated on MRI or MDCT).
- May infiltrate along periodontal ligament spaces, with irregular widening and destruction of the lamina dura.
- May infiltrate into the follicular spaces of developing teeth, displacing the calcified structures and destroying the follicular cortices.
- Some demonstrate irregular widening of the mandibular canal with destruction of the borders.
- May be associated with variable soft tissue mass (as demonstrated on MDCT or MRI).
- Periosteal response is sometimes seen. May be lamina or spiculated.

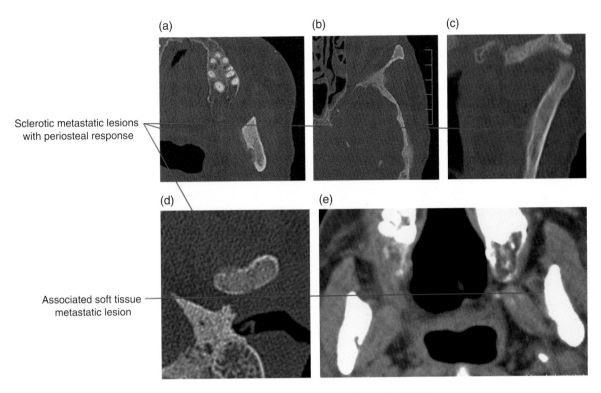

Sclerotic metastatic lesions with periosteal response

Associated soft tissue metastatic lesion

Figure 11.3 Metastatic prostate carcinoma: axial (a,b,d) and coronal (c) bone and axial soft tissue (e) MDCT images.

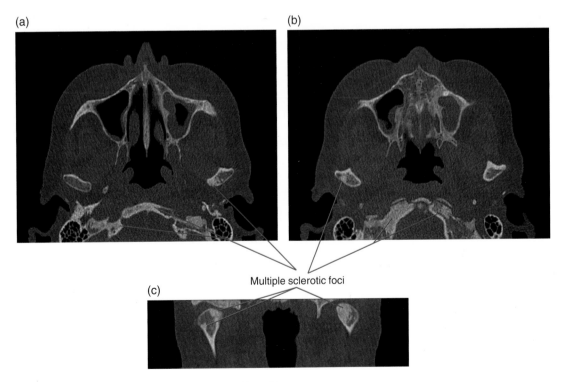

Multiple sclerotic foci

Figure 11.4 Metastatic breast carcinoma: axial (a,b) and coronal (c) MDCT images.

Irregular widening of the 17, 16, 15 and 14 periodontal ligament
spaces indicative of the infiltrative nature of this lesion. Note the
destruction of the buccal cortex and maxillary antral floor

(a)   (b)   (c)

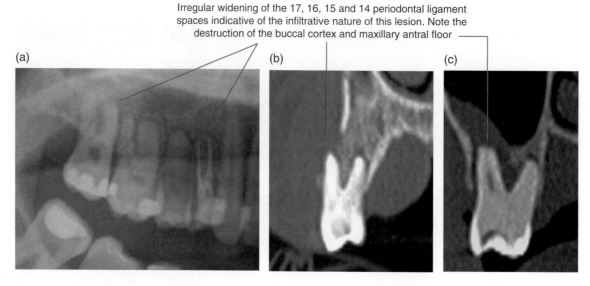

Figure 11.5 Lymphoma involving the right maxilla: cropped panoramic radiograph (a) and cross-sectional MDCT images (b,c).

Lytic ill-defined lesion with destruction of the left maxillary
antral cortical floor. Soft tissue density at the left maxillary
antral base represents the tumour mass

(a)   (b)   (c)

Figure 11.6 Lymphoma: cropped panoramic radiograph (a) and corrected sagittal (b) and cross-sectional (c) CBCT images.

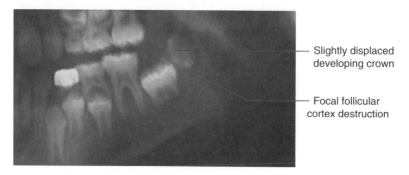

Slightly displaced
developing crown

Focal follicular
cortex destruction

Figure 11.7 Leukaemia: cropped panoramic image.

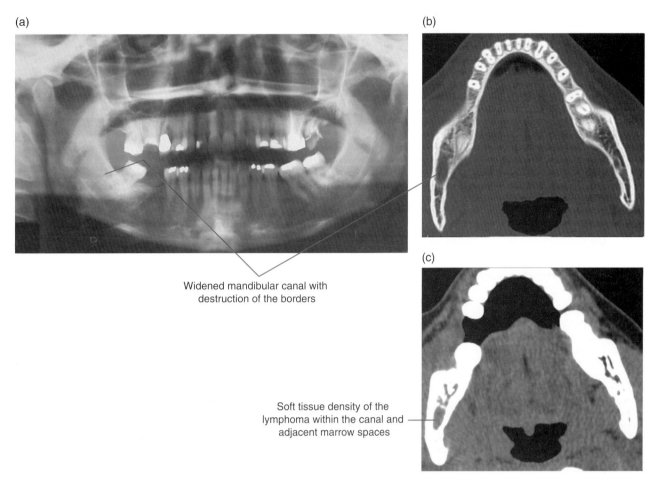

Widened mandibular canal with destruction of the borders

Soft tissue density of the lymphoma within the canal and adjacent marrow spaces

Figure 11.8 Lymphoma: panoramic radiograph (a) and axial bone (b) and soft tissue (c) MDCT images.

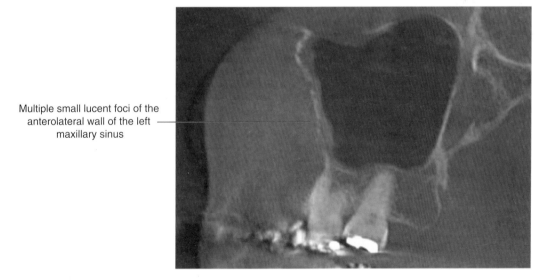

Multiple small lucent foci of the anterolateral wall of the left maxillary sinus

Figure 11.9 Lymphoma: corrected sagittal CBCT image.

(a)　　　　　　　　　　　　　　　　　　(b)

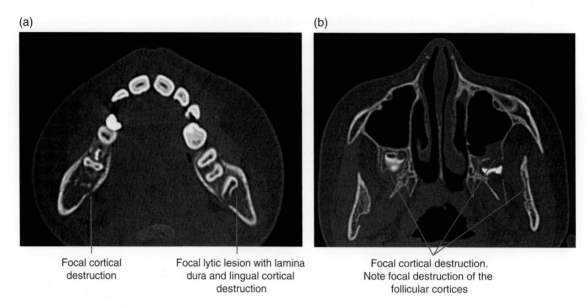

Focal cortical
destruction

Focal lytic lesion with lamina
dura and lingual cortical
destruction

Focal cortical destruction.
Note focal destruction of the
follicular cortices

Figure 11.10 Leukaemia: axial MDCT images (a,b).

- Osteosarcoma (Figure 11.11).
  - *Synonym*: osteogenic sarcoma.
  - This bone-forming malignant tumour is rarely seen in the jaws.
  - Usually presents as a lesion with aggressive permeative borders and cortical destruction.
  - Internally, it is variable, ranging from being lucent to various abnormal patterns of internal opacities which reflect tumour bone and related calcifications.

  - There is usually a prominent periosteal response, the 'sunburst' spiculated appearance being classically described. A Codman triangle (refer to section 11.2) is sometimes seen. Laminated periosteal reaction is less common.
  - When teeth are involved, there may be infiltrative irregular widening of the periodontal ligament spaces.
  - Usually associated with an enhancing soft tissue mass.

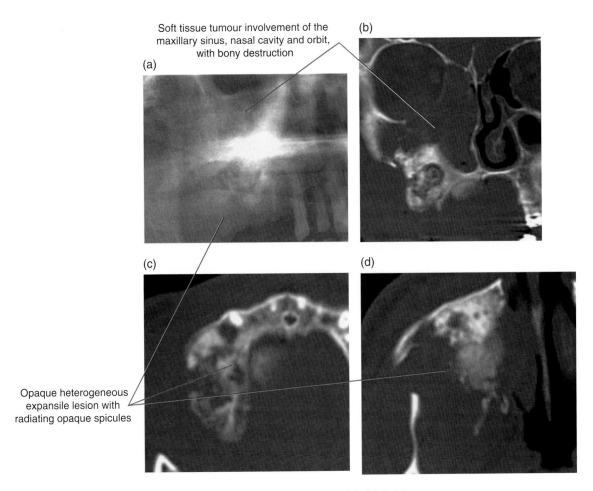

Soft tissue tumour involvement of the maxillary sinus, nasal cavity and orbit, with bony destruction

(a)

(b)

(c)

(d)

Opaque heterogeneous expansile lesion with radiating opaque spicules

Figure 11.11 Osteosarcoma: cropped panoramic radiograph (a) with coronal (b) and axial (c,d) MDCT images.

- Chondrosarcoma (Figure 11.12).
  - *Synonym*: chondrogenic sarcoma.
  - Malignant cartilaginous tumour, rarely seen in the jaws.
  - Variable radiological appearances depending on subtypes and grade.
  - May be quite benign in appearance with well-defined, even corticated borders. The expanded jaw cortices may be preserved. Higher grade lesions demonstrate invasive borders.
  - Internally may be lytic. Some demonstrate internal ring/arc-shaped calcifications and the classically described 'popcorn' appearance. Others demonstrate multiple internal sclerotic-appearing foci which may be irregular.
  - When affecting the teeth, tooth displacement and root resorption may be seen. Infiltrative irregular widening of the periodontal ligament spaces may be seen.
  - May involve adjacent muscles.

(a)　　　　　　　　　　　　　　　(b)

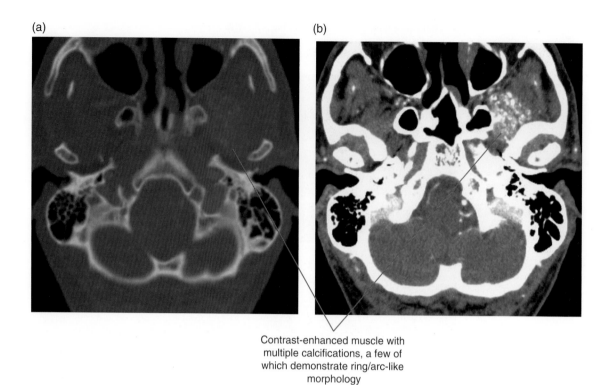

Contrast-enhanced muscle with
multiple calcifications, a few of
which demonstrate ring/arc-like
morphology

Figure 11.12 Chondrosarcoma from the skull base involving the left lateral pterygoid muscle: postcontrast axial bone (a) and soft tissue (b) MDCT images.

- Mucoepidermoid carcinoma (involving the jaws) (Figures 11.13 and 11.14).
  - Usually occurs in the salivary glands.
  - Rarely arises from within bone (central). Lesions arising from the major and minor salivary glands may invade the adjacent jaws.

- Unlike most malignant lesions, this malignancy can demonstrate benign features.
- Often presents as a multilocular expansile lesion with sclerotic or heavily corticated borders. Can be very similar in appearance to the ameloblastoma but root resorption is less commonly seen with the mucoepidermoid carcinoma.

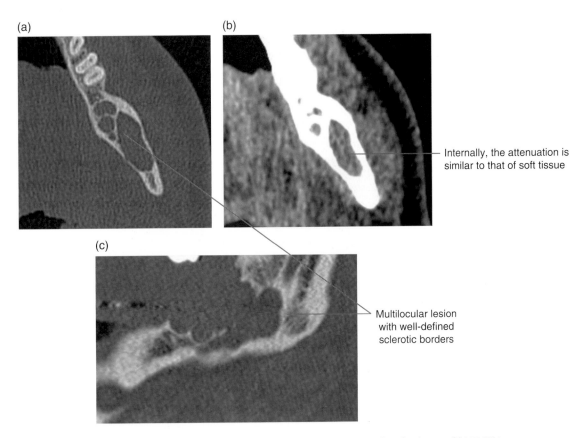

Figure 11.13 Intraosseous mucoepidermoid carcinoma: axial and corrected sagittal bone (a,c) and axial soft tissue (b) MDCT images.

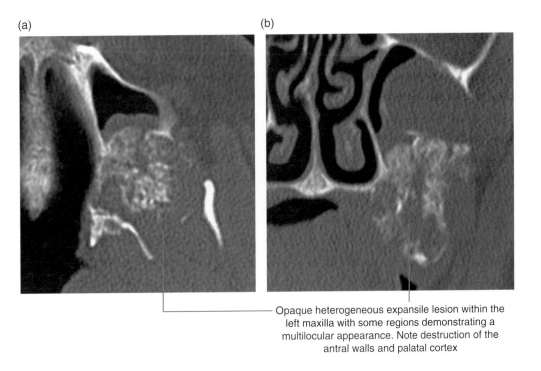

Figure 11.14 Intraosseous mucoepidermoid carcinoma: axial (a) and coronal (b) MDCT images.

- Multiple myeloma (Figures 11.15 and 11.16).
  - A malignancy of the plasma cells.
  - Most common primary malignant neoplasm of bone.
  - In the jaws, most commonly seen in the posterior mandible.
  - Classically presents as multiple 'punch-out' lytic lesions with borders which demonstrate variable degrees of invasive features. May coalesce in severe cases, and may appear multilocular on 2D radiography.

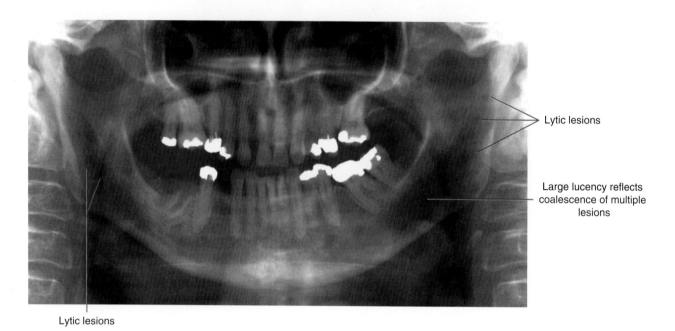

Lytic lesions

Large lucency reflects coalescence of multiple lesions

Lytic lesions

Figure 11.15 Multiple myeloma: panoramic radiograph.

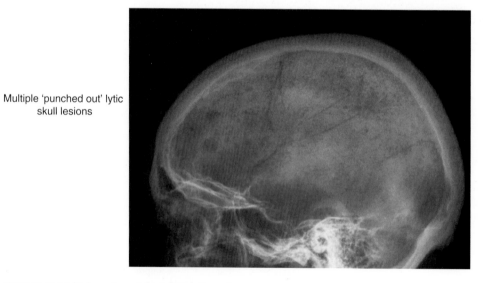

Multiple 'punched out' lytic skull lesions

Figure 11.16 Multiple myeloma: lateral skull radiograph.

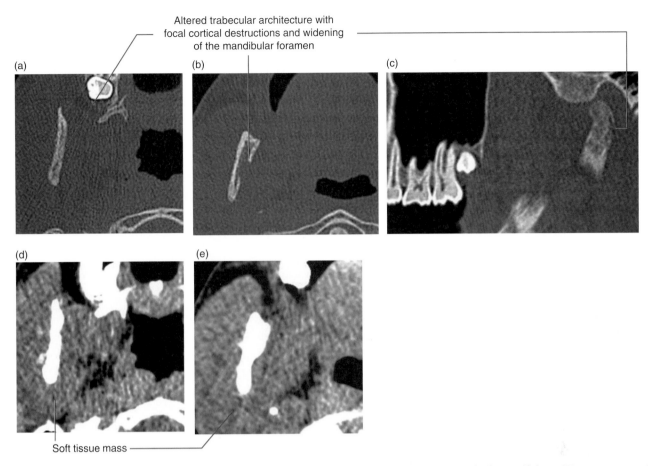

Figure 11.17 Ewing's sarcoma of the right ramus and condyle: axial (a,b) and corrected sagittal (c) bone and axial soft tissue (d,e) MDCT images.

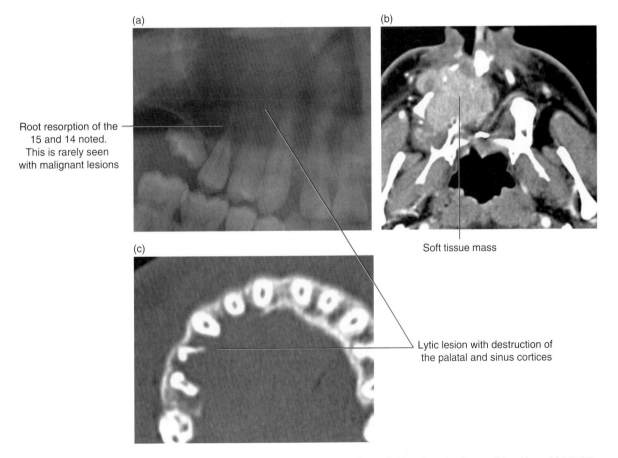

Figure 11.18 Malignant fibrous histiocytoma of the right maxilla: cropped panoramic radiograph (a) with axial soft tissue (b) and bone (c) MDCT images.

Differential diagnosis (non-malignant lesions)

Key radiological differences

Periapical inflammatory lesions	May appear similar. Inflammatory lesions are usually centred at the apical foramen (occasionally related to a lateral canal on other root surfaces). In contrast, malignancies demonstrate irregularly widened periodontal ligament spaces or periradicular lucencies, which tend to occur at any of the root surfaces. There are often infiltrative margins. There may be relatively normal-appearing periodontal ligament space and lamina dura between abnormal foci.
Vascular malformations	May appear aggressive, especially larger lesions. Abnormal vascular channels at cortices may give the impression of an invasive or infiltrative lesion.
Osteomyelitis	May appear similar, especially when acute. Malignancies (e.g. SCCa) tend to demonstrate more aggressive borders. Periosteal response is often seen in osteomyelitis but it can also be present in some malignancies, and oral malignancies which are exposed to the oral cavity are often secondarily infected.
Osteoradionecrosis	May appear similar. Malignant borders demonstrate more invasive features. Irregularly widened periodontal ligament spaces may be seen in osteoradionecrosis and also some malignant lesions.
Fibrous dysplasia	May rarely appear similar to osteosarcoma and chondrosarcoma. Fibrous dysplasia demonstrates a more benign appearance. When teeth are involved, fibrous dysplasia usually thins and/or alters the architecture of the lamina dura, while malignant lesions usually variably destroy the lamina dura.
Ossifying fibroma	May appear similar to osteosarcoma and chondrosarcoma. Ossifying fibroma demonstrates a more benign appearance.

CHAPTER 12
Vascular Anomalies of the Mid- and Lower Face

Michael Bynevelt, Andrew Thompson and Bernard Koong

Vascular anomalies comprise two broad categories: vascular tumours (proliferative neoplasms) and vascular malformations. Ultrasound and magnetic resonance angiography (MRA) can assist in characterising the vascular flow dynamics.

VASCULAR TUMOURS (PROLIFERATIVE NEOPLASMS)

12.1 Haemangioma (Figures 12.1 and 12.2)

- Most common lesion in this grouping of true vascular neoplasms.
- Can be subcategorised into infantile and congenital types.
  - Infantile.
    - Present in the postnatal period or first 6 months of life with approximately two-thirds arising in the head and neck region; commonly involving the parotid glands, orbits, nasal cavity, subglottis, anterior and posterior regions of the neck.
    - Demonstrate a triphasic growth pattern with proliferative, plateau and involution phases, reaching a maximum size between 3 and 5 months.
    - Lesions usually begin to involute by 1 year. Approximately half of these lesions will show near complete resolution by 5 years.
  - Congenital; present at birth and further classified as:
    - Non-involuting congenital haemangioma: grow proportionally with the growth of the patient.
    - Rapidly involuting congenital haemangioma: maximal in size at birth but involute in the first 12–18 months.
- First-line treatment is medical, utilising propranolol, with surgery reserved for complicated (ulcerating, bleeding) or refractory lesions.

Radiological features
- The purpose of imaging is to characterise, locally stage for the deep extent and assess for multiplicity.
- Haemangiomas present clinically as a raised 'strawberry-like' plaque, which may be classified as cutaneous, subcutaneous, visceral or mixed. Assessment of deep lesions and definition of locoregional extent in children should be undertaken with ultrasound and magnetic resonance imaging (MRI).
- During the proliferating phase, haemangiomas are well defined but of mixed echogenicity on ultrasound with low-resistance high flows on Doppler studies.
- On MRI haemangiomas are of heterogeneous and usually slightly hyperintense signal relative to muscle on T2-weighted imaging, with flow voids and intense contrast enhancement.
- MRA may show associated anomalies such as in PHACES (posterior fossa malformations–haemangiomas–arterial anomalies–cardiac defects–eye abnormalities–sternal cleft and supraumbilical raphe) syndrome.

Differential diagnosis

	Key radiological differences
Venocavernous malformation	Insinuating, trans-spatial, variable enhancement, phleboliths.
Arteriovenous malformation	Flow voids, minor soft tissue component.
Hypervascular primary neoplasms	Avidly contrast enhancing, flow voids.
Hypervascular metastases	Avidly contrast enhancing, flow voids, known primary tumour.

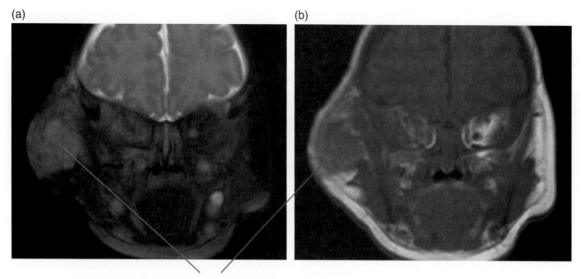

Extensive trans-spatial lesion involving the right side of the face, masticator space and right orbit. Clinical appearances and ultrasound appearances were consistent with an infantile haemangioma

Figure 12.1 Infantile haemangioma: fat-saturated T2-weighted (a) and T1-weighted (b) coronal MRI.

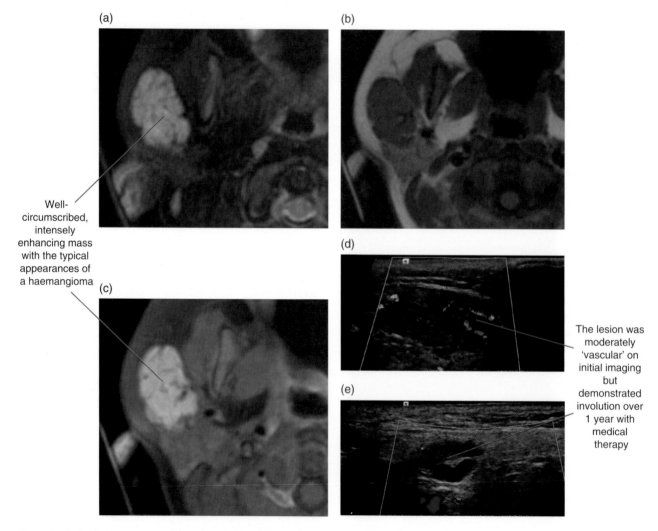

Well-circumscribed, intensely enhancing mass with the typical appearances of a haemangioma

The lesion was moderately 'vascular' on initial imaging but demonstrated involution over 1 year with medical therapy

Figure 12.2 Infantile haemangioma of the right parotid and buccal spaces: fat-saturated T2-weighted axial MRI (a); T1-weighted axial MRI (b); fat-saturated gadolinium-enhanced T1-weighted axial MRI (c); Doppler ultrasound of the lesion at diagnosis (d); and 12 months post treatment (e).

12.2 Other lesions included in this grouping

- Tufted angioma.
- Kaposiform and spindle cell haemangioendotheliomas.
- Pyogenic granulomas.
- Haemangiopericytoma.

VASCULAR MALFORMATIONS

- A spectrum of non-proliferative lesions resulting from errors in vascular formation. Uncomplicated lesions increase in size proportionally with patient growth.
- Can be grouped according to the morphology of their constituent vascular structures (capillary, venous, cavernous, lymphatic, arterial or combined).
- Lesions with metameric associations can be grouped as a craniofacial arteriovenous or craniofacial venous metameric syndrome.
- Intralesional blood flow rates, demonstrated on colour Doppler ultrasound, facilitate categorisation.

Complications
- Often cause any of these lesions to rapidly increase in size, become painful and may compromise adjacent structures. These include:
  ◦ intralesional thrombosis
  ◦ inflammation and infection
  ◦ haemorrhage – importantly, possible intraosseous and transosseous communications are a consideration prior to local surgical procedures, including local anaesthetic injections and dentoalveolar/orofacial procedures.
  ◦ Kasabach–Merritt syndrome: a consumptive coagulopathy and thrombocytopenia.

12.3 Low-flow lesions

Venolymphatic malformations or lymphangiomas (Figure 12.3)

- Congenital lesions consisting of malformed lymphatic channels, the majority of which are found in the head and neck region, most commonly in the posterior triangle. The lesions can also be found in the orbit, floor of the mouth and in the oral tongue.
- Usually present before 2 years old as a compressible swelling with a yellow-red discoloration of the overlying skin when presenting as a mucosal lesion.

- Slow growing unless complicated by infection, inflammation or haemorrhage, when they can suddenly increase in size.
- Aside from conservative management, which may be employed for small microcystic lesions, treatment options include percutaneous sclerotherapy and surgery.

Radiological features
- The purpose of imaging is to characterise, locally stage for the deep extent and assess for multiplicity.
- Structurally are cystic, with variable signal on MRI reflecting cyst content, which may be haemorrhagic or proteinaceous.
- Septated macrocystic lesions (>1 cm) are more commonly present at birth, in contrast to the more prevalent microcystic (<1 cm) lesions that present later in age.
- Variable enhancement is observed following intravenous contrast administration; pure lymphangiomas are non-enhancing.
- Appearances on ultrasound and MRI vary in accordance with the size of the constituent cysts. The microcystic type is diffusely hyperechoic on ultrasound without demonstrable flow, hypointense on T1- and hyperintense on T2-weighted MRI. The macrocystic subtype are septated anechoic structures, which may reveal fluid–fluid levels, but no flow with Doppler interrogation.
- Computed tomography (CT) is often the imaging modality of choice if the patient presents urgently with a complication, potentially requiring urgent therapeutic intervention.

Differential diagnosis

	Key radiological differences
Branchial cleft cyst	Location: in the region of the angle of mandible.
Ranula	No contrast enhancement.
Dermoid cyst	High T1 signal.
Thyroglossal duct remnant	Related to hyoid and midline position.

Capillary malformations

- These lesions are clinically readily apparent and, although typically isolated, have important syndromic associations such as Sturge–Weber syndrome (with a 'trigeminally' distributed lesion or 'port-wine stain' on the face, with leptomeningeal, choroidal and oral mucosal lesions) and Klippel–Trénaunay syndrome.
- Treatment includes pulsed laser therapy.

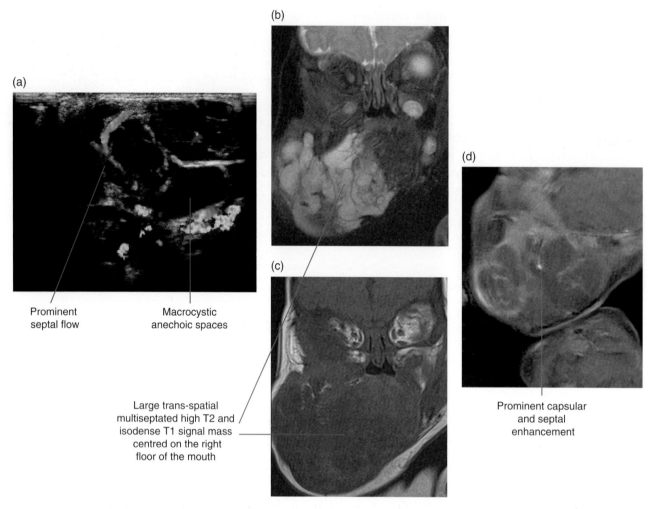

(a)

(b)

(c)

(d)

Prominent
septal flow

Macrocystic
anechoic spaces

Large trans-spatial
multiseptated high T2 and
isodense T1 signal mass
centred on the right
floor of the mouth

Prominent capsular
and septal
enhancement

Figure 12.3 Inflamed lymphangioma: Doppler ultrasound of the lesion (a); fat-saturated T2-weighted coronal MRI (b); T1-weighted coronal MRI (c); and fat-saturated gadolinium-enhanced T1-weighted coronal MRI (d).

Venocavernous malformations (Figures 12.4–12.8)

- Composed of dilated dysplastic venous spaces, which may be focal and encapsulated or diffuse with trans-spatial insinuation.
- Often extend around a neurovascular bundle, along and through the fascial planes, and into deep anatomic subsites in the neck, such as the masticator and parapharyngeal spaces. Lesions can be in part or entirely intraosseous.
- The patient may have multiple cutaneous and mucosal venous malformations as part of an inherited disorder such as the blue rubber naevus syndrome.
- Lesions are bluish, may be compressible and/or expand on Valsalva manoeuvre.
- Percutaneous sclerotherapy is the primary treatment option. Focal lesions are typically sequestered but drain into normal adjacent veins. Diffuse lesions may have extensive regional venous drainage, which, if not recognised, may cause systemic toxicity with sclerotherapy.

Radiological features

- The purpose of imaging is to characterise, locally stage for the deep extent and assess for multiplicity. Cone beam computed tomography (CBCT) is insufficient.
- MRI characteristics of these lesions include high signal on T2-weighted imaging and isointense on T1-weighted imaging relative to skeletal muscle.
- Fat-saturated T2-weighted imaging provides the best information related to the local extent of lesions, their intrinsic flow rates and soft tissue/calcified components.
- Large lesions are often cystic, exhibiting prominent vascular channels, and are hyperintense with septations. Small lesions reveal less prominent vascular channels and tend to be more 'solid' with intermediate signal intensities.
- On T1-weighted imaging lesions are lobulated and associated localised fat hypertrophy has been described.
- With intravenous contrast medium, homogeneous or heterogeneous enhancement patterns are seen.

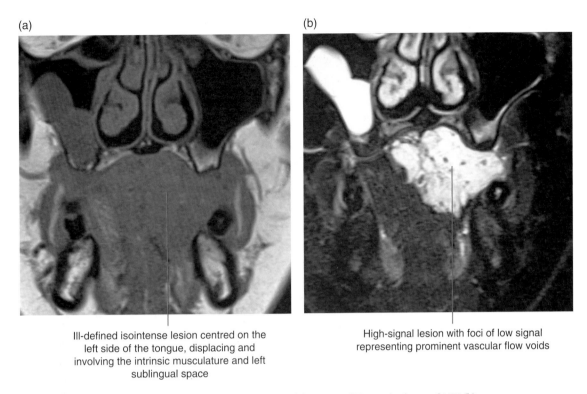

Ill-defined isointense lesion centred on the left side of the tongue, displacing and involving the intrinsic musculature and left sublingual space

High-signal lesion with foci of low signal representing prominent vascular flow voids

Figure 12.4 Venocavernous malformation: T1-weighted coronal MRI (a) and fat-saturated T2-weighted coronal MRI (b).

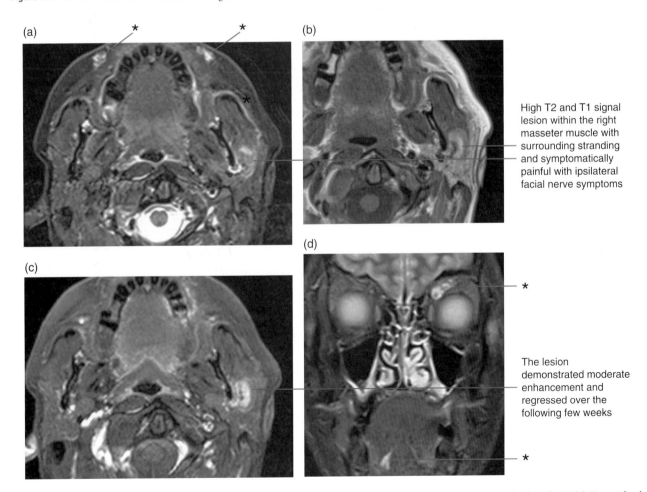

High T2 and T1 signal lesion within the right masseter muscle with surrounding stranding and symptomatically painful with ipsilateral facial nerve symptoms

The lesion demonstrated moderate enhancement and regressed over the following few weeks

Figure 12.5 Thrombosed venocavernous malformation, multifocal venous malformations (asterisks): fat-saturated T2-weighted axial MRI (a); T1-weighted coronal MRI (b); fat-saturated gadolinium-enhanced T1-weighted axial MRI (c); and fat-saturated T2-weighted coronal MRI (d).

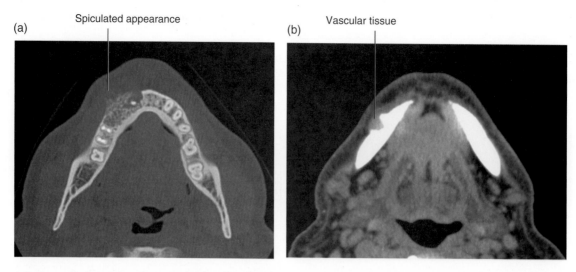

Figure 12.6 Right mandibular low-flow vascular malformation: non-contrast axial bone (a) and soft tissue (b) MDCT images. (Courtesy of Professor Paul Monsour, School of Dentistry, The University of Queensland, Australia.)

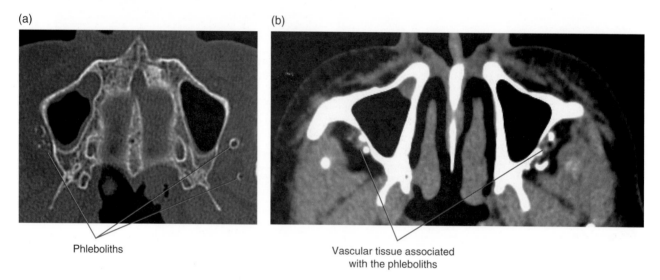

Figure 12.7 Bilateral low-flow vascular malformations adjacent to the maxilla: non-contrast axial bone (a) and soft tissue (b) MDCT images.

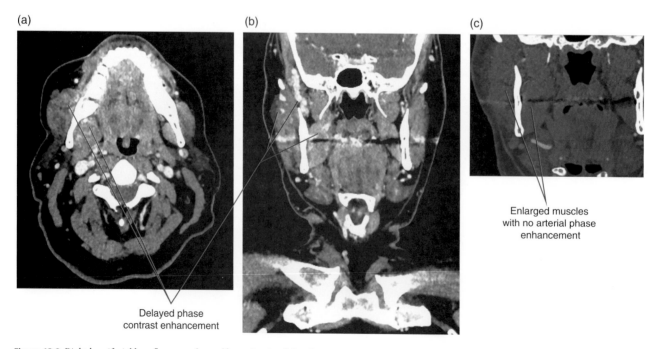

Figure 12.8 Right hemifacial low-flow vascular malformation involving the masticatory muscles: postcontrast axial (a) and coronal (b,c) MDCT images.

- MRA and magnetic resonance venography (MRV) may reveal localised and remote associated vascular changes and multi-focal lesions. An associated enlarged draining vein or anomalous venous drainage may be seen.
- When involving the bones of the jaw, CT may demonstrate a well-marginated or ill-defined lesion. A variety of bone changes can be seen in the lesion, which have been described as 'lace like', 'sunburst', 'soap bubble', 'honeycomb' or 'tennis racket'. A periosteal reaction may also be seen.
  Prominent feeding and draining vessels may result in curvilinear or serpiginous lucencies within the mandible and may enlarge the mandibular canal.
- When involving teeth, there is usually root resorption and tooth displacement.
- Phleboliths may also be demonstrated.
- Multidetector computed tomography (MDCT) angiography may also assist with lesion characterisation and staging.
- Doppler ultrasound assists in the portrayal of vascular channels and their associated flow rates. Lesions with smaller vascular channels are generally of increased echogenicity and are less compressible. Phleboliths appear as echogenic foci that cause posterior acoustic shadowing.
- The general appearance of the lesion is often quite 'aggressive' when inflamed or with superimposed thrombosis. Malignancy and inflammatory lesions are a necessary consideration in this setting.
- MDCT is often the imaging modality of choice if the patient presents as an emergency with a complication, potentially requiring urgent therapeutic intervention.

Differential diagnosis

	Key radiological differences
Haemangioma	High T2 signal, avidly enhancing, clinical.
Lymphatic malformation	No contrast enhancement, fluid–fluid levels.
Arteriovenous malformation (slow flow)	Flow voids, minor soft tissue component.

12.4 High-flow lesions

Arteriovenous malformations (Figure 12.9)

- Composed of single or multiple arteriovenous fistulae bypassing the normal highly resistive capillary bed, are often traumatic but also present at birth, arising in the face or cavernous sinus region. The associated vessels in this category possess a true vessel wall structure.
- Despite the rapid flows, a lesion may not be apparent clinically prior to detailed clinical and radiological investigation.

- Clinically they are pink/blue lesions, often exhibiting a palpable thrill or audible bruit, and may grow in stages enlarging from quiescence to that which causes systemic cardiovascular decompensation.

Radiological features

- The purpose of imaging is to characterise, locally stage for the deep extent and assess for multiplicity. CBCT is insufficient.
- Jaw based lesions usually present as a lucent (unilocular) or variably multilocular well-defined corticated lesion and most commonly these are seen in the posterior mandible. Occasionally, the borders are ill defined in appearance, especially on intraoral and panoramic radiographs.
- Mandibular canal and associated foramina are often enlarged and are curvilinear or serpiginous in outline.
- Small lucent channel-like lucencies at the jaw cortices are often present.
- Occasionally, a spiculated periosteal response is seen and intralesional phleboliths may be identified.
- When involving teeth, there is usually root resorption and tooth displacement.
- MDCT angiography provides a structural anatomical assessment. Similarly, MRI, MRA and MRV demonstrate a tangled mesh of dilated arteries and veins, containing flow voids. Susceptibility-weighted sequences can demonstrate associated haemorrhagic foci and contrast studies will highlight some components of slow flow and tissue injury.
- Conventional or catheter angiography (internal and external carotid artery) can confirm the suspected diagnosis, providing more refined information as regards arterial 'feeders', draining veins, flow characteristics, nidal configuration as well as collateral vessels which may contain dangerous anastomoses.
- MDCT is often the imaging modality of choice if the patient presents as an emergency with a complication, potentially requiring urgent therapeutic intervention.
- Doppler ultrasound demonstrates high systolic and diastolic flow, and arteriovenous shunting with arterial waveforms in veins.
- Lesions often appear quite 'aggressive' when inflamed or with superimposed thrombosis.

Differential diagnosis

	Key radiological differences
Haemangioma	High T2 signal, avidly enhancing, clinical.
Lymphatic malformation	No contrast enhancement, fluid–fluid levels.
Venocavernous malformation	Insinuating, trans-spatial, variable enhancement, phleboliths.
Vascular tumour	Avidly contrast enhancing, flow voids.
Hypervascular metastases	Avidly contrast enhancing, flow voids, known primary tumour.

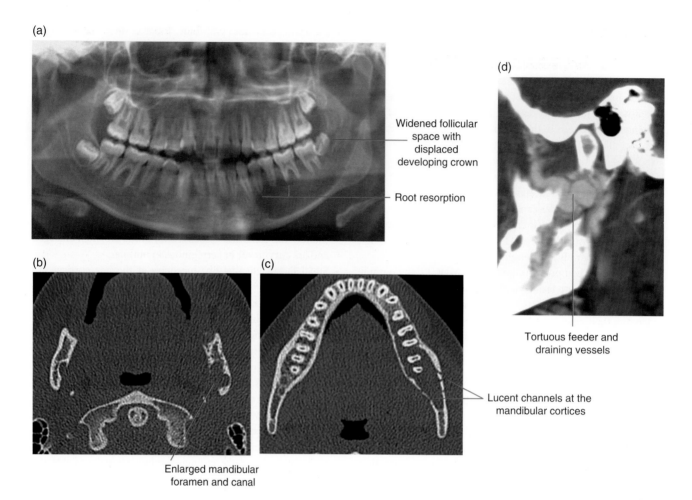

(a)

Widened follicular space with displaced developing crown

Root resorption

(b)

Enlarged mandibular foramen and canal

(c)

Lucent channels at the mandibular cortices

(d)

Tortuous feeder and draining vessels

Figure 12.9 Left mandibular arteriovenous malformation: panoramic radiograph (a), axial non-contrast MDCT (b,c) and corrected sagittal MDCT angiogram (d) images.

CHAPTER 13
Other Diseases Affecting the Jaws

Bernard Koong and Tom Huang

13.1 Central giant cell granuloma
(Figures 13.1–13.5)

- *Synonyms*: CGCG, giant cell reparative granuloma.
- A non-neoplastic lesion consisting of vascular tissue and multinucleated giant cells. Generally considered to be reactive or reparative in nature.
- Most commonly occurs in the jaws, especially the mandible.
- Most often presents in the second and third decades of life. When seen in the older person, hyperparathyroidism should be considered (brown tumour).
- While not a tumour, it often presents with tumour-like clinical features.
- Usually surgical removal. Recurrence is relatively rare.

Radiological features
- Multidetector computed tomography (MDCT) is the preferred imaging modality. However, cone beam computed tomography (CBCT) may be sufficient for some cases. Magnetic resonance imaging (MRI) can be useful for further characterisation, especially in differentiating from the aneurysmal bone cyst.
- Well-defined multilocular expansile lesion. The septa are typically extremely fine, which may be difficult to identify, especially on 2D radiography and CBCT. These septa are often more obvious in soft tissue windows (MDCT). In the classical lesion, one or two of these septa can be seen at right angles to the expanded jaw cortices. The appearances of these septa are similar to those of the aneurysmal bone cyst.
- Expanded cortices often demonstrate a lobulated appearance. The expanded cortices are often largely preserved, although focal cortical effacements are not uncommon, especially with maxillary lesions.
- Sometimes, the margins may be poorly defined, especially in the maxilla, resulting in a more aggressive appearance.
- Can be unilocular, especially small lesions.
- When sufficiently large, tooth displacement and root resorption are often seen.

Differential diagnosis

Key radiological differences

Other lesions which may appear to be multilocular, including:

Ameloblastoma Odontogenic myxoma	Thick and curved internal septa. Presence of one or a few straight septa is a feature. Typically demonstrates mild expansion for size.
Aneurysmal bone cyst (ABC)	Fine internal septa can appear very similar to the CGCG. However, the ABC is typically extremely expansile. MDCT soft tissue windows may demonstrate focal regions of fluid attenuation. The characteristic fluid–fluid level is a feature of the ABC which is well demonstrated on MRI, and occasionally appreciated on MDCT (narrow width soft tissue window).
Brown tumour	Can be identical radiologically and histologically. The brown tumour is related to hyperparathyroidism and the associated osteopenic changes may be seen.

Atlas of Oral and Maxillofacial Radiology, First Edition. Bernard Koong.
© 2017 John Wiley & Sons Ltd. Published 2017 by John Wiley & Sons Ltd.

Cysts	The unilocular CGCG can resemble a cyst, especially the simple bone cyst in the younger patient. However, the simple bone cyst typically does not displace or resorb tooth roots.	Vascular malformation/ haemangioma	Often demonstrates serpiginous appearances. Can appear to be multilocular on 2D radiography. Prebiopsy evaluation with MRI should be considered if this is suspected.
Ossifying fibroma	When this lesion demonstrates internal septa, they tend to be larger.	Cherubism	Can be radiologically identical but cherubism is usually multifocal, occurring posteriorly.
Keratocystic odontogenic tumour	Internal septa are uncommon and this lesion demonstrates only mild expansion for its size.		

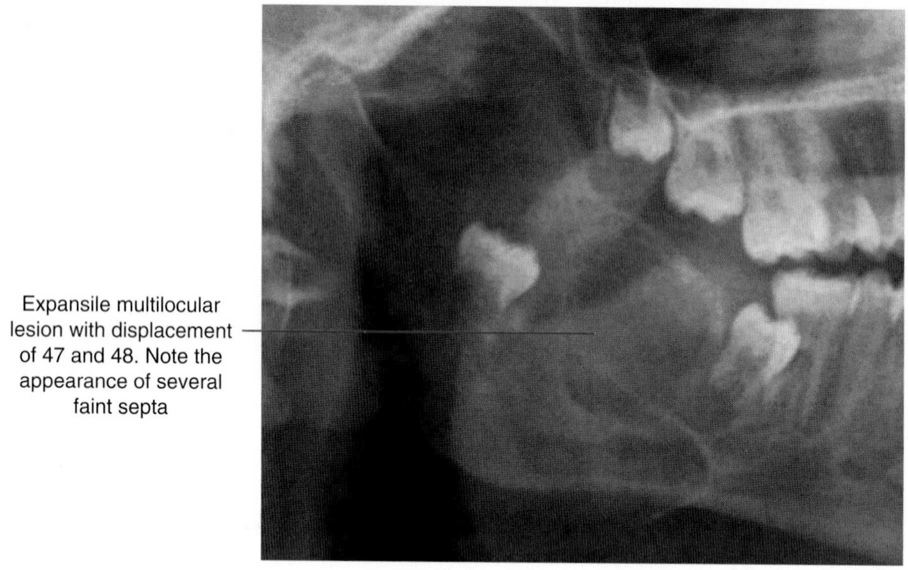

Expansile multilocular lesion with displacement of 47 and 48. Note the appearance of several faint septa

Figure 13.1 Central giant cell granuloma of the right posterior mandible: cropped panoramic radiograph.

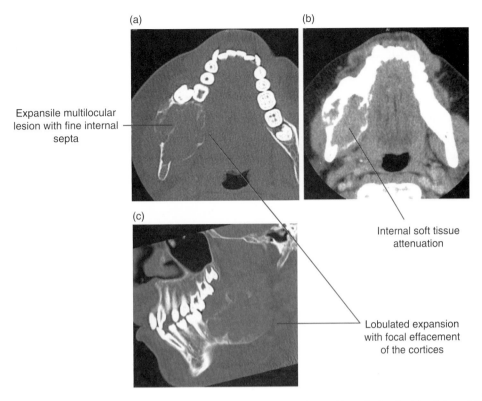

Expansile multilocular lesion with fine internal septa

Internal soft tissue attenuation

Lobulated expansion with focal effacement of the cortices

Figure 13.2 Central giant cell granuloma of the right posterior mandible: axial and corrected sagittal bone (a,c) and axial soft tissue (b) MDCT images.

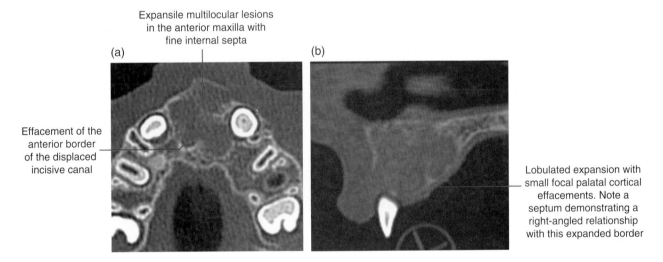

Expansile multilocular lesions in the anterior maxilla with fine internal septa

Effacement of the anterior border of the displaced incisive canal

Lobulated expansion with small focal palatal cortical effacements. Note a septum demonstrating a right-angled relationship with this expanded border

Figure 13.3 Central giant cell granuloma of the anterior maxilla: axial (a) and sagittal (b) MDCT images.

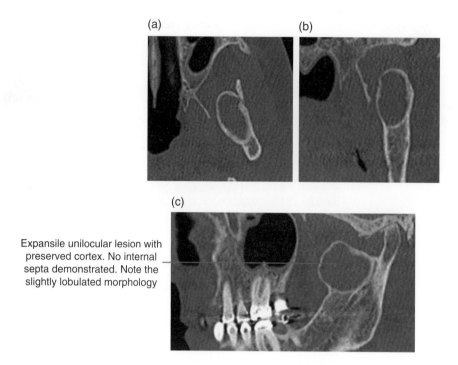

Expansile unilocular lesion with preserved cortex. No internal septa demonstrated. Note the slightly lobulated morphology

Figure 13.4 Central giant cell granuloma of the left coronoid process: axial (a), coronal (b) and corrected sagittal (c) MDCT images.

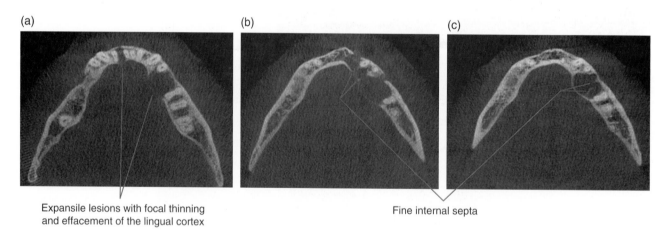

Expansile lesions with focal thinning and effacement of the lingual cortex

Fine internal septa

Figure 13.5 Brown tumours within the mandibular body, related to hyperparathyroidism: axial CBCT images (a–c).

13.2 Cherubism (Figure 13.6)

- *Synonyms*: familial multilocular cystic disease of the jaw, familial fibrous jaw dysplasia.
- Autosomal dominant familial disorder.
- Occurs in the mandible more than in the maxilla.
- Usually presents as a bilateral mandibular enlargement. Expansion related to large maxillary lesions, when present, may cause retraction of the lower eyelids and expose the sclera, resulting in the classically described clinical appearance of upward gaze.
- The lesion usually develops in early childhood and progresses until puberty, when it may regress. After the lesion becomes static, surgery may be required for cosmetic or orthodontic reasons.

Radiological features

- Bilateral, well-defined, expansile, multilocular lesions, usually centred in the posterior mandible and/or maxilla. Occasionally seen anteriorly.
- Internal septa are usually fine and wispy. There may be septa which are thicker and more obvious in appearance.
- Can cause tooth displacement and failure of eruption.

Differential diagnosis

Key radiological differences

Central giant cell granuloma	Similar radiographic appearance but usually not bilateral.
Aneurysmal bone cyst	Similar radiographic appearance but usually not bilateral.

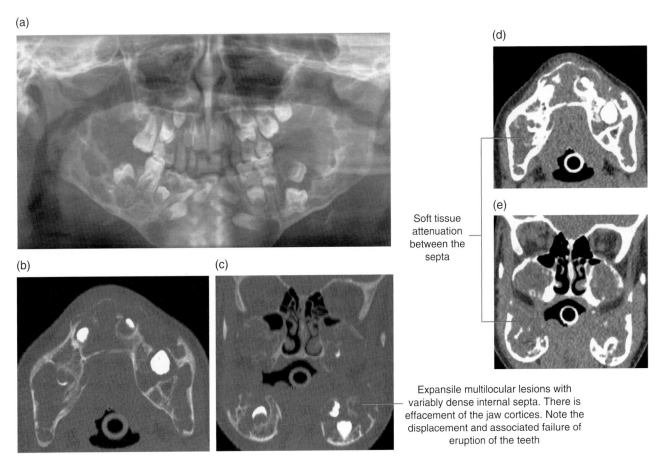

(a)

(b)   (c)

(d)

(e)

Soft tissue attenuation between the septa

Expansile multilocular lesions with variably dense internal septa. There is effacement of the jaw cortices. Note the displacement and associated failure of eruption of the teeth

Figure 13.6 Cherubism: lesions within the mandible (anterior and posterior) and posterior maxilla bilaterally: panoramic radiograph (a) with axial bone (b), coronal bone (c), axial soft tissue (d) and coronal soft tissue (e) MDCT images.

13.3 **Aneurysmal bone cyst** (Figure 13.7)

- *Synonym*: ABC.
- A benign bone lesion composed of non-endothelialised blood-filled spaces separated by septa which consists of fibroblasts, giant cells and reactive bone/osteoid.
- Uncertain aetiology but generally not considered to be a true tumour or cyst. Some consider the ABC to be a reactive lesion.
- May be secondary to an underlying lesion, including fibrous dysplasia, chondroblastoma and giant cell tumour.
- Typically seen in the long bones.
- Usually surgical removal. Recurrence is relatively high. May require resection and/or chemical treatment.

Radiological features

- MDCT is the first imaging modality of choice. However, features on CBCT and 2D radiography may be contributory. MRI can be particularly useful, demonstrating the characteristic fluid–fluid levels.
- Well-defined multilocular expansile lesion. Small lesions can be unilocular.
- The internal septa are typically extremely fine, which may be difficult to identify, especially on 2D radiography and CBCT. These are often more obvious in MDCT soft tissue windows. These septa are similar to those of CGCG. There may also be septa that are at right angles to the expanded jaw cortices, also seen in CGCG.
- MDCT soft tissue windows may demonstrate focal regions of fluid attenuation. Occasionally, fluid–fluid levels can be appreciated when a narrow window width is employed (much better appreciated on MRI).
- Expansion is a feature when large, more than CGCG.
- When sufficiently large, there may be associated tooth displacement and root resorption.
- MRI: when present, fluid–fluid levels are well demonstrated. However, it should be noted that fluid–fluid levels may be seen in other lesions, including the giant cell tumour and rarely the simple bone cyst. Gadolinium-enhanced septa may be seen.

Differential diagnosis

	Key radiological differences
Other lesions which may appear to be multilocular, including:	
Ameloblastoma	Thick and curved internal septa.
Odontogenic myxoma	Presence of one or a few straight septa is a feature. Typically demonstrates mild expansion for size.
Giant cell granuloma	Fine internal septa can appear very similar to the ABC. However, the ABC is typically extremely expansile.
Brown tumour	Essentially radiologically and histologically identical to the CGCG. The brown tumour is related to hyperparathyroidism and associated osteopenic changes may be seen.
Cysts	The small unilocular ABC may resemble a cyst.
Ossifying fibroma	When this lesion demonstrates the appearance of internal septa, they tend to be larger than those seen in the ABC.
Keratocystic odontogenic tumour	Internal septa are uncommon and this lesion demonstrates only mild expansion for its size.
Vascular malformation/ haemangioma	Often demonstrates serpiginous appearances. Can appear multilocular on 2D radiography. Prebiopsy evaluation with MRI should be considered if this is suspected.
Cherubism	Can be radiologically similar but cherubism is usually multifocal, occurring posteriorly.

(a)

(b)

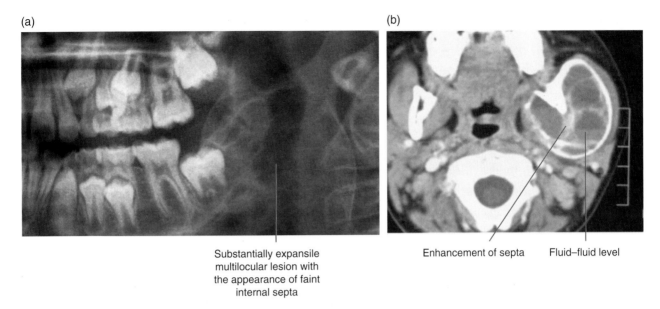

Substantially expansile
multilocular lesion with
the appearance of faint
internal septa

Enhancement of septa   Fluid–fluid level

Figure 13.7 Aneurysmal bone cyst of the left mandible: cropped panoramic radiograph (a) and postcontrast axial soft tissue MDCT image (b). (Courtesy of Professor Paul Monsour, School of Dentistry, The University of Queensland, Australia.)

13.4 Langerhans cell histiocytosis

(Figures 13.8–13.12; see also Figure 20.16)

- *Synonyms*: LCH, histiocytosis X.
- A rare disease involving abnormal clonal proliferation of Langerhans cells (dendritic cells) which clinically manifests according to a number of subtypes which range from a solitary bone lesion to multisystem disease. The course also ranges from spontaneous remissions to aggressive acute disseminated disease.
- Historical subdivision of overlapping clinical variants are controversial, with variation in definitions among clinicians and authors:
  - Eosinophilic granuloma.
    - Some consider this term to refer to the solitary lesion. Others consider it to refer to lesions confined to one organ. Most commonly seen in bone, where it may be monostotic or polyostotic.
    - Most commonly seen in children and younger adults.
    - Prognosis is good when there are only skeletal lesions, especially when solitary.
  - Hand–Schüller–Christian disease.
    - Multiple disseminated lesions. Some consider the term to refer to patients with several lesions within one organ and others accept involvement of multiple organs. Still others have used this term to refer to a triad of multiple bone lesions, diabetes insipidus and exophthalmos.
    - Most commonly seen in children.
  - Letterer–Siwe disease.
    - Disseminated, multisystem, rapidly progressive disease, often considered as the malignant form.
    - Most commonly in children under 2 years old.
    - Poor prognosis.

- More recent classifications involve the extent of disease and also subdivision of non-malignant and malignant forms.
- In the jaws, the lesions may be solitary or multiple.
- Treatment includes surgical excision, radiotherapy and chemotherapy, depending on the extent of disease.

Radiological features (jaw lesions)

- MDCT and MRI are the imaging modalities of choice. However, features on CBCT and 2D radiography may be contributory. Both single-photon emission computed tomography (SPECT) and positron emission tomography (PET) with or without CT may assist in the staging of the disease but there is a significant false-negative rate in bone and gallium scanning. PET imaging findings may also be misleading given the variability in the presentation of the disease.
- Lytic destructive lesion(s). However, the borders range from relatively well defined, including 'punched out' borders, to ill-defined aggressive appearances.
- When involving the alveolar processes, they tend to be multifocal, most commonly involving the posterior mandible. A useful feature is that these lesions are usually centred upon the middle third of the tooth roots. These lesions destroy bone around teeth and may eventually result in the 'floating teeth' appearance.
- Alveolar lesions may be secondarily infected, with associated radiological changes including adjacent reactive sclerosis.
- Elsewhere in the jaws, it destroys jaw cortices and is usually associated with soft tissue mass. The laminar periosteal response is a feature not usually seen with alveolar lesions.
- MRI: low to intermediate T1 signal, intermediate to high T2 and short T1 inversion recovery (STIR) signal. Enhancement is demonstrated with intravenous gadolinium.

Differential diagnosis

Plaque-related inflammatory periodontal bone loss

Key radiological differences

Plaque-related inflammatory periodontal bone loss begins at the alveolar crest and extends apically. LCH lesions involving the alveolar processes are usually centred on the midroot surface, where preservation of the alveolar crests may be seen at the leading edges of the lesion(s).

Malignant lesions, including lymphoma, leukaemia, Ewing sarcoma and metastatic disease. Bony invasion of adjacent soft tissue malignancies (e.g. squamous cell carcinoma) should also be considered

LCH alveolar lesions are usually centred upon the midroot surfaces. Also, these lesions tend to be more well defined in appearance than malignant lesions. When it is seen elsewhere in the jaws, there is usually a laminar periosteal response.

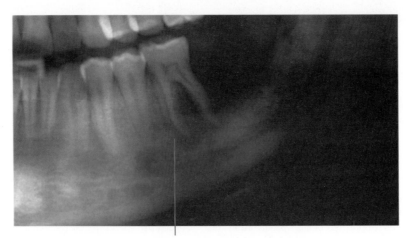

The morphology of the mesial extension of this periradicular lucent defect is not typical of plaque-related periodontal bone loss. Of note is the preservation of the bone at the furcation

Figure 13.8 Langerhans cell histiocytosis of the left mandibular alveolar process: cropped panoramic radiograph.

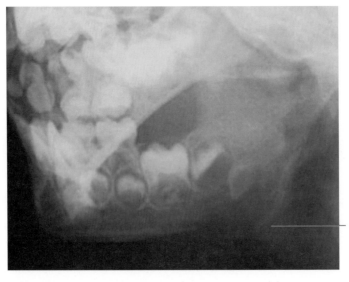

Lytic lesion in the right mandibular angle with inferior lamina periosteal reaction

Figure 13.9 Langerhans cell histiocytosis of the left posterior mandible: oblique mandible radiograph.

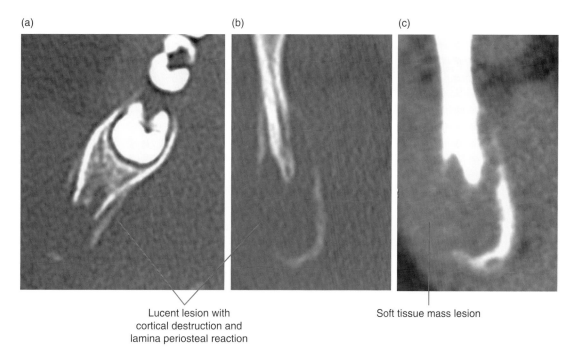

(a)　　　　(b)　　　　(c)

Lucent lesion with
cortical destruction and
lamina periosteal reaction

Soft tissue mass lesion

Figure 13.10 Langerhans cell histiocytosis – solitary lesion at the right-angle of the mandible: axial bone (a), coronal bone (b) and coronal soft tissue (c) MDCT images.

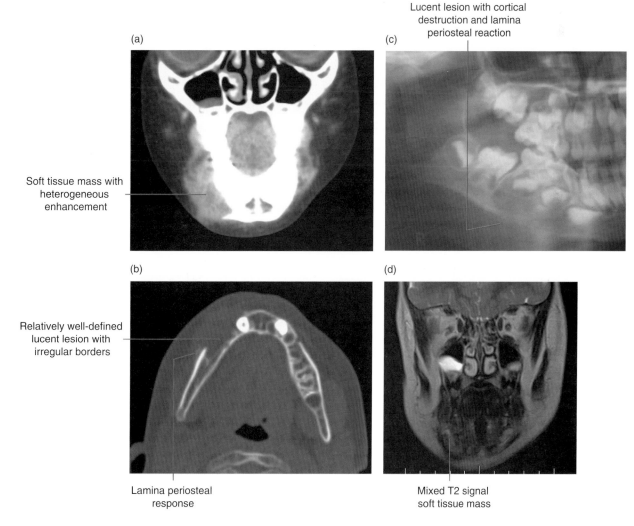

(a)

(c)

Lucent lesion with cortical
destruction and lamina
periosteal reaction

Soft tissue mass with
heterogeneous
enhancement

(b)

(d)

Relatively well-defined
lucent lesion with
irregular borders

Lamina periosteal
response

Mixed T2 signal
soft tissue mass

Figure 13.11 Langerhans cell histiocytosis of the right body of the mandible: coronal postcontrast soft tissue (a) and axial bone (b) MDCT images, cropped panoramic radiograph (c) and coronal T2 MRI image (d).

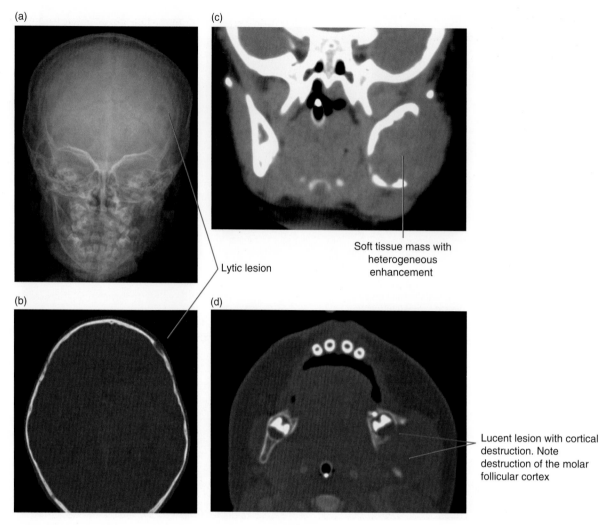

(a)

(c)

Lytic lesion

Soft tissue mass with
heterogeneous
enhancement

(b)

(d)

Lucent lesion with cortical
destruction. Note
destruction of the molar
follicular cortex

Figure 13.12 Langerhans cell histiocytosis of the left mandible and skull: posteroanterior radiograph (a) with axial bone (b,d) and coronal postcontrast soft tissue (c) MDCT images.

13.5 Paget disease of bone (Figure 13.13; see also Figure 20.18)

- *Synonym*: osteitis deformans.
- Chronic disorder of the bone characterised by aberrant bone remodelling and formation of bone that is structurally abnormal, with expansion and deformity.
- Usually presents in the fourth decade of life or beyond.
- While most are symptom free, some present with skeletal deformities and pain and ill-fitting dentures. May also present with associated cranial neuropathies.
- Bones most frequently involved: skull, sacrum, spine, pelvis and lower extremities.
- It is rarely found in the jaws, more often in the maxilla. Usually bilateral.

- Raised serum alkaline phosphatase levels.
- Rarely, other tumours including the osteosarcoma may arise.

Radiological features (jaw lesions)
- In the incipient (lytic) phase, lucent appearances are noted.
- In the intermediate phase (lysis and sclerosis), it is heterogeneous and may demonstrate a 'cotton wool' appearance.
- A later sclerotic stage follows. The trabecular bone may demonstrate homogeneous regions and other regions of coarse trabeculae where a linear pattern may be seen.
- Expansion is also a feature.
- There is usually displacement of teeth and alteration of the lamina dura. Hypercementosis may be seen.

Differential diagnosis

	Key radiological differences
Fibrous dysplasia	Fibrous dysplasia occurs in a younger age group. Ground-glass appearance is seen in the classical fibrous dysplasia. Paget disease is usually bilateral.
Chronic osteomyelitis	A periosteal response is almost always present in chronic osteomyelitis.
Metastatic disease	In the lytic phase, it may be difficult to differentiate. If there is sclerosis without bone expansion, then prostate or breast metastasis is favoured.
Osteopetrosis	Presents in the young. Diffused dense sclerosis.

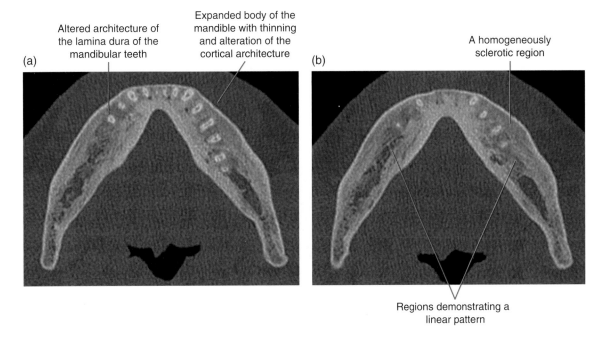

Figure 13.13 Paget disease: axial MDCT images (a,b).

CHAPTER 14
Other Morphological Anomalies Involving the Jaws

14.1 Hemimandibular hyperplasia
(Figures 14.1–14.3)

- Increased development of a hemimandible.
  - Note:
    - Bilaterally and symmetrically relatively prominent mandibles are not infrequently seen, a normal variant (class III relationship).
    - Symmetric abnormal excessive growth of the mandible can be seen in endocrine disorders such as acromegaly.
- Generally considered to be developmental.
  - Note that facial bones are often slightly asymmetric, a normal variant.
- The hyperplasia may involve the entire hemimandible or a part of it. It may be limited to the mandibular condylar (refer to Chapter 18) and/or coronoid (refer to Chapter 18) processes. It can also be limited to the ramus. Other cases involve the ramus and posterior body of the mandible.
- Most common presentation is facial asymmetry.
  - Varying degrees of severity and rates of progression.
  - Growth may occasionally continue past the end of skeletal maturity of other bones.
  - May be more evident in the vertical (craniocaudal) dimension or may be primarily in the transverse dimension, where the mandibular symphysis is located contralateral to the overall facial midline. Various combinations are seen.
  - There are often associated changes to the occlusion, e.g. open bite and cross bite. Canting of the occlusal plane and associated compensatory asymmetry of the maxillary alveolar process is often seen.
- Sometimes, there is associated temporomandibular joint dysfunction and related symptoms.

Radiological features
- When imaging is indicated, multidetector computed tomography (MDCT) or cone beam computed tomography (CBCT) are recommended over 2D radiography. Magnetic resonance imaging (MRI) may be useful if there is associated joint dysfunction or other related symptoms.

- Technetium bone scans, especially single-photon emission computed tomography, may be useful to determine condylar growth activity. However, increased uptake is non-specific and many other conditions, including degenerative changes, can contribute to this. Therefore, evaluation with MDCT or CBCT is recommended prior to bone scans.
- The affected hemimandible demonstrates variably larger condyle, coronoid process, ramus and body of the mandible. This increased dimension may be more evident in one plane than another. For example, a hemimandible (or part of) may be larger craniocaudally (vertically) or longer with asymmetry limited to the transverse dimension or may be larger mediolaterally (buccolingually) or there may be various combinations.
- The condylar neck may be bowed posteriorly and/or laterally and the ramus may be bowed laterally.
- The antegonial notch is usually less obvious or flattened relative to the normal contralateral side. Occasionally, the inferior border of the mandible in this antegonial region may appear convex.
  - Note that there is a large normal variation in the prominence of the antegonial notches, which are sometimes non-existent. However, these appearances should be symmetric.
- There may be remodelling of the glenoid fossa related to condylar hyperplasia.

Differential diagnosis

	Key radiological differences
Contralateral hemimandibular hypoplasia	The morphology typical of hyperplasia or hypoplasia may be helpful. Occasionally, differentiation can be difficult as the hemimandibles are similar in morphology where the difference in size is the only feature.
Conditions contributing to increased size of the condyle or hemimandible	For example, osteochondroma, osteoma, fibrous dysplasia – these conditions present as focal diseases and may be associated with focal bony prominence rather than overall enlargement.

Atlas of Oral and Maxillofacial Radiology, First Edition. Bernard Koong.
© 2017 John Wiley & Sons Ltd. Published 2017 by John Wiley & Sons Ltd.

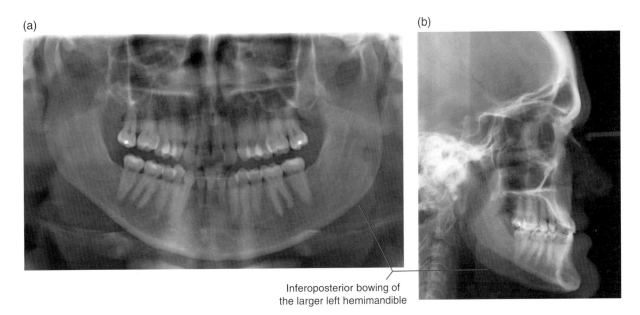

Inferoposterior bowing of
the larger left hemimandible

Figure 14.1 Left hemimandibular hyperplasia: panoramic (a) and lateral (b) radiographs.

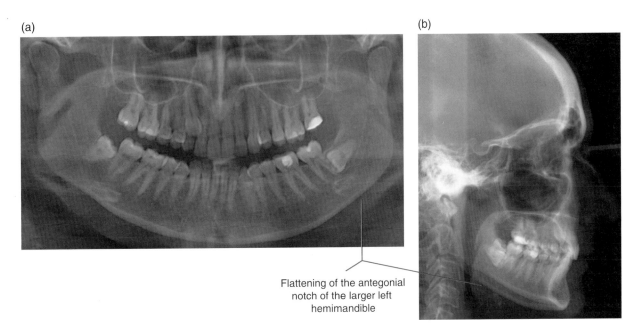

Flattening of the antegonial
notch of the larger left
hemimandible

Figure 14.2 Left hemimandibular hyperplasia: panoramic (a) and lateral (b) radiographs.

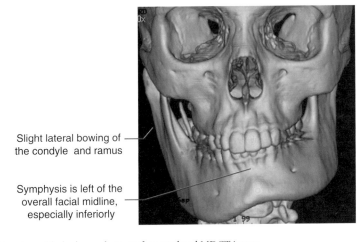

Slight lateral bowing of
the condyle and ramus

Symphysis is left of the
overall facial midline,
especially inferiorly

Figure 14.3 Right hemimandibular hyperplasia: surface-rendered MDCT image.

14.2 Acromegaly

Refer to Chapter 15.

14.3 Mandibular and hemimandibular hypoplasia (Figures 14.4–14.6)

- Reduced development of the affected mandible.
  - Note that facial bones are often slightly asymmetric, a normal variant.
- May be bilateral (mandibular) or unilateral (hemimandibular).
- May be developmental or related to a trauma/condition interrupting mandibular growth (usually the condyle). Occasionally congenital, most of which are related to syndromes, e.g. Pierre Robin syndrome.
- Most cases demonstrate condylar hypoplasia of the affected side. However, hypoplasia can be limited to the condyle (refer to Chapter 18). While generally not considered to be a hypoplastic condition, the bifid condyle (refer to Chapter 18) may result in an overall smaller appearance of the affected condyle, especially on a panoramic radiograph.
- Bilateral cases present with small hypoplastic mandibles, usually symmetric.
- Unilateral cases present with facial asymmetry. Associated canting of the occlusal plane and compensatory asymmetry of the maxillary alveolar process is often seen.
- Sometimes associated with temporomandibular joint dysfunction and related symptoms. Hypoplastic condyles often demonstrate degenerative changes earlier in life.

Radiological features

- When imaging is indicated, MDCT or CBCT are recommended over 2D radiography. MRI may be useful if there is associated joint dysfunction or other related symptoms.
- The affected mandible/hemimandible is smaller than usually expected.
- Almost all cases of mandibular hypoplasia demonstrate condylar hypoplasia (refer to Chapter 18).
- The affected mandible/hemimandible also demonstrates a variably smaller ramus and body of the mandible. This decreased dimension may be more evident in one plane than another. Occasionally, the hypoplasia affects the condyle and ramus much more than the body of the mandible.
- The condylar neck is usually bowed anteriorly and/or medially and the ramus may be bowed medially.
- The antegonial notch is usually more pronounced.
  - It should be noted that there is a large normal variation in the prominence of the antegonial notch, which is sometimes non-existent.

Differential diagnosis

	Key radiological differences
Contralateral hemimandibular hyperplasia in unilateral cases	The morphology typical of hyperplasia or hypoplasia may be helpful. Occasionally, differentiation can be difficult as the hemimandibular difference in size is the only difference.
Normal variant	The mandible can be relatively small in normal persons, and is considered a normal variant (class II relationship).

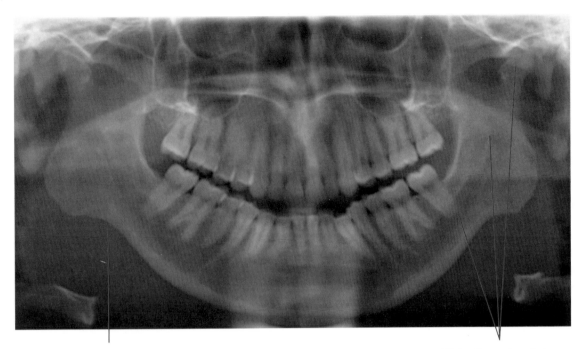

Prominent antegonial
notches bilaterally

Bilaterally small posterior
body, rami and condyles.
Note the short and square
appearance of the rami

Figure 14.4 Mandibular hypoplasia: panoramic radiograph.

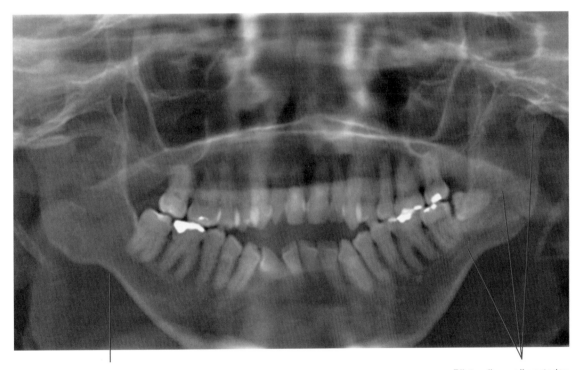

Prominent antegonial
notches bilaterally

Bilaterally small posterior
body, rami and condyles

Figure 14.5 Mandibular hypoplasia: panoramic radiograph.

(a)   (b)

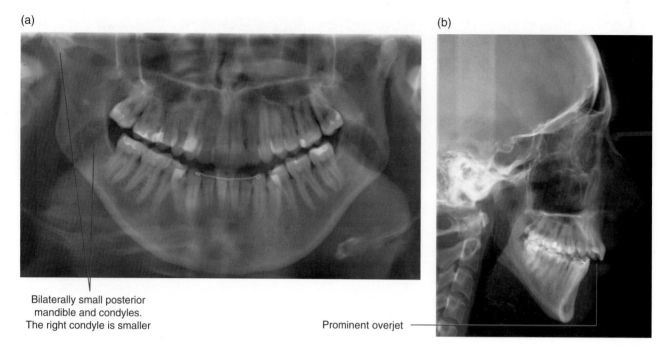

Bilaterally small posterior
mandible and condyles.
The right condyle is smaller   Prominent overjet ——

Figure 14.6 Mandibular hypoplasia: panoramic (a) and lateral (b) radiographs.

14.4 Stafne defect (Figures 14.7–14.9)

- *Synonyms*: lingual salivary gland depression, Stafne cyst, Stafne bone cavity.
- Focal corticated depression at the medial/lingual surface of the mandible.
- Most commonly seen in the posterior mandible inferiorly.
- It is has been historically accepted that these concavities are developmental, related to adjacent submandibular salivary glands. However, this proposed aetiology is questioned.
- These defects have been seen to develop and slowly enlarge in the adult, and the vast majority do not demonstrate presence of salivary gland tissue within the depression.
- Often incidentally identified. Does not require treatment. Radiological examination (optimally MDCT) is usually sufficient, not requiring biopsy.

Radiological features

- When imaging is indicated, MDCT is preferred over CBCT as the soft tissue content within the depression is poorly demonstrated with CBCT. However, CBCT may suffice, especially if there is no access to MDCT.
  - Focal, well-corticated, round, ovoid or lobulated depression at the medial/lingual surface of the mandible. Not infrequently, a cortical lip is seen at the lingual cortical edges of this depression.
  - When located at the inferior body of the mandible, it often involves the lingual/medial aspect of the inferior mandibular cortex, preserving the lateral/buccal aspect of this inferior cortex.
  - The vast majority demonstrate fat within these concavities (MDCT soft tissue window or MRI). Occasionally, a part of a submandibular lymph node or salivary gland is seen within this portion of the concavity.
- In the panoramic radiograph, it classically presents as a lucency with a heavily corticated superior border and a thinner and/or more hypodense inferior border. In a larger defect involving the inferior border of the mandible, the inferior mandibular cortex may appear absent or hypodense in this view.

Differential diagnosis

	Key radiological differences
Cystic lesions	Classically presenting Stafne defects may be sufficiently obvious on a panoramic radiograph. However, unless there is absolute confidence in the nature of the lucency based upon this view, MDCT or at least CBCT is suggested. The Stafne defect is almost always definitively identified on MDCT.

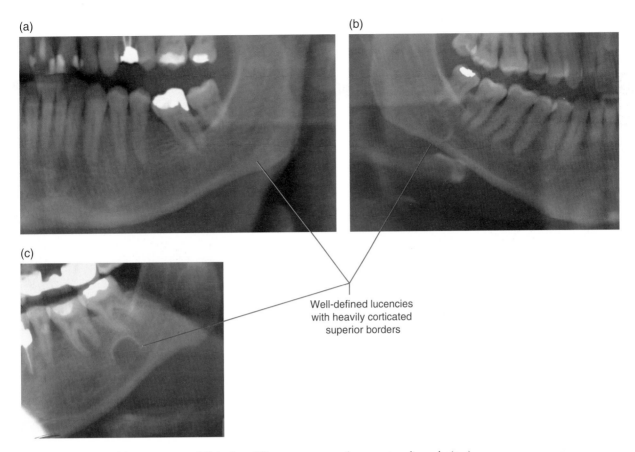

Figure 14.7 Stafne defect of the posterior mandible in three different cases: cropped panoramic radiographs (a–c).

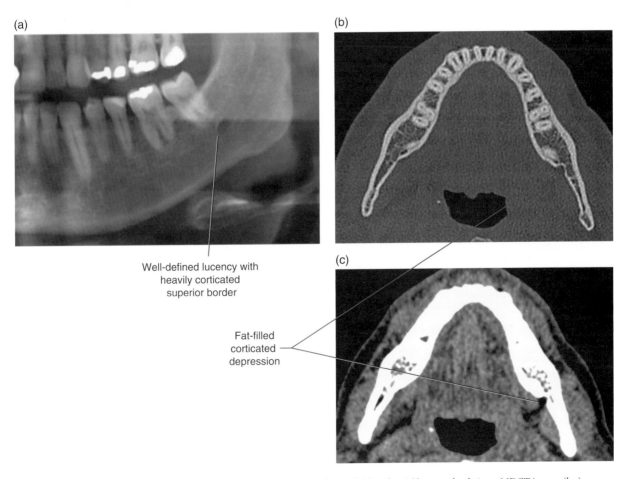

Figure 14.8 Stafne defect of the left posterior mandible: cropped panoramic radiograph (a) with axial bone and soft tissue MDCT images (b,c).

(a)

(b)

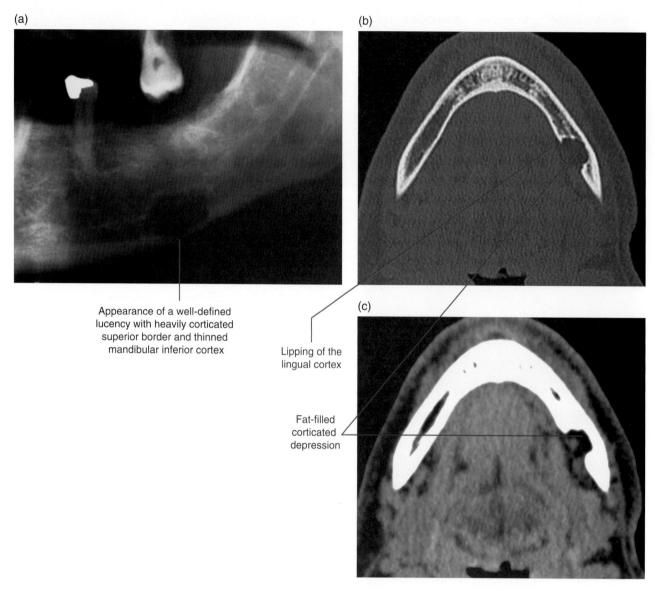

Appearance of a well-defined lucency with heavily corticated superior border and thinned mandibular inferior cortex

Lipping of the lingual cortex

(c)

Fat-filled corticated depression

Figure 14.9 Stafne defect of the left posterior mandible: cropped panoramic radiograph (a) with axial bone and soft tissue MDCT images (b,c).

14.5 Cleft lip and palate (Figures 14.10–14.13)

- A group of developmental anomalies that include cleft lip, cleft palate or both.
- One of the most common facial birth defects.
- Failure of fusion of developmental processes.
- Often divided into two groups, with different aetiologies:
  ○ Cleft lip with or without cleft palate
  ○ Cleft palate.
- Variable severity, ranging from a small unilateral lip cleft to bilateral osseous and soft tissue cleft of the alveolus and also at the palatal midline. The bifid uvula is considered a mild manifestation.
- There are many associated problems including speech, swallowing and increased risks of middle ear infections.

- There are often dental anomalies at the alveolar cleft, including congenital absent, supernumerary, hypoplastic and malformed teeth. Dental anomalies elsewhere are also more commonly seen and there may be a slight delay in the overall dental development.
- The maxilla is often relatively smaller in relation to the mandible and is taken into account as part of the orthodontic and orthognathic evaluation and management.

Radiological features
- When imaging is indicated, MDCT or CBCT are recommended over 2D radiography.
- *In utero* imaging for the presence of cleft lip/palate (antenatal ultrasound) is not within the scope of this atlas.

- The osseous clefts appear as well-defined corticated defects.
  - There may soft tissue bridging these osseous clefts.
  - Where there is oronasal communication an air track (MDCT or CBCT) may be seen within the bony clefts. However, an oronasal communication cannot be excluded when an air track is not seen, as the mucosal lining of the oronasal communication may be in contact.
- Dental anomalies may be seen at the region of the alveolar clefts and/or elsewhere (refer to Chapter 3).

Differential diagnosis

Key radiological differences

Anterior maxillary lucent lesions	On panoramic and intraoral radiographs, the bony clefts may sometimes present as non-specific lucencies. If clinically indicated, the clefts are usually obvious on CBCT and MDCT.

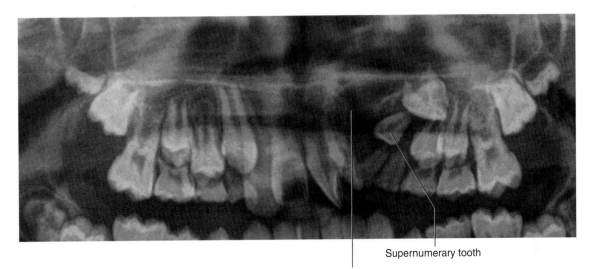

Supernumerary tooth

Lucent cleft defect which is only partly within the focal trough. The corticated mesial border is visualised

Figure 14.10 Left anterior maxillary cleft: cropped panoramic radiograph.

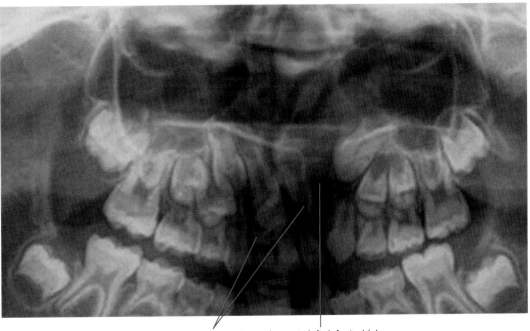

Malformed teeth   Lucent cleft defect which is partly within the focal trough

Figure 14.11 Left anterior maxillary cleft: cropped panoramic radiograph.

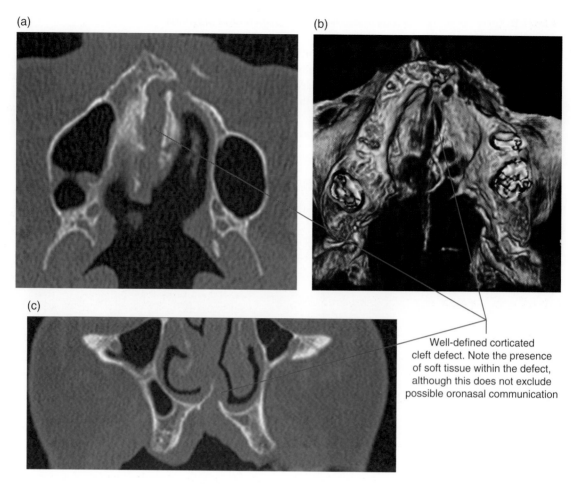

(a)

(b)

(c)

Well-defined corticated
cleft defect. Note the presence
of soft tissue within the defect,
although this does not exclude
possible oronasal communication

Figure 14.12 Palatal and left anterior maxillary cleft: axial and coronal (a,c) and surface-rendered (b) MDCT images.

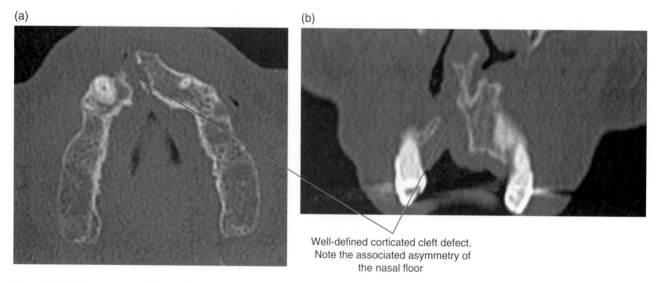

(a)

(b)

Well-defined corticated cleft defect.
Note the associated asymmetry of
the nasal floor

Figure 14.13 Right anterior maxillary cleft: axial (a) and coronal (b) MDCT images.

CHAPTER 15
Other Systemic Disorders that may Involve the Jaws

Alterations of the jaws and teeth in relation to other systemic disorders are occasionally seen radiologically, and are usually non-specific. Rarely, the changes in the jaws identified radiologically may lead to the diagnosis of a condition which is otherwise undetected.

15.1 Osteopenic appearance of the jaws
(Figure 15.1)

- There are normal variations in the cortical and trabecular appearances of the jaws and it is difficult to identify osteoporotic conditions based on diagnostic imaging of the jaws. Also, a patient with known osteoporosis may not demonstrate particularly severe radiological changes in the jaws. However, disease conditions should be considered when there is substantial deviation from normal. Examples include:
  - Hyperparathyroidism, hypothyroidism, hypophosphatasia, hypophosphataemia, Cushing syndrome, sickle cell anaemia, thalassaemia.
    - Hyperparathyroidism (Figure 15.2): may see brown tumours (identical to central giant cell granuloma). Should consider this condition when a central giant cell granuloma is seen in an adult aged over 20 years.

- Bone mineral density measurement.
  - One of the most commonly employed and accepted indirect indicators of osteoporosis. The associated risk of fracture can be calculated.
  - Estimates levels of calcium hydroxyapatite and other minerals in an area of bone.
  - Dual-energy X-ray absorptiometry is most commonly used. Considered to be most reliable. There are other techniques.

Radiological features
- Decreased density appearance of the trabecular bone, which may also appear finer. There may also be alteration of the normal trabecular architecture.
- Hypodense and/or thinner appearances of the jaw cortices, which may not be even.
- Hypodense appearances of the lamina dura of tooth roots may be seen. Occasionally, there may be alteration of the lamina dura architecture such that the lamina dura is not easily identified but the periodontal ligament space remains preserved.
- Teeth appear more obvious because of the decreased density of the surrounding bone.

Atlas of Oral and Maxillofacial Radiology, First Edition. Bernard Koong.
© 2017 John Wiley & Sons Ltd. Published 2017 by John Wiley & Sons Ltd.

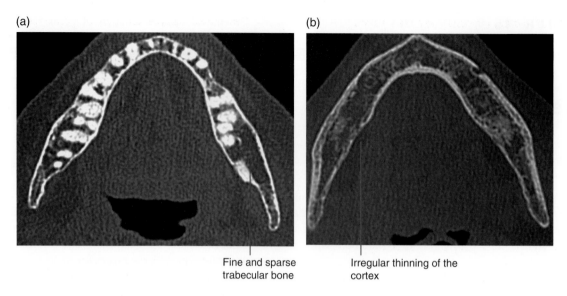

(a)

(b)

Fine and sparse
trabecular bone

Irregular thinning of the
cortex

Figure 15.1 Two cases of known osteoporosis demonstrating slight osteopenic appearance of the mandible: axial MDCT images (a,b).

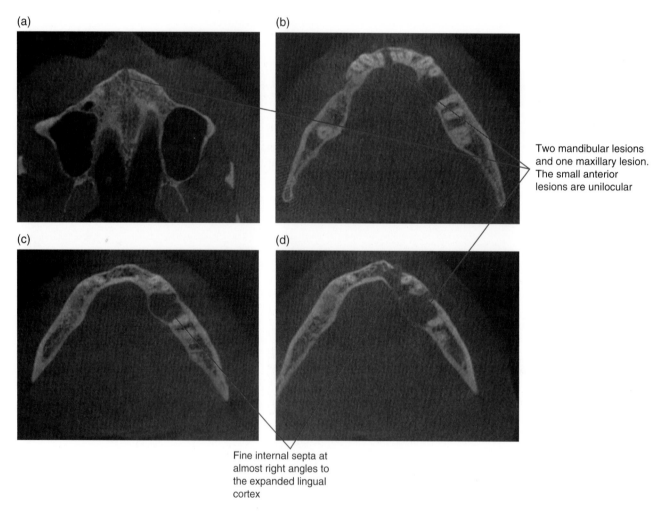

(a)

(b)

(c)

(d)

Two mandibular lesions
and one maxillary lesion.
The small anterior
lesions are unilocular

Fine internal septa at
almost right angles to
the expanded lingual
cortex

Figure 15.2 Multiple brown tumours related to hyperparathyroidism: axial CBCT images (a–d).

15.2 Increased density of the jaws

- Osteopetrosis.
  - Can be extremely dense in appearance.

15.3 Alterations in jaw size

- Larger: may be a normal variant. Consider a pituitary tumour if extreme, e.g. acromegaly (Figure 15.3). Other conditions include thalassaemia and sickle cell anaemia.
- Smaller: may be a normal variant. Many other causes, but consider hypopituitarism if extreme.

15.4 Changes to jaw morphology

- Altered mandibular morphology may be seen in scleroderma, where there is loss of bone at the angles, anterior mandible and condylar and coronoid processes, usually bilateral.
- Expansion with osteopenic appearances; may be related to marrow hyperplasia associated with sickle cell anaemia and thalassaemia.

15.5 Dentoalveolar alterations

- Unexplained non-specific alteration in the density and/or morphology of multiple teeth should raise the possibility of a systemic cause.
- Eruption and exfoliating times.
  - Note large variation in the timing of normal eruption and exfoliating of teeth in relation to age.
  - Generalised delayed eruption of permanent teeth with delayed exfoliation of deciduous dentition may be seen in hypopituitarism, hypothyroidism, hypoparathyroidism and rickets.
  - Generalised early deciduous exfoliation and early eruption of permanent teeth may be related to hyperthyroidism and Cushing syndrome.
- Tooth density and morphology.
  - Generalised hypoplasia and/or hypocalcification of enamel may be seen in rickets, hypophosphatasia, hypophosphataemia and renal osteodystrophy.
  - Unexplained generalised large pulps may be seen in hypophosphatasia and hypophosphataemia.
  - Hypercementosis may be seen in hyperpituitarism.
  - Teeth can appear more obvious because of the decrease in the density of the surrounding bone.
- Lamina dura of tooth roots.
  - Hypodense appearances of the lamina dura may be seen in relation to osteopenia. Occasionally, the architecture of the lamina dura is altered, and the lamina dura is not easily identified although the periodontal ligament space remains preserved.
  - Absence of the lamina dura may be seen in several conditions, including hyper/hypothyroidism, hypophosphatasia, hypophosphataemia and renal osteodystrophy.
- Widened periodontal ligament spaces.
  - There are many causes.
  - It may be useful to consider scleroderma when there is unexplained generalised widening of the periodontal ligament spaces in the presence of unusual remodelling of the mandible (refer to section 15.4).

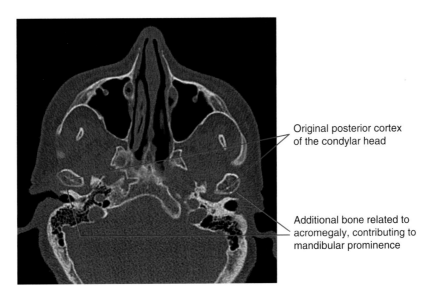

Original posterior cortex of the condylar head

Additional bone related to acromegaly, contributing to mandibular prominence

Figure 15.3 Acromegaly: axial MDCT image.

CHAPTER 16

Common Opacities in the Orofacial Soft Tissues

Bernard Koong and Tom Huang

16.1 Tonsillar calcifications (Figures 16.1–16.3)

- *Synonym*: tonsillolith.
- Quite commonly seen with the palatine (faucial) tonsils. Occasionally the adenoids and, rarely, the lingual tonsils.
- The vast majority are post inflammatory, not requiring treatment. Rarely, these may be related to granulomatous disease or malignancies including lymphoma.

Radiological features

- If imaging is clinically indicated, multidetector computed tomography (MDCT) is recommended over cone beam computed tomography (CBCT).
  - Poorly depicted on a panoramic radiograph, although faucial (palatine) tonsillar calcifications are often fortuitously demonstrated in these views.
- Irregular well-defined foci of calcifications within or around the tonsillar crypts. May be solitary or large in numbers. Also variable in size.

On the panoramic radiograph, faucial (palatine) tonsillar calcifications are usually projected over the region of the mandibular ramus, sometimes posterior and rarely anterior to it.

Differential diagnosis

Key radiological differences

Lymph node calcifications	Calcifications are usually larger and occur where lymph nodes are expected to exist.
Sialolith	Usually more ovoid and smooth and located within the duct. Classically demonstrates internal laminated appearance.
Parotid parenchymal calcifications	Usually smaller, rounded. On the panoramic radiograph, these are usually projected over the posterior aspect of the ramus and/or posterior to the ramus.
Bone island	Occasionally, differentiation can be difficult on a panoramic or lateral radiograph. MDCT or CBCT may be indicated.
Phlebolith	Often lucent centrally. MDCT and/or magnetic resonance imaging (MRI) should be considered if a vascular lesion is suspected (refer to Chapter 12).
Tumours	Calcifications can be associated with tumours. If there is clinical suspicion for the presence of a tumour, MDCT is recommended over CBCT.

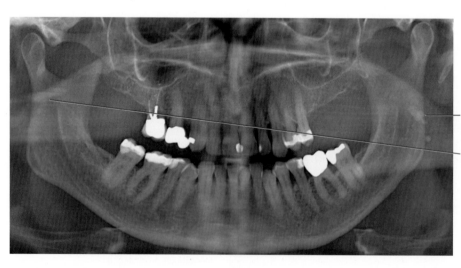

Opacities superimposed over the left ramus. The appearance of 'ghost images' of these left-sided opacities over the right ramus favours the medial location of these opacities relative to the ramus

Figure 16.1 Palatine tonsillar calcifications: panoramic radiograph.

Atlas of Oral and Maxillofacial Radiology, First Edition. Bernard Koong.
© 2017 John Wiley & Sons Ltd. Published 2017 by John Wiley & Sons Ltd.

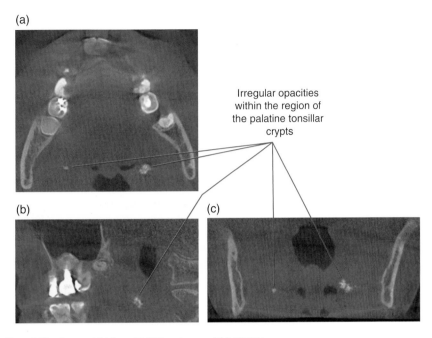

Figure 16.2 Palatine tonsillar calcifications: axial (a), sagittal (b) and coronal (c) CBCT images.

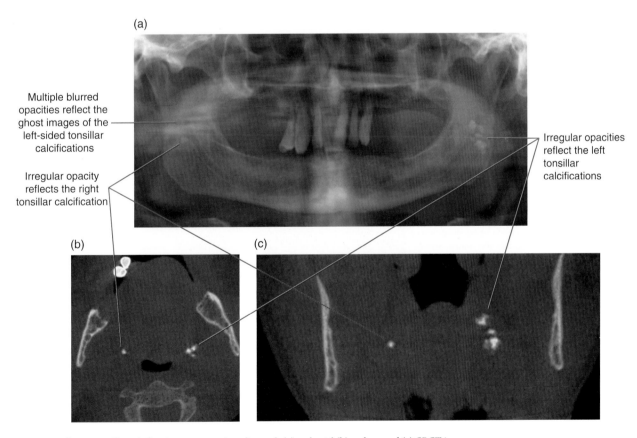

Figure 16.3 Palatine tonsillar calcifications: panoramic radiograph (a) and axial (b) and coronal (c) CBCT images.

16.2 Lymph node calcifications

(Figures 16.4–16.6)

- Cervical lymph node calcifications are rare.
- Isolated lymph node calcification in the level I lymph nodes is usually related to postinflammatory calcification.
- More extensive neck lymph node calcifications are often related to chronic inflammatory diseases, especially granulomatous diseases, including tuberculosis and histoplasmosis. Non-infectious conditions such as sarcoidosis should also be considered.
- Occasionally related to malignant diseases, such as squamous cell carcinoma and treated lymphoma.

Radiological features

- If imaging is clinically indicated, MDCT is recommended over CBCT.
  - Poorly depicted on a panoramic radiograph, although these views may incidentally demonstrate the presence of these calcifications.
- Well-defined irregular opacities appear at sites where lymph nodes are expected. The appearance, number and size of these calcifications are not related to the nature of the primary cause of these calcifications. The classically described 'cauliflower-like' appearance is sometimes seen.
- Occasionally affects the deep cervical chain, resulting in the appearance of a series of calcifications along this chain.
- On the panoramic radiograph lymph node calcifications are usually projected posteroinferiorly to the angle of the mandible. Sometimes these may be projected over the posterior mandibular body or even posterior to the ramus.

Differential diagnosis

	Key radiological differences
Sialolith	Usually more ovoid and smooth and located within the duct or the region where the duct would be expected. Classically demonstrates internal laminated appearance.
Phlebolith	Often lucent centrally. MDCT and/or MRI should be considered if a vascular lesion is suspected (refer to Chapter 12).

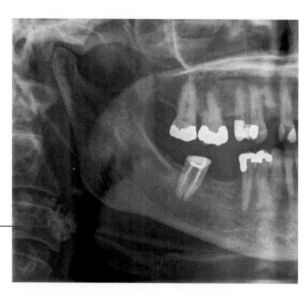

Irregular opacities projected over the anterior C3. The larger opacity demonstrates a 'cauliflower' appearance

Figure 16.4 Lymph node calcifications: cropped panoramic radiograph.

(a)   (b)

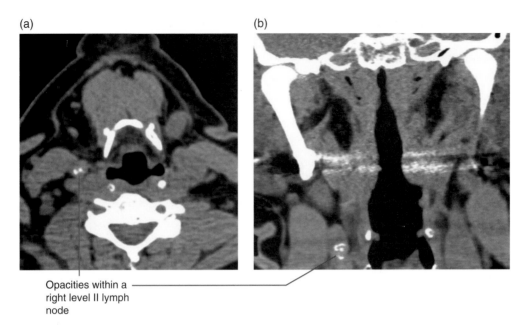

Opacities within a ——
right level II lymph
node

Figure 16.5 Lymph node calcifications: axial (a) and coronal (b) soft tissue MDCT images.

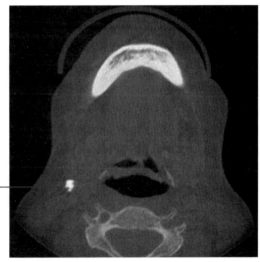

Opacity in the region of a right
level II lymph node. The lymph
node is not visualised in this
scan – note that soft tissues are
poorly examined with CBCT

Figure 16.6 Lymph node calcification: axial CBCT image.

16.3 Stylohyoid ligamentous ossification
(Figures 16.7 and 16.8)

- Often seen and variable in extent.
- Generally considered to be a normal variant. The vast majority are asymptomatic and do not require any management.
- There is essentially no correlation of the appearance and extent of stylohyoid ligamentous ossification with symptoms associated with Eagle syndrome.

Radiological features

- Usually obvious on MDCT and CBCT. Often incidentally identified on the panoramic radiograph.
- Presents as a well-defined cylindrical opacity of variable length with bone-like appearance anywhere along the stylo-hyoid ligament.
- The ossification can be solitary or multiple, unilateral or bilateral.
- Segments of ossification may form pseudoarthroses with each other or with the styloid process.

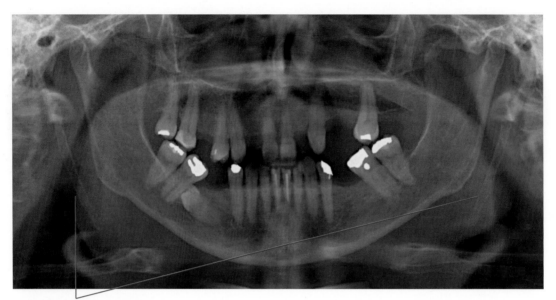

Cylindrical bone-like opacities
corresponding with the location
of the stylohyoid ligaments

Figure 16.7 Stylohyoid ligament ossification: panoramic radiograph.

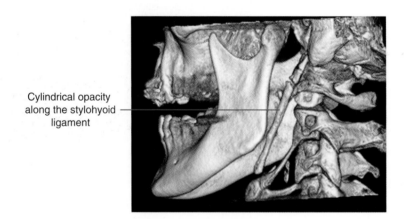

Cylindrical opacity
along the stylohyoid
ligament

Figure 16.8 Stylohyoid ligament ossification: surface-rendered CBCT image.

16.4 Thyroid and triticeous cartilage calcifications (Figures 16.9–16.11)

- Often seen, a normal variant.

Radiological features
- Usually obvious on MDCT and CBCT.
- In the panoramic radiograph, the triticeous cartilage calcification is often partly seen inferior to the greater cornu of the hyoid bone at approximately the level of the superior aspect of C4, classically demonstrating a 'grain of rice' appearance.

Naturally, ossification of the superior cornu of the thyroid cartilage is seen slightly inferior to this.

Differential diagnosis

	Key radiological differences
Carotid atheromatous plaque calcification	May project in the similar regions of the panoramic radiograph. The location and morphology usually assist in differentiation.

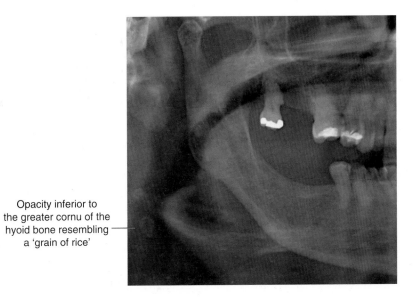

Opacity inferior to
the greater cornu of the
hyoid bone resembling
a 'grain of rice'

Figure 16.9 Triticeous cartilage calcification: cropped panoramic radiograph.

(a)

(b)

(c)

Bone-like
appearance of the
partly visualised
ossified greater
cornu bilaterally

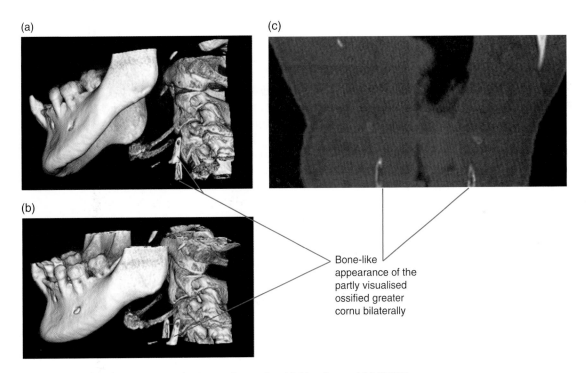

Figure 16.10 Thyroid cartilage greater cornu ossification: surface-rendered (a,b) and coronal (c) CBCT images.

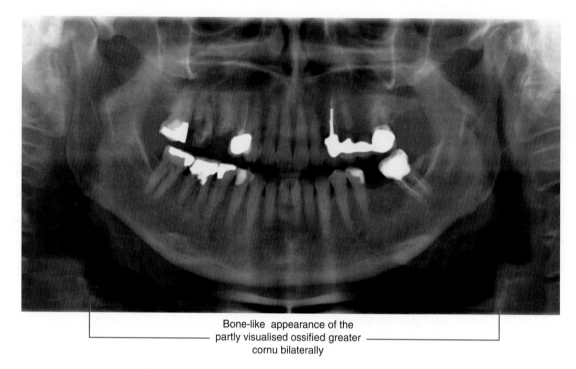

Bone-like appearance of the partly visualised ossified greater cornu bilaterally

Figure 16.11 Thyroid cartilage greater cornu ossification: panoramic radiograph.

16.5 Arterial calcifications related to arteriosclerosis (Figures 16.12–16.16)

- Calcifications or calcified plaques are the by-product of vessel wall chronic inflammation. They arise from non-calcified atheromatous plaques within the vessel wall and are a marker of the pathological process of arteriosclerosis.
- In the orofacial region these vessel calcifications are:
  - Most commonly seen at the carotid artery bifurcation. Carotid vessel atheromatous plaques are associated with an increased risk of cerebrovascular occlusive and embolic events.
  - Sometimes seen in the facial arteries.
- More commonly seen in older persons, those with diabetes and those with renal disease and hypertension.
- Incidental identification of these calcifications should prompt consideration for further clinical evaluation and required tests, especially:
  - smaller arterial calcifications such as the facial artery
  - when seen in the younger patient
  - substantial carotid calcifications.

Radiological features

- In the orofacial region, these are most commonly seen as well-defined calcification(s) within the carotid arteries, usually at the bifurcation. Larger calcifications may demonstrate a circumferential or tubular appearance.
  - Often projected posteroinferiorly to the angle of the mandible on a panoramic radiograph.
  - From an imaging perspective, further evaluation with Doppler ultrasound is suggested for more substantial calcifications.
- Facial artery calcifications are often present as diffused circumferential opacities within the vessel walls.

Differential diagnosis

	Key radiological differences
Triticeous cartilage calcifications	May be mistaken for carotid vessel atheromatous plaque calcifications on panoramic radiographs. The morphology usually aids in differentiating these calcifications.

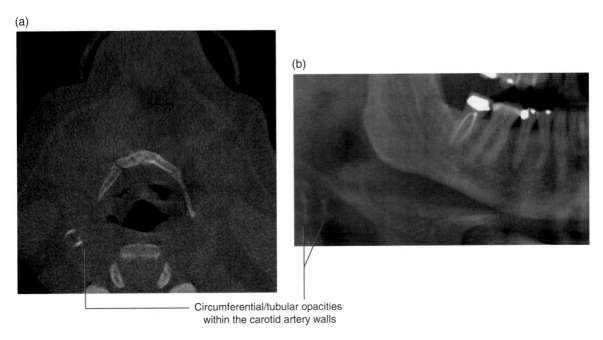

(a)

(b)

Circumferential/tubular opacities
within the carotid artery walls

Figure 16.12 Arteriosclerotic calcifications right external carotid artery: axial CBCT image (a) and cropped panoramic radiograph (b).

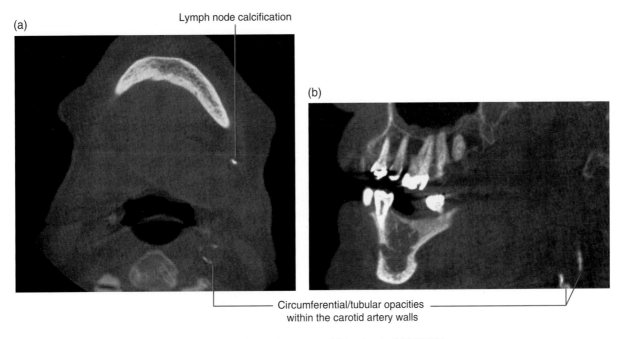

Lymph node calcification

(a)

(b)

Circumferential/tubular opacities
within the carotid artery walls

Figure 16.13 Arteriosclerotic calcifications of the left external carotid artery: axial (a) and sagittal (b) CBCT images.

(a)

(b)

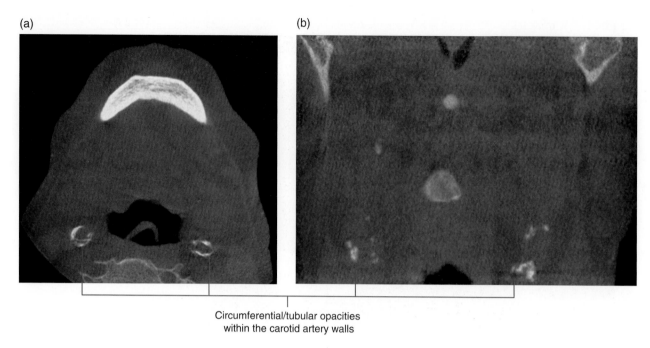

Circumferential/tubular opacities
within the carotid artery walls

Figure 16.14 Bilateral arteriosclerotic calcifications of the external carotid arteries: axial (a) and coronal (b) CBCT images.

(b)

(a)

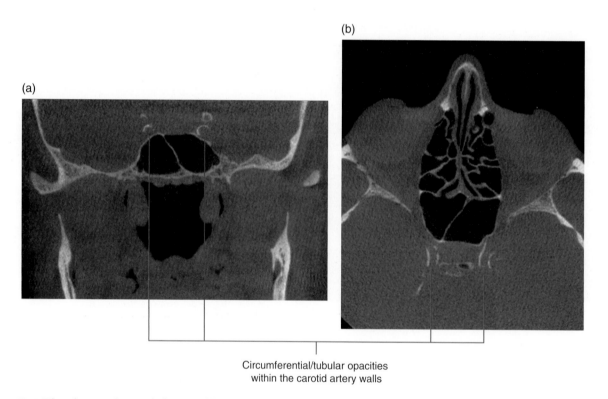

Circumferential/tubular opacities
within the carotid artery walls

Figure 16.15 Bilateral arteriosclerotic calcifications of the internal carotid arteries: coronal (a) and axial (b) CBCT images.

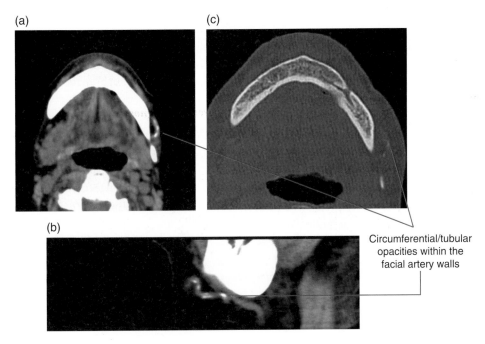

(a)   (c)

(b)

Circumferential/tubular
opacities within the
facial artery walls

Figure 16.16 Arteriosclerotic calcifications of the left facial artery: axial and sagittal soft tissue (a,b) and axial bone (c) MDCT images.

16.6 Phlebolith (see Figure 12.7)

- Calcified thrombi.
- In the orofacial region, these are usually related to vascular malformations (refer to Chapter 12).

Radiological features

- Since most phleboliths in the orofacial region are related to vascular lesions, MDCT is recommended over CBCT and MRI is often necessary (refer to Chapter 12).
- Classically present as well-defined opacities with a circumferential or ovoid appearance with central lucency. Small phleboliths present as fine, small opacities and larger ones may appear quite elongated.
- Variable in numbers. When multiple, they often present in clusters.

Differential diagnosis

	Key radiological differences
Other soft tissue calcifications	The morphology of phleboliths and the often clustered presentation assists in differentiation. If orofacial phleboliths are suspected, MDCT and/or MRI should be considered (refer to Chapter 12).

16.7 Sialoliths (Figures 16.17–16.22; see also Figures 16.23–16.26)

- Calcifications may occur within the salivary gland ductal systems and/or the parenchyma. It may be useful to consider employing the term 'ductal sialolith' to discern these from 'parenchymal calcifications'.
  - Parenchymal calcifications (Figure 16.23) may be related to a previous inflammatory condition or may reflect ongoing chronic sialadenitis such as Sjögren syndrome.
- 80–90% of ductal sialoliths occur within the ductal system of the submandibular salivary glands.
- Single or multiple stones are possible.
- Around 20% of ductal sialoliths have very low mineral content.
- May present with swelling and pain in the area of the gland/duct, typically related to meals. Many are asymptomatic and incidentally identified at imaging.
- MDCT is the most sensitive test for detecting sialoliths and demonstrates the associated salivary gland. CBCT will demonstrate most sialoliths.
  - Note that an MDCT sialogram is optimal for studying flow obstructions/compromise. Some sialoliths demonstrate low mineral content and the calcified component represents only a small portion of the entire sialolith. Other causes of flow obstruction/compromise include mucus plugs/non-calcified sialoliths (Figure 16.24),

acute bends (Figure 16.25), stenosis (Figure 16.26) and presence of soft tissue mass lesions. CBCT sialograms may be sufficient although the soft tissues are not well demonstrated.

Radiological features

- Well-defined opacity with variable size, morphology and internal architecture. The classical sialolith is ovoid/elongated with an internal laminated appearance.
- Most commonly seen within the duct of the submandibular salivary gland, often occurring proximally where the duct curves around the posterior border of the mylohyoid muscle.
- Ductal sialoliths tend to be elongated due to the fluid flow characteristics.
- Sialoliths located in the hilum region tend to be more oval in appearance and may grow larger before becoming symptomatic.

- Parenchymal calcifications usually present as small opacities varying from one or a few within a focal region of the salivary gland to widespread opacities throughout the gland.
- Ductal sialolithiasis may contribute to sialodochitis, sialadenitis, cellulitis and atrophy of the salivary gland.

Differential diagnosis

Key radiological differences

Calcified lymph node	Classically demonstrates a cauliflower-like appearance. May be difficult to distinguish on plane film but this appearance is usually demonstrated on MDCT or CBCT.
Phlebolith	Classically presents as an opaque ring with a lucent centre giving a 'target' appearance. With MDCT, associated soft tissue density of the vascular anomaly is demonstrated.

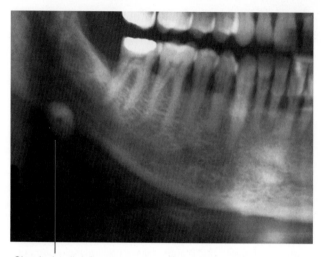

Classical well-defined ovoid laminated opacity projected over the inferior body of the mandible posteriorly. This is likely to be located within the proximal duct of the submandibular salivary gland duct

Figure 16.17 Ductal sialolith related to the right submandibular gland: cropped panoramic radiograph.

(a) (b)

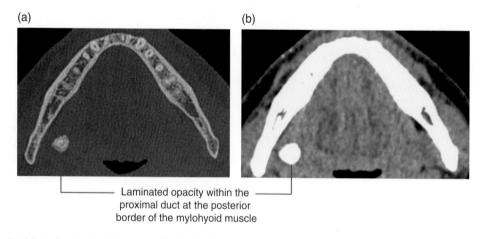

Laminated opacity within the proximal duct at the posterior border of the mylohyoid muscle

Figure 16.18 Ductal sialolith related to the right submandibular gland: axial bone (a) and soft tissue (b) MDCT images.

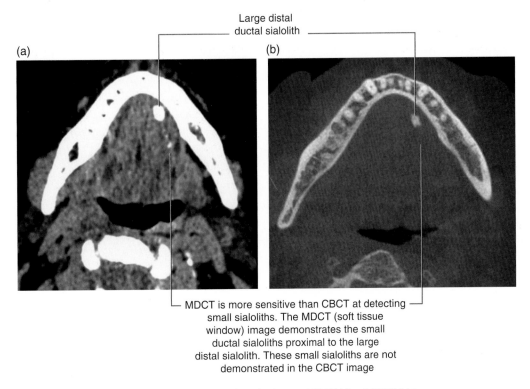

Large distal
ductal sialolith

(a)

(b)

MDCT is more sensitive than CBCT at detecting
small sialoliths. The MDCT (soft tissue
window) image demonstrates the small
ductal sialoliths proximal to the large
distal sialolith. These small sialoliths are not
demonstrated in the CBCT image

Figure 16.19 Ductal sialoliths related to the left submandibular gland: axial soft tissue MDCT (a) and CBCT (b) images.

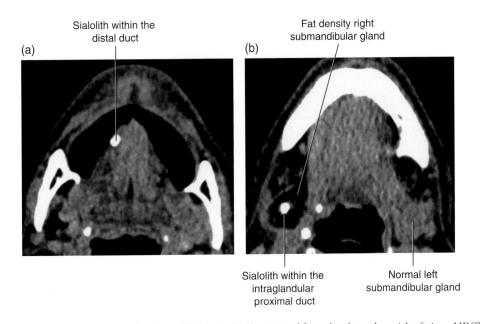

Sialolith within the
distal duct

Fat density right
submandibular gland

(a)

(b)

Sialolith within the
intraglandular
proximal duct

Normal left
submandibular gland

Figure 16.20 Two ductal sialoliths related to the right submandibular gland with associated fat-replaced atrophy: axial soft tissue MDCT images (a,b).

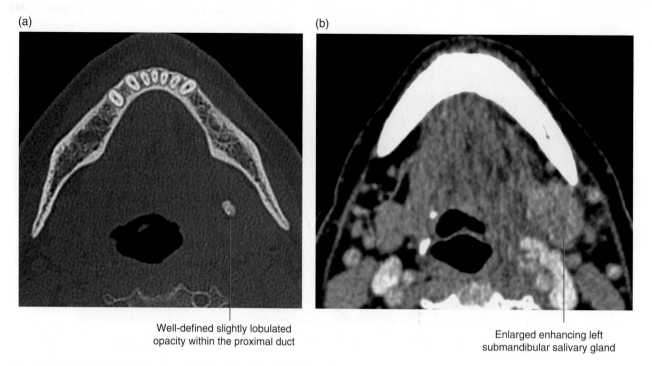

(a)

(b)

Well-defined slightly lobulated
opacity within the proximal duct

Enlarged enhancing left
submandibular salivary gland

Figure 16.21 Sialadenitis of the left submandibular salivary gland related to a ductal sialolith: precontrast axial bone (a) and post-intravenous contrast soft tissue (b) MDCT images.

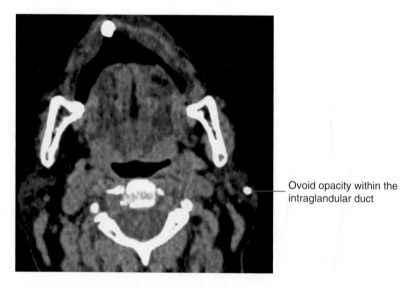

Ovoid opacity within the
intraglandular duct

Figure 16.22 Ductal sialolith in the left parotid gland: axial soft tissue MDCT image.

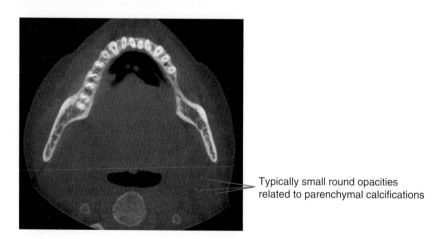

Typically small round opacities
related to parenchymal calcifications

Figure 16.23 Focal parenchymal calcifications within the left parotid related to previous sialadenitis: axial CBCT image.

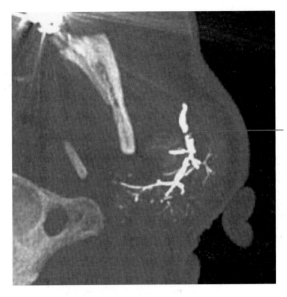

Flow void within the proximal duct reflects either a mucus plug or a non-calcified ductal sialolith. This would not be identified without a sialogram

Figure 16.24 Mucus plug/non-calcified ductal sialolith related to the left parotid gland (recurrent swelling related to meals): axial maximum intensity projection MDCT sialogram image.

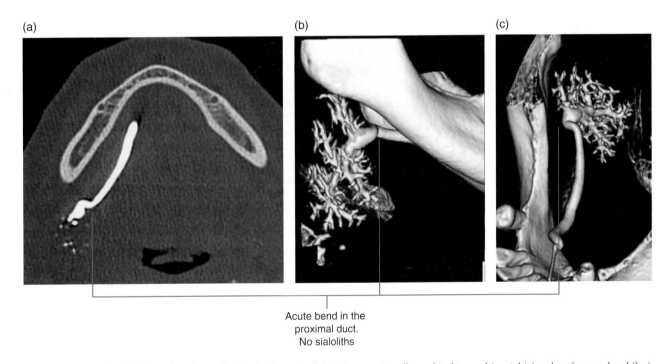

Acute bend in the proximal duct. No sialoliths

Figure 16.25 Acute bend of the right submandibular gland proximal duct (recurrent swelling related to meals): axial (a) and surface-rendered (b,c) MDCT sialogram images.

Stenosis of the distal
duct. No sialoliths

(a)

(b)

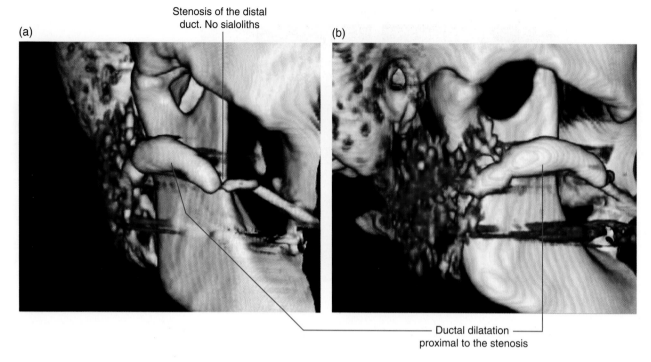

Ductal dilatation
proximal to the stenosis

Figure 16.26 Ductal stenosis of the right parotid duct (recurrent swelling related to meals): surface-rendered MDCT sialogram images (a,b).

16.8 Paranasal and nasal calcifications
(see Figure 19.19)

- Calcifications are sometimes seen within the maxillary sinuses, most often related to chronic inflammatory disease, and may indicate fungal infection.
- Nasal calcifications are rare and appearances are often non-specific.

Radiological features
- If imaging is indicated, MDCT is recommended over CBCT (refer to Chapter 19).

16.9 Myositis ossificans (Figure 16.27)

- Benign ossification within muscles, tendons and ligaments.
  - Traumatic myositis ossificans (myositis ossificans circumscripta/traumatica):
    - Related to trauma.
    - Usually larger muscles. Rarely seen in the muscles of the head and neck, usually the masseter and sternomastoid muscles. Myositis ossificans following trauma related to local anaesthetic injections for dental procedures and masticatory muscle injections is occasionally seen.
  - Progressive myositis ossificans (myositis ossificans progressiva):

- Rare hereditary condition. Spontaneous mutation is extremely rare. Involves multiple muscles, tendons, ligaments, fascia and aponeuroses with muscle atrophy. Often fatal.
- Muscle pain and swelling.

Radiological features
- When suspected, MDCT is the imaging modality of choice. CBCT usually demonstrates the opacity(s) unless subtle. Early ossifications may not be seen on MRI.
- Well-defined opacity within muscle with variably more hypodense appearance centrally (the ossification begins from the border proceeding centrally). The initial peripheral ossification is often seen 3–6 weeks after trauma. In time, the opacity typically increases in density as it matures. Eventually, usually after approximately 6 months, it usually decreases in size.
- The opacity is variable in morphology and may be irregular, ovoid, elongated or occasionally linear in appearance running along the muscle fibres.
- Associated swelling of the muscle may be demonstrated.
- The ossifications related to progressive myositis ossificans are similar but are multiple.

Differential diagnosis

	Key radiological differences
Parosteal osteosarcoma	Calcifies from the centre outwards to the periphery.

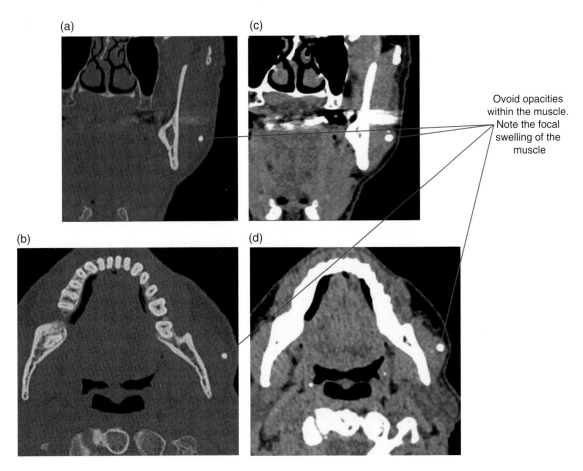

Ovoid opacities within the muscle. Note the focal swelling of the muscle

Figure 16.27 Traumatic myositis ossificans of the left masseter muscle: coronal and axial bone (a,b), coronal and axial soft tissue (c,d) MDCT images.

CHAPTER 17

Trauma and Fractures

Tom Huang

TEETH AND SUPPORTING STRUCTURES

- Acute traumatic injuries to the teeth and jaws are best examined with cone beam computed tomography (CBCT) or multidetector computed tomography (MDCT) although intraoral radiography may suffice in cases where the trauma is minor, at least initially. Many of the radiological features described may not be evident on intraoral and panoramic radiographs.

17.1 Subluxation (Figure 17.1; see Figure 17.6)

- Tooth loosening related to acute trauma, without displacement from the socket.

Radiological features
- Variable widening of the periodontal ligament (PDL) space. May not be appreciated with 2D radiography when centred palatally/lingually or labially.

Differential diagnosis

	Key radiological differences
During and following recent orthodontic therapy	History of orthodontic treatment. Teeth involved in treatment will demonstrate widening of the PDL spaces, related to the forces exerted and tooth movement in orthodontic therapy
Periodontal disease	There should also be evidence of periodontal bone loss in addition to the appearance of widened PDL spaces. These widened PDL spaces usually reflect increased mobility, related to the loss of bony support of the teeth.
Bruxism/increased loading on teeth	Involved teeth may demonstrate widened PDL spaces.

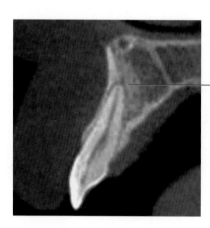

Slight widening of the periodontal ligament space

Figure 17.1 Subluxation: corrected sagittal CBCT image.

Atlas of Oral and Maxillofacial Radiology, First Edition. Bernard Koong.
© 2017 John Wiley & Sons Ltd. Published 2017 by John Wiley & Sons Ltd.

17.2 Luxation (Figures 17.2–17.4)

- Tooth is pushed out of the socket following acute trauma.
- Tooth is mobile and displaced.
- Can be intrusive (apical direction – into the alveolar bone), extrusive (coronal direction – away from the alveolar process) or lateral ('sideways').

Radiological features

- Tooth is displaced from the socket.
- There may be evidence of an expanded tooth socket with/without alveolar fracture (see Figures 17.3, 17.4 and 17.14), including the adjacent alveolar cortices; best demonstrated with MDCT or CBCT if indicated.

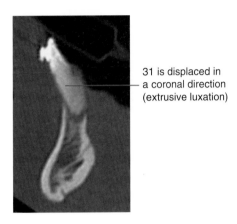

31 is displaced in a coronal direction (extrusive luxation)

Figure 17.2 Luxation, 31: corrected sagittal MDCT image.

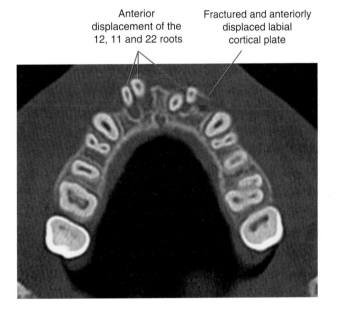

Anterior displacement of the 12, 11 and 22 roots

Fractured and anteriorly displaced labial cortical plate

Figure 17.3 Luxation, 12, 11 and 22: axial MDCT image.

Intrusive (apical direction)
and labial displacement

(a)   (b)

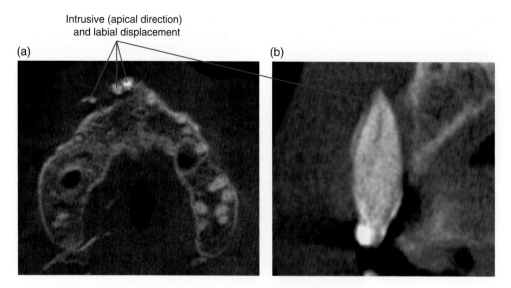

Figure 17.4 Luxation, 13, 12 and 11: axial (a) and corrected sagittal (b) CBCT images.

17.3 Avulsion (Figure 17.5)

- Tooth completely displaced from the socket as a result of acute trauma.
- May be dislodged into surrounding soft tissue.

Radiological features
- Empty socket, which may be expanded.

- There may be fracture of the alveolus and adjacent alveolar cortices; best demonstrated with MDCT or CBCT if indicated.
- If the location of the tooth is unknown, dislodgement into the adjacent soft tissues should be considered. When imaging is indicated, MDCT is optimal.
- Inhalation or swallowing of an entire tooth is rare. A chest radiograph could be considered in the appropriate clinical setting.

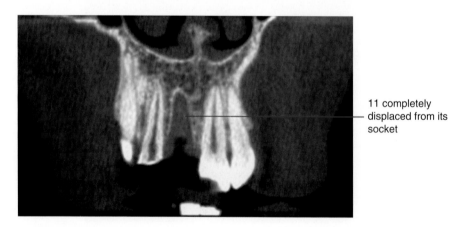

11 completely
displaced from its
socket

Figure 17.5 Avulsion, 11: corrected coronal CBCT image.

17.4 Fracture of teeth (Figures 17.6–17.13)

- While this chapter largely discusses acute trauma-related fractures, it should be noted that tooth fractures may be related to acute trauma, chronic increased occlusal loading (e.g. clenching and/or bruxism) or normal occlusal forces exerted upon a tooth which is structurally compromised (e.g. endodontically treated and/or heavily restored teeth). Tooth fracture can also be related to a combination of these potential causes.
- The fracture may involve the crown, root, or both the crown and root.
- Uncomplicated fractures do not involve the pulp and/or root canal(s). Complicated fractures involve the pulp and/or root canal(s).
- Alveolar fracture may be seen in association with tooth fractures related to acute trauma.
- Acute traumatic tooth fractures usually involve the anterior teeth. Posterior tooth fractures may also be seen following acute trauma, typically when there is impact on the jaws/head such that the maxillary and mandibular teeth contact with significant force.

Radiological features

- Where there is no loss of tooth structure, the fracture appears as a narrow well-defined lucent line involving the crown and/or root, with/without displacement of the tooth fragments.
  - These fracture lines are only demonstrated on periapical and panoramic radiography when the plane of the fracture is coincident with the projection angle of the X-ray beam. That is, tooth fractures may not be demonstrated with periapical and panoramic radiography, especially when undisplaced.

The presence, orientation and extent of tooth fractures are best demonstrated with CBCT or MDCT.
  - Tooth fractures related to acute trauma are almost always demonstrated with CBCT and MDCT.
  - Undisplaced tooth fractures related to chronic increased occlusal loading and/or weakened tooth structure are not infrequently subresolution and not appreciated, even with CBCT and MDCT. However, longstanding undisplaced fractures may be associated with a chronic inflammatory vertical periodontal bone defect or longitudinally widened periodontal ligament space, best demonstrated with CBCT and MDCT
- There may be associated loss of coronal fragment of the fracture. If the location of this coronal fragment is unknown, dislodgement into the adjacent soft tissue should be considered. A chest radiograph should be considered if there is suspicion of inhalation of the fragment.
- When there is a crown and root or root fracture, the fragments may remain largely *in situ*, held by the periodontium. The coronal fragment is usually mobile.
- There may be associated alveolar fractures (Figures 7.3 and 17.14); best demonstrated with MDCT or CBCT if indicated.

Differential diagnosis

	Key radiological differences
Longstanding root fracture following previous acute trauma	Lucent fracture line of the root is seen without recent history of acute trauma. The fracture line often demonstrates a more rounded appearance at the edges.

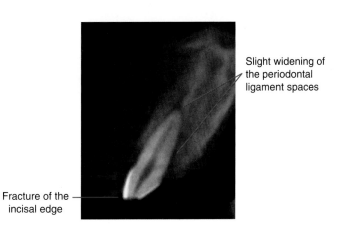

Slight widening of the periodontal ligament spaces

Fracture of the incisal edge

Figure 17.6 Acute traumatic crown fracture with subluxation, 13: corrected sagittal CBCT image.

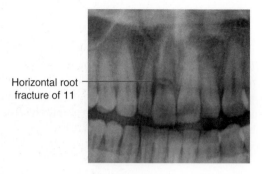

Horizontal root
fracture of 11

Figure 17.7 Acute traumatic root fracture, 11: cropped panoramic radiograph.

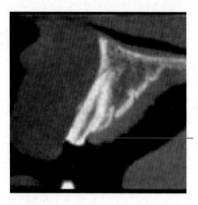

Crown fracture
extends to involve
the cervical aspect of
the root palatally.
The coronal fragment
is absent

Figure 17.8 Acute traumatic crown–root fracture, 21: corrected sagittal CBCT image.

(a) (b)

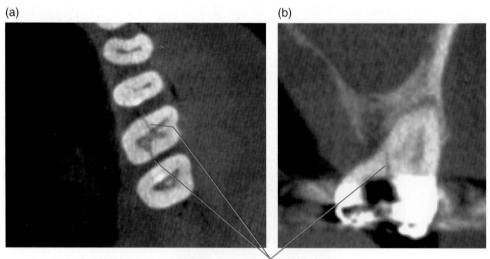

Vertical fracture of the crown and root. The fracture line runs
mesiodistally, extending from the occlusal aspect coronally to the
palatal surface radicularly. Note the large restoration

Figure 17.9 Crown–root fracture related to a combination of increased occlusal loading and compromised tooth structure, 26: axial (a) and corrected coronal (b) CBCT images.

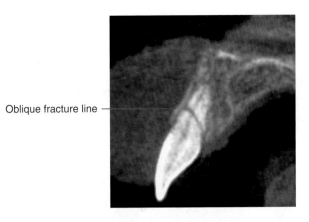

Oblique fracture line —

Figure 17.10 Oblique root fracture related to acute trauma, 11: corrected sagittal CBCT image.

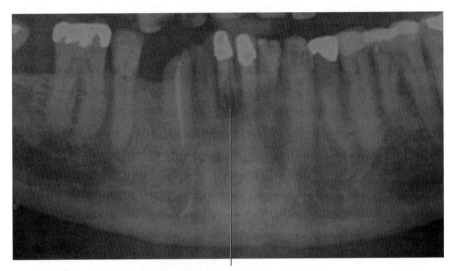

Displaced vertical root fracture of the
endodontically treated 41. The central
linear opacity represents the endodontic
obturation material (gutta percha)

Figure 17.11 Vertical root fracture related to compromised tooth structure, 41: cropped panoramic radiograph.

(a) (b)

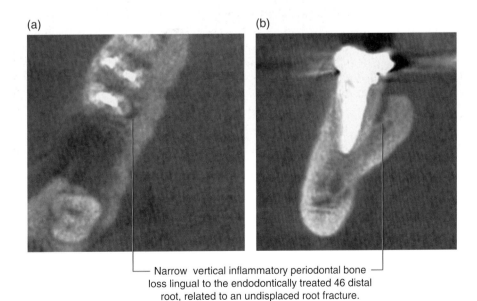

— Narrow vertical inflammatory periodontal bone —
loss lingual to the endodontically treated 46 distal
root, related to an undisplaced root fracture.
The root fracture is subresolution

Figure 17.12 Root fracture related to compromised tooth structure, 46: axial (a) and corrected coronal (b) CBCT image.

(a)   (b)

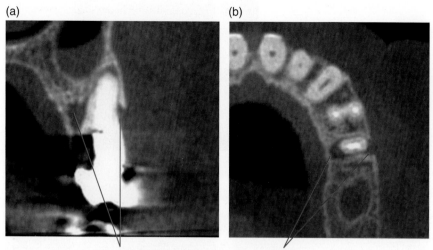

Buccal and palatal lucent inflammatory lesions
related to an undisplaced root fracture,
which is subresolution. Note the
presence of a post and crown associated
with this endodontically treated tooth

Figure 17.13 Root fracture related to compromised tooth structure, 25: corrected coronal (a) and axial (b) CBCT image.

Alveolar cortical fracture. Note the
widened periodontal ligament spaces
of the involved teeth, related to
subluxation and luxation

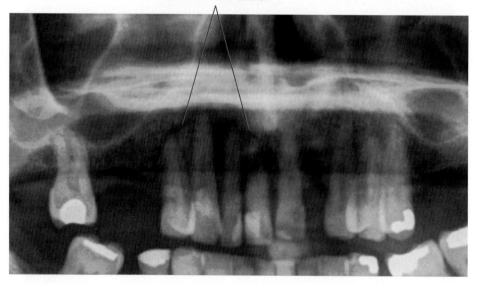

Figure 17.14 Alveolar fracture, 14–11 segment: cropped panoramic radiograph.

FACIAL BONES

- Obvious on computed tomography (CT). MDCT is generally the imaging modality of choice, which may demonstrate important associated soft tissue findings. CBCT may suffice in some cases.
- On plain film (2D radiograph):
  - A thin lucent line represents the fracture.
  - When displaced, this may present with cortical discontinuity with a 'step' defect.
  - When displaced and overlapping, this may appear as a region of increased density.

17.5 Mandibular fractures (Figures 17.15–17.18)

- Mandibular fractures are often caused by assaults, sports or motor vehicle accidents.
- Patients usually present with pain and swelling. Contusion is usually seen at the floor of the mouth when there is a fracture of the mandibular body. There may be malocclusion, limited or unusual jaw movements, laceration to the skin and chin paraesthesia.
- Angle > body > condyle > parasymphyseal region > ramus > coronoid process.
- While most mandibular fractures are unilateral, bilateral fractures are not uncommon.

Radiological features

- MDCT is optimal where mandibular fractures are suspected, especially condylar fractures. Associated soft tissue changes may not be demonstrated with CBCT but this technique may suffice in many cases, and could be considered where there is no access to MDCT. Plain 2D radiography may be sufficient in some cases although it must be recognised that some fractures may not be demonstrated in these views, especially condylar fractures and undisplaced fractures.
- Discontinuity of the bone with/without displacement.
- Bone overlap resulting in an increased density appearance on 2D radiography.

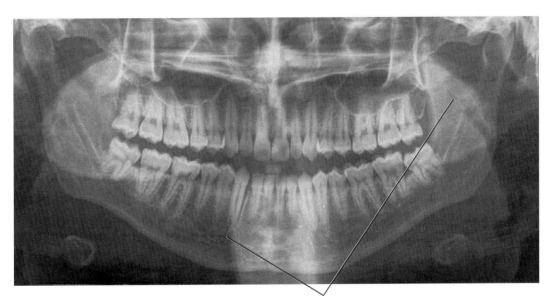

Well-defined narrow lucencies related
to undisplaced fractures

Figure 17.15 Undisplaced right parasymphyseal and left ramus mandibular fractures: panoramic radiograph.

Increased density reflects the overlap of the ends
of the displaced right condylar neck fracture

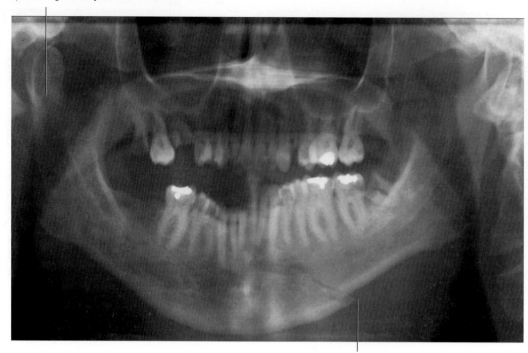

'Step defect' in the left
parasymphyseal region

Figure 17.16 Displaced right condylar neck and left parasymphyseal mandibular fractures: panoramic radiograph.

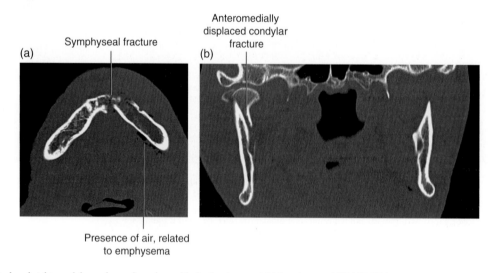

Figure 17.17 Displaced right condylar and symphyseal mandibular fractures: axial (a) and coronal (b) MDCT images.

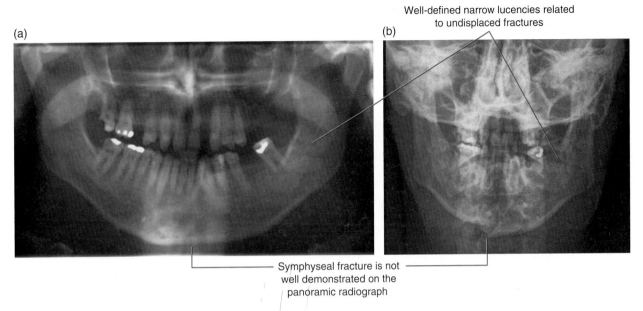

(a)

(b)

Well-defined narrow lucencies related to undisplaced fractures

Symphyseal fracture is not well demonstrated on the panoramic radiograph

Figure 17.18 Symphyseal and left angle mandibular fractures: panoramic (a) and posteroanterior mandible (b) radiographs.

17.6 Nasal fracture (Figure 17.19)

- Common facial fracture.
- Lateral impact injuries are the most common type of injury leading to fracture.
- Imaging may not alter patient management.

- The worst outcome occurs when septal haematoma develops, leading to necrosis, with loss of nasal support and development of saddle nose. Intracranial spread of infection has also been reported.
- Best examined with MDCT. CBCT may be sufficient if there is no clinical suspicion for complications or other facial fractures.

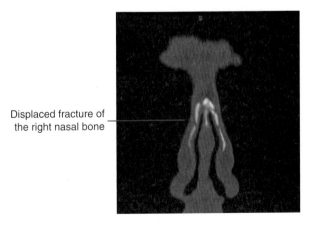

Displaced fracture of the right nasal bone

Figure 17.19 Nasal bone fracture: coronal MDCT image.

17.7 Zygomaticomaxillary complex fracture (Figure 17.20)

- Relatively common facial fracture.

- Fracture variably involves the zygomatic arch, floor and lateral wall of the orbit and the anterolateral and posterolateral walls of the maxillary sinus.
- MDCT is the modality of choice.

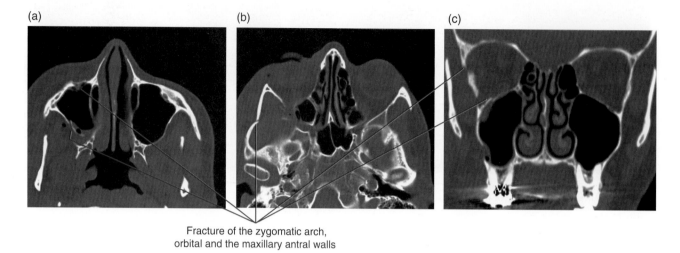

(a)   (b)   (c)

Fracture of the zygomatic arch,
orbital and the maxillary antral walls

Figure 17.20 Zygomaticomaxillary complex fracture: axial (a,b) and coronal (c) MDCT images.

17.8 Orbital blow-out fracture (Figure 17.21)

- Caused by trauma to the orbit by an object too large to enter the orbit.
  - Usually fractures the orbital floor, but the medial, lateral and superior walls may also be involved. Typically, the orbital rim remains undamaged.

  - Medial wall fractures accompany approximately 50% of orbital floor fractures.
- Herniation of the inferior rectus and inferior oblique muscles and orbital fat may occur, with occasional muscle entrapment.
  - Results in diplopia on upward gaze.
- MDCT is the modality of choice.

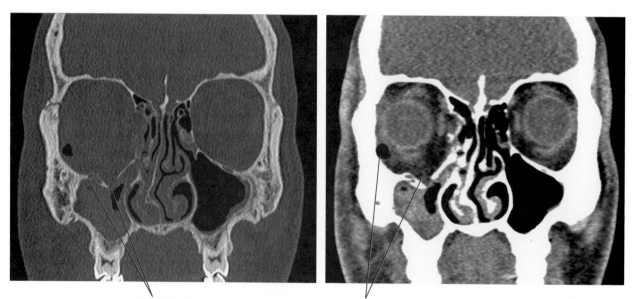

Inferiorly displaced fractured right orbital floor involving
the infraorbital canal, with herniation of orbital fat. Note the
presence of gas/air within the extraconal fat

Figure 17.21 Orbital blow-out fracture: coronal bone and soft tissue MDCT images (a,b).

17.9 Le Fort fractures

- Usually associated with major trauma.
- A combination of these fractures may occur.
- MDCT is the modality of choice.

Le Fort I

- Horizontal fracture separating the palate, alveolar process and teeth from the upper face.
- Fracture line runs above the nasal floor, through the inferior nasal septum, inferior aspect of the maxillary sinus walls and part of the pterygoid plates.

Le Fort II

- Pyramidal fracture, with the region of the nasofrontal suture representing the apex and the alveolar process/dental arch at the base of the pyramid.
- Fracture line involves the lacrimal bones and medial orbital walls and then extends laterally to the root of the nose.

It continues to the floor of the orbit near the infraorbital canal and continues down the zygomaticomaxillary suture and the anterior wall of the maxilla. Posteriorly, the fracture involves the infratemporal surface of the maxilla and the inferior pterygoid plates.

Le Fort III

- Dislocation of the facial bones from the skull base.
- Fracture line runs through the root of the nose, lacrimal bones, medial orbital walls, floors of the orbit, lateral orbital walls and the zygomaticofrontal sutures and zygomatic arches. The fracture line extends to the posterior maxilla and the lower portions of the pterygoid plates.

17.10 Other complex facial fractures
(Figure 17.22)

- Includes variable combinations of fractures of multiple bones, often with comminuted fractures.

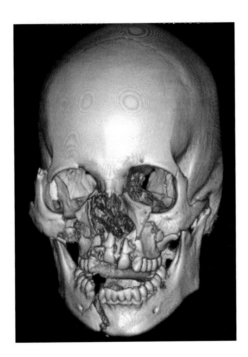

Figure 17.22 Complex facial fractures: surface-rendered MDCT image.

CHAPTER 18
Temporomandibular Joints

18.1 Imaging the temporomandibular joints

Panoramic radiograph

- Arthropathy cannot be excluded with this technique (see Figures 18.20–18.22). Moderate to gross osseous abnormalities may be identified but this technique is neither sensitive nor specific for temporomandibular joint (TMJ) bony abnormalities.
- Tomographic views obtained by panoramic machines usually have the same limitations as panoramic radiographs and do not offer additional value.
- Because of the oblique projection, condylar positions cannot be evaluated from studies obtained by panoramic machines.
- May be a useful supplementary study, when an initial overview of the teeth and jaws is also required.

Other plain film studies and dedicated conventional tomography

- Have substantial limitations and have largely been replaced by more advanced techniques.

Cone beam computed tomography (CBCT)

- For evaluation of the osseous structures.
- Substantial variation in image quality between machines should be considered. Subtle osseous changes may not be detected, often related to beam hardening (which is not usually seen in multidetector CT).
- Variation in radiation dose levels delivered between machines is also noted.
- Soft tissues are not sufficiently well demonstrated.

Multidetector (multislice) computed tomography (MDCT)

- The best modality for evaluation of the osseous structures.
- Adjacent soft tissues are also visualised, which may demonstrate clinically significant findings.

- The articular disc positions may be demonstrated on MDCT studies when appropriate protocols are employed for modern scanners. It should be noted that the articular disc is not always demonstrated with MDCT and MRI is the imaging modality of choice for this.

Magnetic resonance imaging (MRI)

- The best modality for the evaluation of the soft tissues, including the articular disc.
- Also useful to evaluate for the presence of joint effusion and synovitis, distension of the joint spaces and marrow oedema as well as changes in the adjacent soft tissues including the masticatory muscles. These features can be critical in diagnosis, including explanation for pain (e.g. marrow oedema), and also identifying conditions which are not easily identified with CBCT and MDCT (e.g. active inflammatory/erosive arthropathies).
- Subtle osseous changes may be subresolution. Calcified loose joint bodies are usually not detected.
- No ionising radiation.

18.2 Condylar hyperplasia (Figures 18.1 and 18.2; see also Figures 14.1–14.3 and 15.3)

- Most commonly refers to the increased development of one mandibular condyle.
- Several proposed aetiological factors.
- May be associated with hemimandibular hyperplasia (refer to Chapter 14).
- Most common presentation is facial asymmetry:
  - Varying degrees of severity.
  - Progresses at various rates.
  - Growth may occasionally continue past the end of skeletal maturity of other bones.
  - The contribution to mandibular asymmetry may be limited to the vertical (craniocaudal) dimension or may be primarily in the transverse dimension, where the mandibular symphysis is located contralateral to the overall facial midline. Various combinations are also seen.

Atlas of Oral and Maxillofacial Radiology, First Edition. Bernard Koong.
© 2017 John Wiley & Sons Ltd. Published 2017 by John Wiley & Sons Ltd.

○ There are often associated changes to the occlusion, e.g. open bite and cross bite. Canter of the occlusal plane and associated compensatory asymmetry of the maxillary alveolar process is often seen.

- Sometimes, there is associated TMJ dysfunction and related symptoms.
- Symmetric abnormal excessive condylar growth can be seen in endocrine disorders such as acromegaly (refer to Chapter 14).

Radiological features

- When imaging is indicated, MDCT or CBCT are recommended over 2D radiography. MRI may be useful if there is associated joint dysfunction or other related symptoms.
- Technetium bone scans, especially single-photon emission computed tomography (SPECT), may be useful to determine growth activity. However, increased uptake is non-specific and many other conditions, including degenerative changes, can contribute to this. Therefore, evaluation with MDCT or CBCT is recommended prior to bone scans.
- The affected condyle is larger than the contralateral condyle.
- The morphology may be normal or altered. The anterior surface of the condylar head is often directed (rotated) more anteriorly than the normal anteromedial orientation.
- The condylar neck may be bowed posteriorly and/or laterally.
- There may be remodelling of the glenoid fossa.

Differential diagnosis

Contralateral condylar hypoplasia

Ipsilateral hemimandibular hyperplasia

Degenerative hyperplastic response

Osteochondroma and osteoma

Key radiological differences

The condylar morphology and orientation of the condylar head may assist. Occasionally, differentiation can be difficult as size is the only difference between the condyles.

The hyperplasia is not limited to the condyle. The ipsilateral body and ramus of the mandible are larger and there may be a less pronounced antegonial notch.

A severe hypertrophic response is sometimes associated with degenerative disease beyond osteophytic lipping (which is more commonly seen). In these cases, the condyle can appear larger. Occasionally, it can be difficult to differentiate from the hyperplastic condyle with degenerative disease.

These are usually associated with the appearance of a focal bony prominence rather overall enlargement of the condyle.

(a)

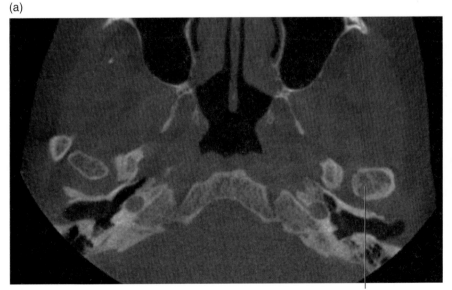

Left condyle is larger than the right and is oriented more anteriorly

(b) Larger left condylar head

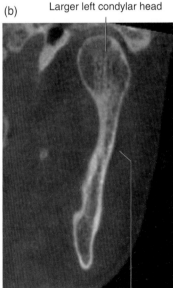

Slight lateral bowing of the condyle

Figure 18.1 Left condylar hyperplasia: axial (a) and coronal (b) CBCT images.

(a)   (b)

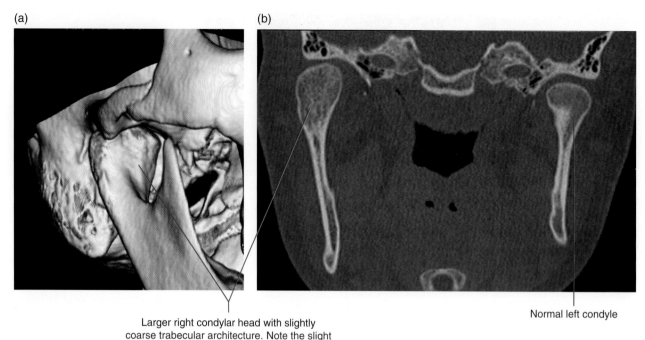

Larger right condylar head with slightly
coarse trabecular architecture. Note the slight
lateral bowing of the condylar neck

Normal left condyle

Figure 18.2 Right condylar hyperplasia: surface-rendered (a) and coronal (b) MDCT images.

18.3 Coronoid hyperplasia (Figure 18.3)

- Rare increased dimensions of the coronoid process in the absence of a focal mass lesion.
- May be bilateral or unilateral. Most are considered to be developmental.
- May be associated with hemimandibular hyperplasia (refer to Chapter 14).
- Often presents with TMJ hypomobility (reduced mouth opening and lateral movements).
  - Generally considered to be related to impingement of the hyperplastic coronoid process on the zygoma.
- Sometimes, there is associated TMJ dysfunction and related symptoms.

Radiological features
- Best examined with MDCT, although CBCT may be sufficient if there is no suspicion for soft tissue lesions.

- Larger than normal coronoid process(es). The morphology may alter slightly, appearing elongated or more rounded, but the cortical and trabecular architecture are within normal limits.

Differential diagnosis

	Key radiological differences
Normal variant	It can be difficult to differentiate this from the bilateral cases. Generally considered to be a normal variant unless it contributes to reduced mandibular movement or the processes are overtly enlarged.
Osteochondroma and osteoma	Presence of a tumour mass (refer to Chapter 10 for osteoma).

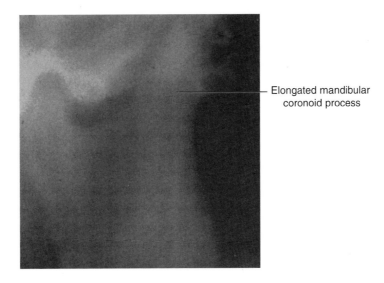

— Elongated mandibular
coronoid process

Figure 18.3 Right coronoid hyperplasia: cropped panoramic radiograph.

18.4 Condylar hypoplasia (Figures 18.4–18.6)

- Reduced development of the mandibular condyle(s).
- Most are generally considered to be developmental or related to childhood conditions and trauma which may affect condylar growth. Occasionally may be related to other conditions, e.g. hemifacial microsomia.
- May be unilateral or bilateral.
- Quite commonly associated with mandibular hypoplasia (refer to Chapter 14).
- Bilateral cases present with small, usually symmetric, mandibles.
- Unilateral cases present with facial asymmetry. Associated canter of the occlusal plane and compensatory asymmetry of the maxillary alveolar process is often seen.
- Sometimes associated with TMJ dysfunction and related symptoms. Hypoplastic condyles usually demonstrate degenerative changes earlier in life.

Radiological features
- When imaging is indicated, MDCT or CBCT are recommended over 2D radiography. MRI may be useful if there is associated joint dysfunction or other related symptoms.
- The affected condyle is smaller than usually expected. The condylar neck is usually correspondingly small.

- The anterior surface of the condylar head is often directed more medially than the usual anteromedial orientation.
- The morphology of the small condyle may otherwise be:
  - Normal.
  - Altered. The morphology of the condylar head may demonstrate an elongated appearance and the short condylar neck may be bowed/angled posteriorly.
- The glenoid fossa is often normal, giving an appearance of a disproportionately small condylar head within the fossa.

Differential diagnosis

	Key radiological differences
Contralateral condylar hyperplasia	The condylar morphology (when altered) and orientation of the condylar head may assist. Occasionally, differentiation can be difficult as size is the only difference between the condyles.
Juvenile rheumatoid arthritis	The condyle usually demonstrates an irregular morphology, and variable erosive destruction of the articular eminence is usually seen in rheumatoid arthritis.

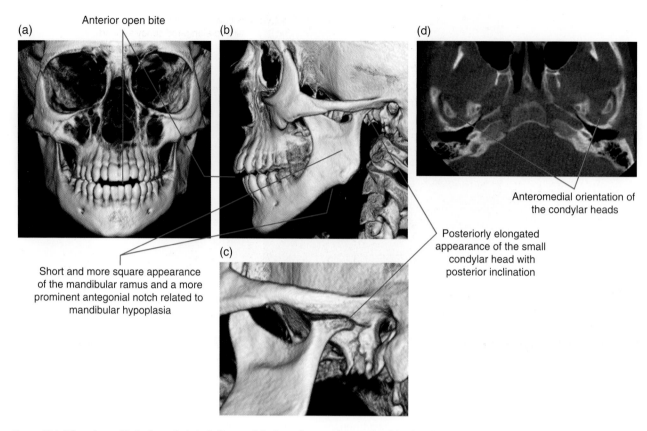

Anterior open bite

(a)

(b)

(d)

Anteromedial orientation of
the condylar heads

Posteriorly elongated
appearance of the small
condylar head with
posterior inclination

(c)

Short and more square appearance
of the mandibular ramus and a more
prominent antegonial notch related to
mandibular hypoplasia

Figure 18.4 Bilateral mandibular hypoplasia including condylar hypoplasia: surface-rendered (a–c) and axial (d) CBCT images.

Slight anteroposterior elongated appearance of the
small condylar head with posterior inclination

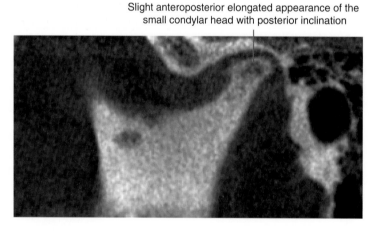

Figure 18.5 Condylar hypoplasia: corrected sagittal CBCT image.

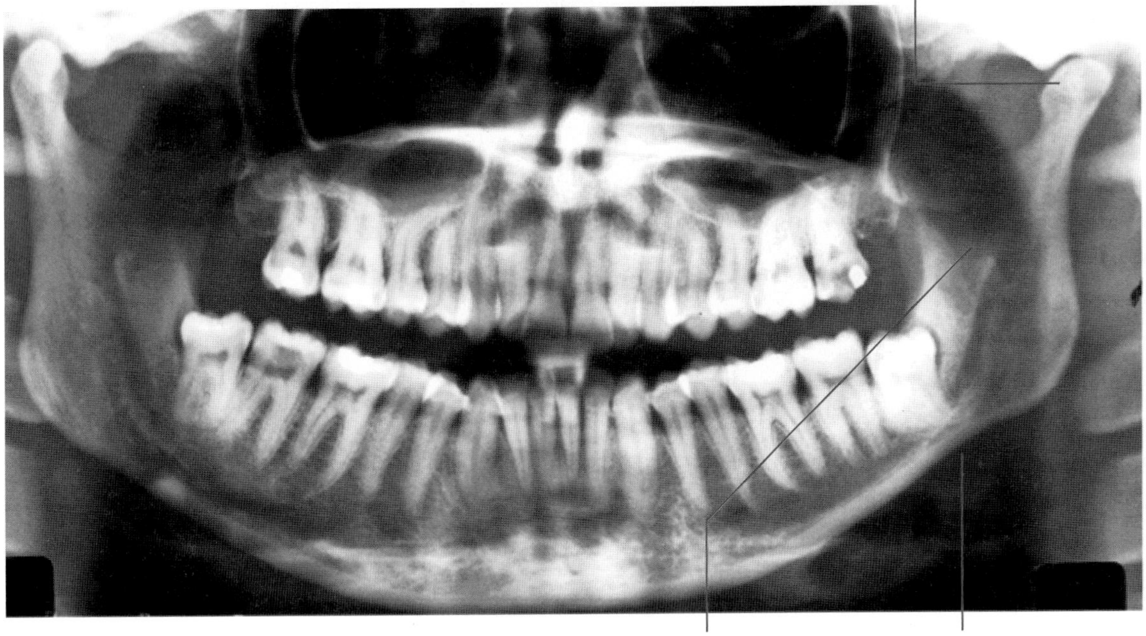

Hypoplastic condyle with appearances of slight posterior tilt and elongated condylar head

Short and squarer appearance of the mandibular ramus

Prominence of the antegonial notch

Figure 18.6 Left hemimandibular hypoplasia including condylar hypoplasia: panoramic radiograph.

18.5 Bifid condyle (Figure 18.7)

- A deep groove or cleft dividing the condylar head is classical although rare. Most cases seen are fruste forme, demonstrating superior or posterosuperior depressions/clefts of varying depths, rather than a deep, near complete, division of the condylar head.
- May be unilateral or bilateral.
- Often considered to be developmental but may also be related to childhood trauma.
- Occasionally associated with TMJ dysfunction and related symptoms.

Radiological features

- When imaging is indicated, MDCT or CBCT are recommended over 2D radiography. MRI may be useful if there is associated joint dysfunction or other related symptoms.
- Variable corticated depression or cleft at the superior or posterosuperior aspect of the condylar head.

Differential diagnosis

Key radiological differences

Normal variant	It can be difficult to differentiate this from the fruste forme cases as there is a large variation in normal condylar morphology.

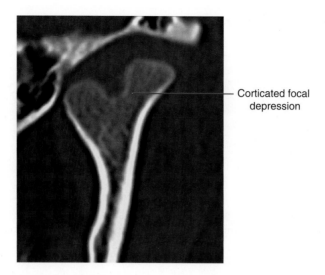

Corticated focal depression

Figure 18.7 Left bifid condyle: corrected coronal MDCT image.

18.6 Internal derangements of the temporomandibular joint

(Figures 18.8–18.17)

- Dysfunction of the articular disc, usually referring to discal displacement and/or abnormality and the related soft tissue changes.
- Most commonly presents with joint noises. There may be pain and/or restricted mobility.
- May be bilateral or unilateral.
- Not all disc displacements are related to pain or clinically identifiable dysfunction.
  - Some argue that, in the absence of symptoms, disc displacements may be a normal variant. Others consider that disc displacements predispose to joint dysfunction and associated degenerative changes.

Radiological features

- When imaging is indicated, MRI is the modality of choice. MDCT studies, with appropriate protocols, often demonstrate disc displacement although MDCT should be employed primarily for evaluation of the osseous structures as it does not reliably demonstrate the articular discs.
- The articular disc is not seen on CBCT and plain 2D radiography.
  - It has been suggested that a posterior position of the condylar head (with teeth maximally occluded) is associated with anterior disc displacement but this is not reliable.
  - Hypomobility may sometimes be related to non-reducing disc displacements. Importantly, internal derangement does not account for all hypomobile joints. In addition,

there may be a normal range of condylar movement in cases with non-reducing disc displacements.
  - 2D radiography is insufficient when TMJ dysfunction is clinically suspected.
- The disc is normally a biconcave low-signal structure in T2, T1 and proton density (PD) sequences. Classically described as demonstrating a bow tie appearance on corrected (oblique) sagittal images.
- In the normal position, the intermediate zone of the disc (thinner portion between the anterior and posterior bands) is located at the narrowest region between the condylar head and articular eminence.
  - In these normal cases, the posterior band often sits superior to the condylar head. However, the posterior band may be slightly anterosuperior or posterosuperior to the condylar head, depending on the bony morphology of the joint and the relative size and morphology of the articular disc.
- Articular discs can be displaced in any direction, although anterior displacements are most commonly seen, followed by anteromedial displacements. Medial displacements are sometimes seen. Lateral displacements are uncommon and posterior displacements are extremely rare.
- Displaced discs may be:
  - Non-recaptured, remaining displaced. In these cases, the disc may fold or is otherwise further distorted at maximal opening.
  - Recaptured/reduced (moves back into a normal position between the condyle and articular eminence) upon varying degrees of opening.
  - When recaptured, this can occur early (at the early part of condylar translation) or late (close to or at maximal opening).
  - Partial or incomplete re-captures are sometimes seen.

- The discal morphology may be abnormal, to varying extents. Two common changes are:
  - Thickening of the posterior band. This may contribute to non-reduction upon opening.
  - Thickening of the intermediate zone, resulting in a flat or biconvex appearance of the disc, which is normally biconcave.
- Discal degeneration.
  - Most commonly seen in the posterior band, which demonstrates an intermediate T1 or PD signal, rather than the normally low signal of the articular disc.
- Fibrotic changes in the retrodiscal tissues.
  - Often seen as a focal low signal of the retrodiscal tissues immediately posterior to the posterior band of the articular disc. This fibrotic change is generally thought to be related to chronic non-reducing disc displacement.
- Effusion and synovitis.
  - Effusion may be seen in relation to internal derangements although this is also a feature of inflammatory/erosive arthropathies and trauma.
    - Homogeneously hyperintense T2 signal. This can be seen within the superior and/or inferior joint spaces. Sometimes limited to the anterior or posterior recesses.
    - Substantial effusion may result in distension of the joint space(s), which may distort adjacent soft tissues, e.g. superficial tissues and adjacent masticatory muscles.

- Synovitis
  - Intermediate T1 signal.
  - When effusion is present, there is almost certainly synovitis. However, the synovitis may not be appreciated if it is minimal.
- Perforation.
  - Most commonly seen in the retrodiscal tissues rather than in the disc, usually with non-reducing disc displacements. Perforation at the intermediate zone is less common.
  - Can be difficult to identify on MRI. Arthrography usually demonstrates this.
  - Where there is bony contact of the condyle with the articular eminence of the glenoid fossa, there is almost certainly perforation of the disc or retrodiscal tissues.
- Adhesions.
  - May be seen in cases with, although not limited to, internal derangements.
  - Difficult to identify on MRI.
- Marrow oedema.
  - May be seen in a wide range of joint conditions including internal derangement, degenerative disease, trauma, erosive/inflammatory arthropathies, etc.
  - Increased T2 signal within the marrow spaces.
  - Usually correlates with pain.
- Associated bony degenerative changes of the joints may be seen (see section 18.8).

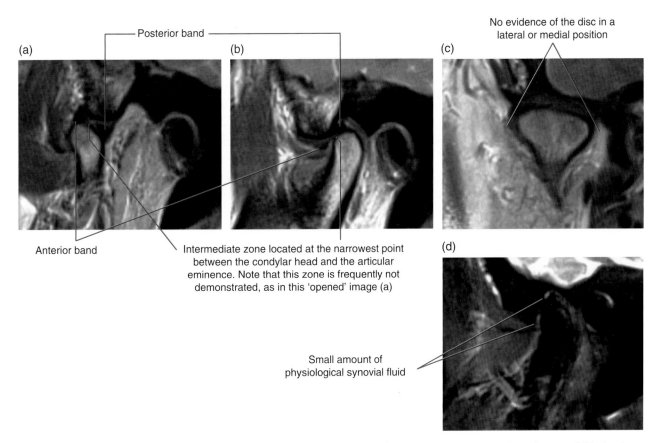

Figure 18.8 Normal articular disc and normal osseous structures of the TMJ: MRI; corrected sagittal opened (at maximal mouth opening) (a), closed (with teeth in occlusion) (b) and coronal closed (c) PD images. Corrected sagittal T2 image (d).

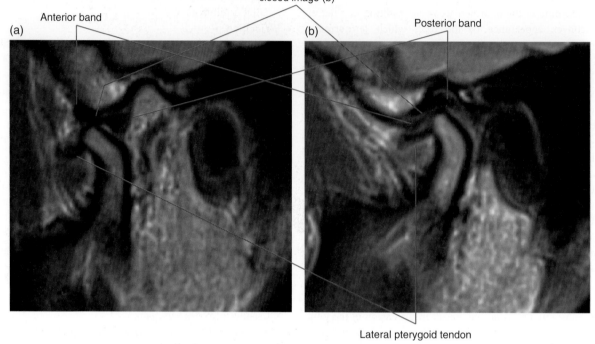

Figure 18.9 Normal articular disc and normal osseous structures of the TMJ: MRI; corrected opened (a) and closed (b) PD images.

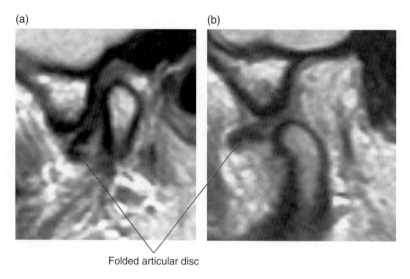

Folded articular disc

Figure 18.10 Non-reducing moderate anterior displacement of a folded articular disc: MRI; corrected sagittal closed (a) and opened (b) PD images.

(a)   (b)

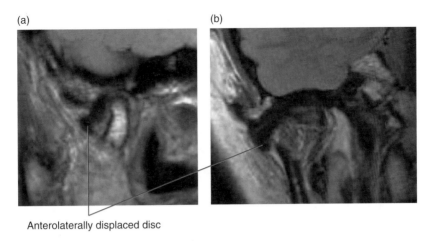

Anterolaterally displaced disc

Figure 18.11 Moderate anterolaterally displaced articular disc: MRI; corrected sagittal (a) and corrected coronal (b) PD images with teeth in occlusion.

(a)   (b)

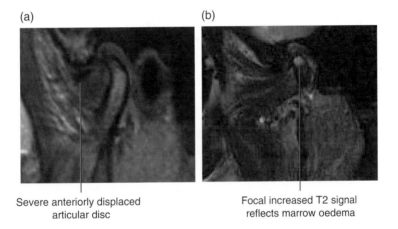

Severe anteriorly displaced
articular disc

Focal increased T2 signal
reflects marrow oedema

Figure 18.12 Severe anterior articular disc displacement and condylar marrow oedema: MRI; corrected sagittal closed PD (a) and T2 (b) images with teeth in occlusion.

Homogeneously bright effusion
within the superior joint space
(a)   (b)   (c)

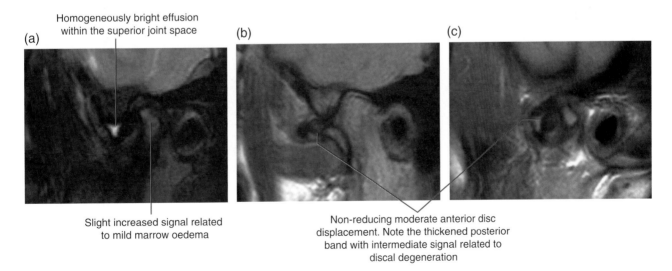

Slight increased signal related
to mild marrow oedema

Non-reducing moderate anterior disc
displacement. Note the thickened posterior
band with intermediate signal related to
discal degeneration

Figure 18.13 Non-reducing moderate anterior articular disc displacement with thickened degenerating posterior band and effusion. There is mild condylar marrow oedema: MRI; corrected sagittal closed T2 (a), corrected sagittal opened PD (b) and corrected sagittal closed PD (c) images.

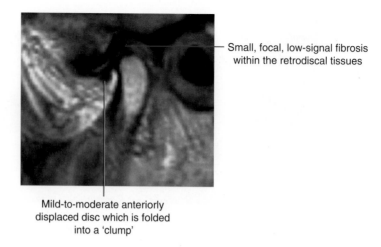

Small, focal, low-signal fibrosis
within the retrodiscal tissues

Mild-to-moderate anteriorly
displaced disc which is folded
into a 'clump'

Figure 18.14 Folded mild-to-moderate anterior articular disc displacement with focal fibrosis of the retrodiscal tissues related to chronicity: MRI; corrected sagittal closed PD image.

(a)   (b)

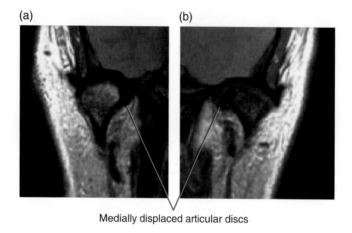

Medially displaced articular discs

Figure 18.15 Bilateral medial articular disc displacements: MRI; corrected coronal PD images of the right (a) and left (b) joints.

(a)   (b)   (c)

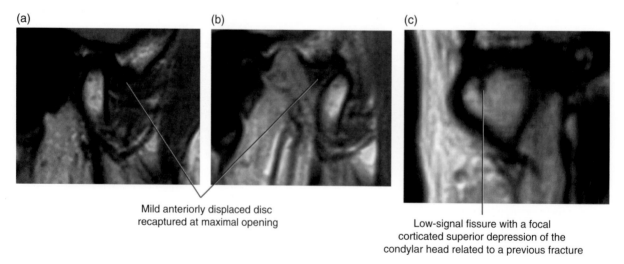

Mild anteriorly displaced disc
recaptured at maximal opening

Low-signal fissure with a focal
corticated superior depression of the
condylar head related to a previous fracture

Figure 18.16 Reducing mild anterior articular disc displacement. Previously fractured condyle: MRI; corrected sagittal closed (a) and opened (b), and corrected coronal closed (c) PD images.

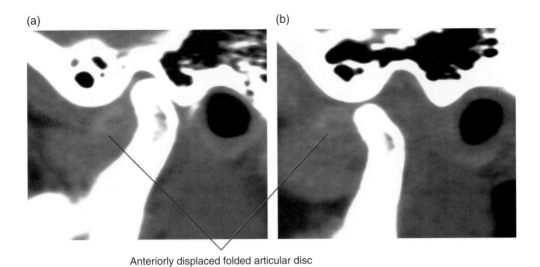

Anteriorly displaced folded articular disc

Figure 18.17 Non-reducing moderate anterior displacement of a folded articular disc: corrected sagittal soft tissue window MDCT images with teeth in occlusion (a) and at maximal opening (b).

18.7 Ganglion cysts (Figures 18.18 and 18.19)

- *Synonym*: synovial cyst.
- Aetiology is unclear. May be related to synovial herniation, leakage of synovial fluid from a joint into the adjacent tissues or degenerative cysts. Not related to the neural ganglion.
- Can be associated with trauma.

- Most commonly seen in the hands and feet. Occasionally seen at the TMJs.

Radiological features
- Usually seen as a lobular, well-defined fluid (homogeneous increased T2 signal) focus, resembling an 'outpouching' at the joint capsule.

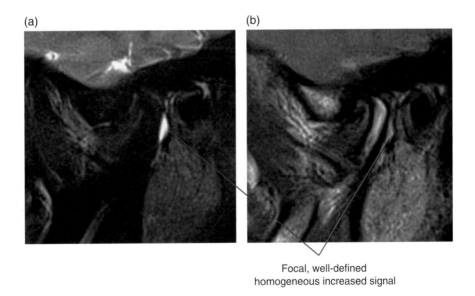

Focal, well-defined
homogeneous increased signal

Figure 18.18 Ganglion cyst related to the left mandibular condyle: MRI; corrected sagittal T2 (a) and PD (b) images.

(a)   (b)

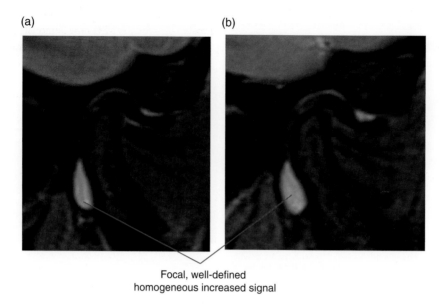

Focal, well-defined
homogeneous increased signal

Figure 18.19 Ganglion cyst related to the right mandibular condyle: MRI; corrected sagittal T2 images (a,b).

18.8 Degenerative joint disease

(Figures 18.20–18.30)

- *Synonyms*: DJD, osteoarthritis (OA).
- A joint condition characterised by flattening, loss of articular cartilage, subchondral sclerosis, bony defects, osteophytosis and decreased joint space. Generally thought to be primarily a non-inflammatory process, related to 'wear and tear' where there is microtrauma over extended periods.
- Several conditions are considered to predispose TMJs to degenerative joint disease, including acute trauma, parafunction (grinding and clenching of teeth), internal derangements, erosive arthropathies and condylar hypoplasia.
- The most common bony arthropathy affecting the TMJ.
- May not be symptomatic.

Radiological features

- When imaging is indicated, MDCT or CBCT are recommended. MDCT is generally more sensitive and subtle bony changes may not be appreciated on some CBCT scans (see section 18.1).
- 2D radiography is usually insufficient when arthropathy is clinically suspected.
- MRI may be useful if there is clinical suspicion for internal derangement. Minor bony changes may be subresolution on MRI. However, MRI may demonstrate marrow oedema, which typically correlates well with pain.
- Flattening of the articular surface of the condylar head and articular eminence.
- Subchondral sclerosis: sclerotic response of the subcortical bone.

- In the absence of other features, mild flattening and subchondral sclerosis are usually considered to reflect remodelling. There is some subjectivity as to the degree to which these changes reflect degenerative joint disease.
- Subarticular pseudocysts: small subcortical cyst-like lucencies of variable sizes. MRI: well-defined, homogeneous T2 hyperintense foci. Not true cysts. May coalesce. As the disease progresses, the overlying cortices are destroyed and these lesions then present as bony defects rather than having cystic appearances.
- Osteophytosis:
  - Formation of osteophytes is seen in many cases. Osteophytes are classically described as lipping, appearing as such; most commonly seen at the anterior aspect of the condylar head. It is also seen elsewhere: relatively common at the lateral aspect of the articular eminence.
  - Osteophytes may separate and appear as opacified loose joint bodies.
  - Occasionally, the hypertrophic response can be exuberant and osteophytes can be larger than the commonly seen lipping appearance. In some cases, the condyle can appear larger than normal. Rarely, a hypertophic response is seen at the base of the glenoid fossa.
- Decreased joint space.
  - This is often seen in association with internal derangement.
  - In severe cases, there may be bony contact of the condyle with the articular eminence. In these cases, there is almost certainly perforation of the articular disc or retrodiscal tissues.

Differential diagnosis

Key radiological differences

Normal variant and remodelling	Occasionally, it can be difficult to differentiate these from very early degenerative joint disease. There is a large variation in normal condylar morphology. There is subjectivity in interpretation of the degree of mild flattening and subchondral sclerosis related to remodelling, as these are also features of degenerative disease.
Opacified loose joint bodies	Other conditions such as chondrocalcinosis, synovial chondromatosis and tumours (see sections 18.13, 18.12 and 18.11, respectively) may present with opacified loose joint bodies. However, differences in the number, pattern and distribution of the opacities as well as other associated changes usually assist in differentiating these entities from separated osteophytes.
Erosive arthropathies	MRI best demonstrates the differences between active inflammatory/erosive arthropathies and degenerative disease. MDCT and CBCT may demonstrate: • Erosive bony defects, which are more irregular and ill defined. • Joint flattening and subchondral sclerosis. These are not features of erosive arthropathy. However, secondary degenerative disease is often seen following the period(s) of acute erosive changes.
Condylar hyperplasia	When present, a substantial degenerative hypertophic response may resemble condylar hyperplasia.
Osteochondroma and osteoma	Osteophytosis, although it can be exuberant, does not usually present as a tumour mass lesion.

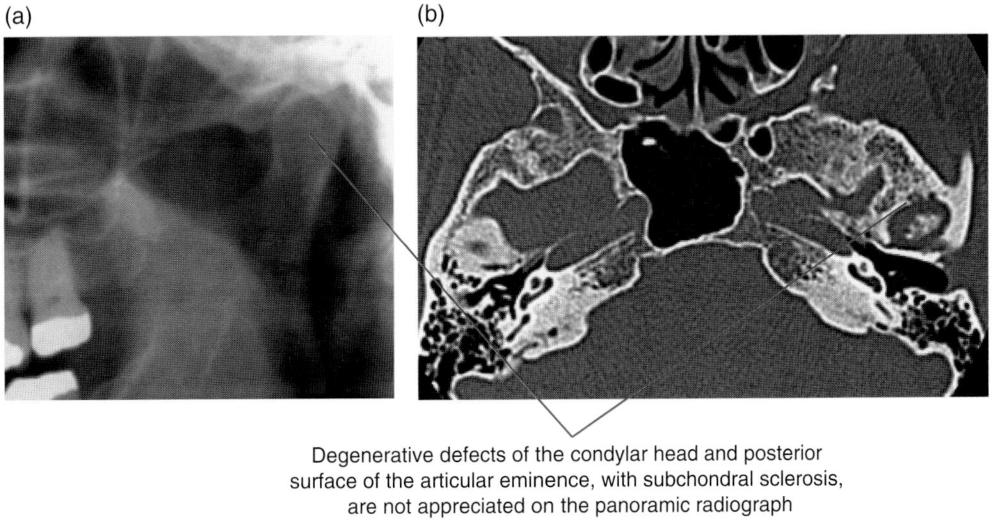

(a)   (b)

Degenerative defects of the condylar head and posterior surface of the articular eminence, with subchondral sclerosis, are not appreciated on the panoramic radiograph

Figure 18.20 Left TMJ degenerative disease not demonstrated on the panoramic radiograph: panoramic radiograph (a) and axial MDCT image (b).

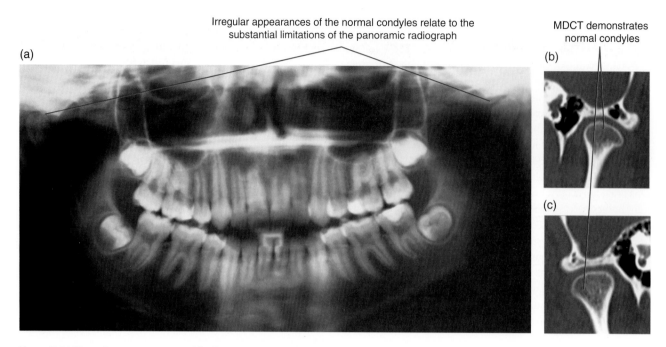

Irregular appearances of the normal condyles relate to the substantial limitations of the panoramic radiograph

MDCT demonstrates normal condyles

(a)

(b)

(c)

Figure 18.21 Normal osseous structures of the TMJs: panoramic radiograph (a) and corrected coronal MDCT images of the left (b) and right (c) joints.

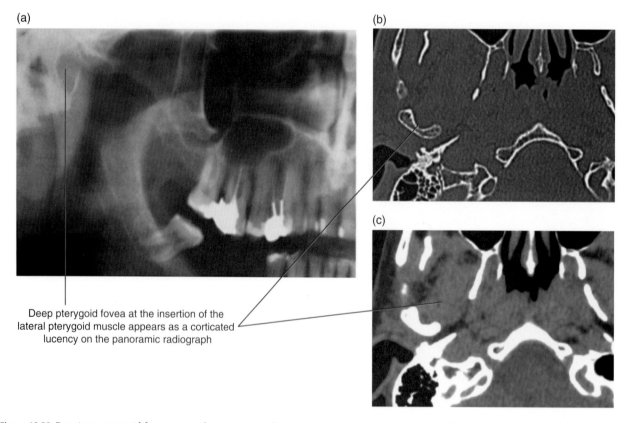

(a)

(b)

(c)

Deep pterygoid fovea at the insertion of the lateral pterygoid muscle appears as a corticated lucency on the panoramic radiograph

Figure 18.22 Prominent pterygoid fovea, a normal variant: cropped panoramic radiograph (a) and axial bone (b) and soft tissue (c) MDCT images.

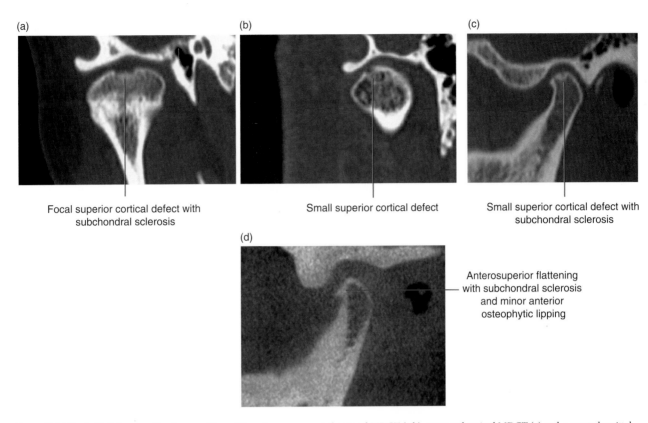

(a)

Focal superior cortical defect with
subchondral sclerosis

(b)

Small superior cortical defect

(c)

Small superior cortical defect with
subchondral sclerosis

(d)

Anterosuperior flattening
with subchondral sclerosis
and minor anterior
osteophytic lipping

Figure 18.23 Early TMJ degenerative disease of four different cases: corrected coronal MDCT (a,b), corrected sagittal MDCT (c) and corrected sagittal CBCT (d) images.

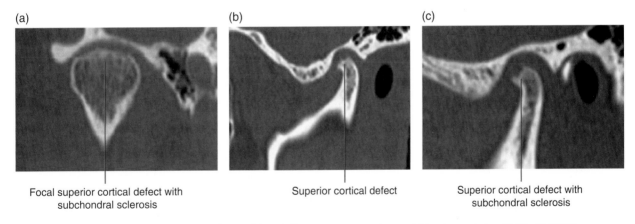

(a)

Focal superior cortical defect with
subchondral sclerosis

(b)

Superior cortical defect

(c)

Superior cortical defect with
subchondral sclerosis

Figure 18.24 Early-to-moderate TMJ degenerative disease of three different cases: corrected coronal (a) and corrected sagittal (b,c) MDCT images.

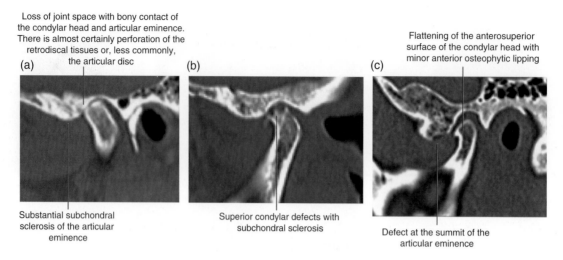

Loss of joint space with bony contact of the condylar head and articular eminence. There is almost certainly perforation of the retrodiscal tissues or, less commonly, the articular disc

Flattening of the anterosuperior surface of the condylar head with minor anterior osteophytic lipping

Substantial subchondral sclerosis of the articular eminence

Superior condylar defects with subchondral sclerosis

Defect at the summit of the articular eminence

Figure 18.25 Moderate TMJ degenerative disease of three different cases: corrected sagittal MDCT images (a–c).

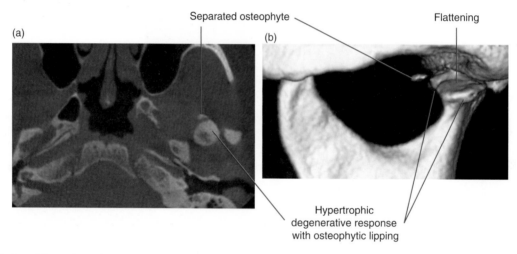

Separated osteophyte

Flattening

Hypertrophic degenerative response with osteophytic lipping

Figure 18.26 Left condylar moderate degenerative disease with separated osteophyte: axial (a) and surface-rendered (b) CBCT images.

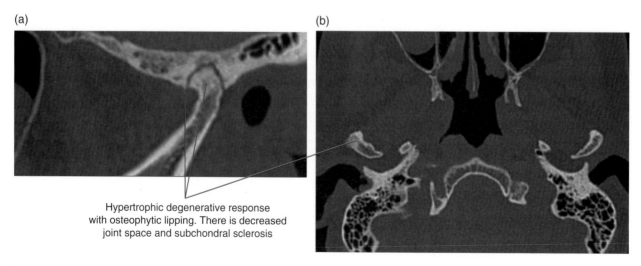

Hypertrophic degenerative response with osteophytic lipping. There is decreased joint space and subchondral sclerosis

Figure 18.27 Right condylar moderate-to-severe degenerative disease: corrected sagittal (a) and axial (b) MDCT images.

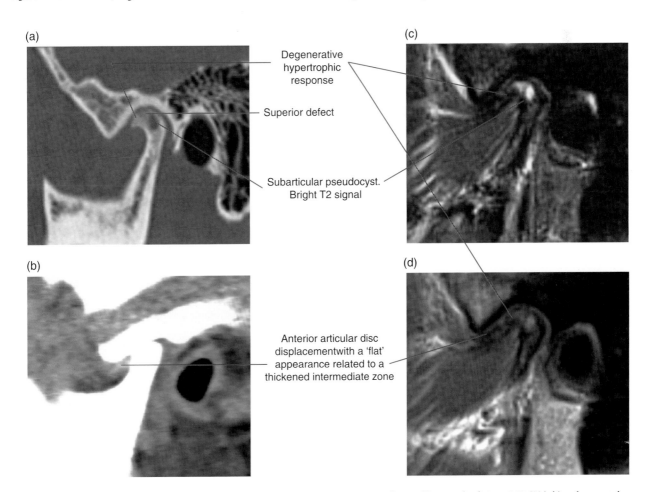

Flattening of the anterosuperior surface of the condylar head and posterior surface of the articular eminence, with subchondral sclerosis. Note the loss of joint space with bony contact. There is almost certainly perforation at the retrodiscal tissues or, less commonly, the articular disc

Separated osteophyte

(a)

(b)

(c)

Large osteophyte

Moderately large defects of the condylar head and posterior aspect of the articular eminence with subchondral sclerosis and an anterior osteophyte. There is bony contact. Therefore, there is almost certainly perforation at the retrodiscal tissues or, less commonly, the articular disc

Figure 18.28 Severe TMJ degenerative disease of three different cases: corrected sagittal MDCT images (a–c).

(a)

(c)

Degenerative hypertrophic response

Superior defect

Subarticular pseudocyst. Bright T2 signal

(b)

(d)

Anterior articular disc displacementwith a 'flat' appearance related to a thickened intermediate zone

Figure 18.29 Severe degenerative disease with anterior articular disc displacement: corrected sagittal bone and soft tissue MDCT (a,b) and corrected sagittal T2 (c) and PD (d) MRI images.

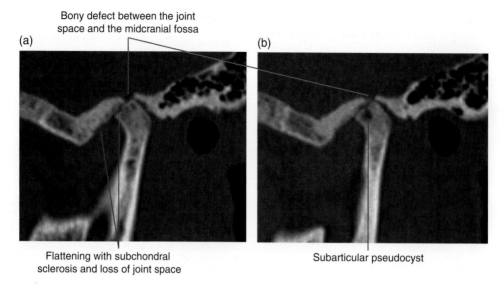

Figure 18.30 Severe degenerative disease with focal bony discontinuity between the joint space and the midcranial fossa: corrected sagittal MDCT images (a,b).

18.9 Inflammatory and erosive arthropathies (Figures 18.31–18.34)

- Generally immune related and include a group of diseases, most commonly:
  - Rheumatoid arthritis
  - Psoriatic arthritis
  - Ankylosing spondylitis.
- The TMJ changes are very similar for this group of conditions.

Radiological features

- When imaging is indicated, MRI should be considered: soft tissue alterations precede osseous changes and osseous changes can be delayed by disease-modifying drugs.
- MDCT is useful in demonstrating bony changes but usually does not demonstrate the soft tissue changes typical of inflammatory arthropathies sufficiently well. CBCT will essentially only demonstrate the osseous changes. 2D radiography is generally considered insufficient when arthropathy is clinically suspected.
- MRI features include:
  - Proliferative synovitis and formation into pannus.
  - Occasionally, the articular disc is no longer identifiable.
  - Effusion.
  - Joint space distension.
  - Marrow oedema.
  - Bony erosive lesions are usually irregular and may demonstrate less well-defined borders than the bony defects seen in degenerative disease. The erosion usually begins at the anterior aspect of the condylar head and posterior aspect of the articular eminence.
  - Pre-erosive subchondral cyst-like appearance:
    - May resemble those of degenerative disease but usually enhance (gadolinium).
  - Decreased joint space.
  - Severe cases may effectively completely destroy the condylar head and articular eminence. Sometimes, the severely affected condyle takes on a sharp pointed morphology.
  - Joint flattening and subchondral sclerosis is not a feature of erosive arthropathies, although it is not uncommon to see secondary degenerative disease following the active phase.
  - Fibrous and bony ankylosis can be seen following the active phase (see section 18.14).
- MDCT and CBCT may demonstrate the erosive bony changes described above.
- MDCT may demonstrate some of the soft tissues changes such as joint space distension and substantial pannus formation.
- In severe cases with substantial bony destruction, the residual condyle is located more anterosuperiorly, resulting in development of an anterior open bite which was not previously present.
  - Anterior open bite:
    - Maxillary and mandibular anterior teeth do not contact when the patient bites, with only the posterior teeth in occlusion.
    - Not all anterior open bites are related to TMJ arthropathy. Indeed, erosive arthropathies are not common causes of anterior open bites.

- Juvenile rheumatoid arthritis (juvenile arthritis):
  - Because of the early onset, mandibular growth is often affected and results in varying degrees of mandibular hypoplasia (refer to Chapter 14). Mandibular asymmetry is seen when the TMJs are affected asymmetrically.

Differential diagnosis

Key radiological differences

Degenerative joint disease

From an imaging perspective, MRI could be considered to assist in the differentiation of these conditions.

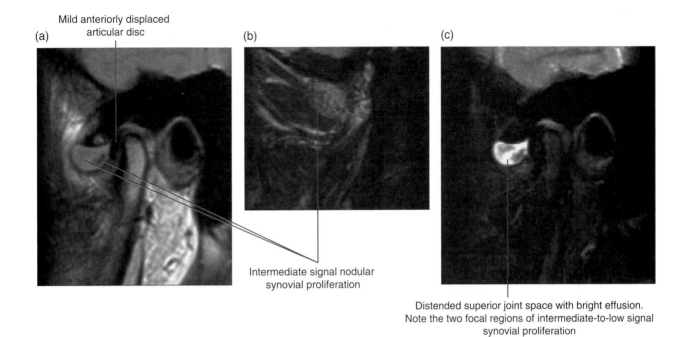

Mild anteriorly displaced articular disc

(a)   (b)   (c)

Intermediate signal nodular synovial proliferation

Distended superior joint space with bright effusion. Note the two focal regions of intermediate-to-low signal synovial proliferation

Figure 18.31 Distension of the superior joint space with synovial proliferation and effusion related to rheumatoid arthritis: corrected sagittal PD (a,b) and T2 (c) MRI images.

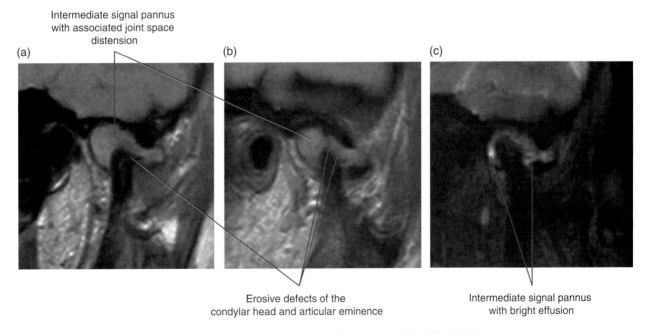

Intermediate signal pannus with associated joint space distension

(a)   (b)   (c)

Erosive defects of the condylar head and articular eminence

Intermediate signal pannus with bright effusion

Figure 18.32 Pannus and bony erosions related to rheumatoid arthritis: corrected sagittal PD (a,b) and T2 (c) MRI images.

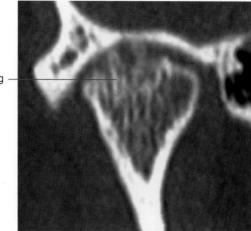

Irregular defects extending into the condylar head

Figure 18.33 Erosive/inflammatory arthropathy: corrected coronal MDCT image.

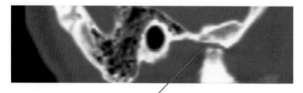

The condylar head and a large portion of the articular eminence are essentially absent. The residual condyle is located at the residual articular eminence in this closed position. There is associated anteroinferior rotation of the mandible and an anterior open bite is likely

Figure 18.34 Juvenile rheumatoid arthritis: corrected sagittal MDCT image with teeth in occlusion.

18.10 Osteochrondroma (Figure 18.35)

- A benign tumour characterised by a bony prominence with a cartilaginous cap. Some consider this as a hamartoma rather than a true benign tumour.
- Most commonly affects long bones. Occasionally involves the mandibular condyle.
- Most solitary lesions are not treated. Occasional radiological review may be useful. Local surgical resection may be required if symptomatic.
- Malignant change is rare; generally considered to be highly unlikely when it involves the mandibular condyle.

Radiological features
- CBCT may be sufficient in most cases, although MDCT demonstrates possible associated soft tissue changes/mass.
- Irregular bony prominence associated with the mandibular condyle. Most often originating at the anterior surface of the condyle. Sometimes extends along the lateral pterygoid muscle.

- Often internally heterogeneous in appearance, with sclerotic regions.
- The cartilaginous caps associated with the mandibular condylar lesions are usually not demonstrated, presumably because they are subresolution.

Differential diagnosis

	Key radiological differences
Degenerative joint disease	Degenerative hypertophic response and large osteophytes can resemble the osteochondroma. The osteochondroma has more of a tumour-like growth morphology.
Osteoma	Usually demonstrates a smoother and more convex morphology than the usually irregular bony prominence of the osteochondroma.

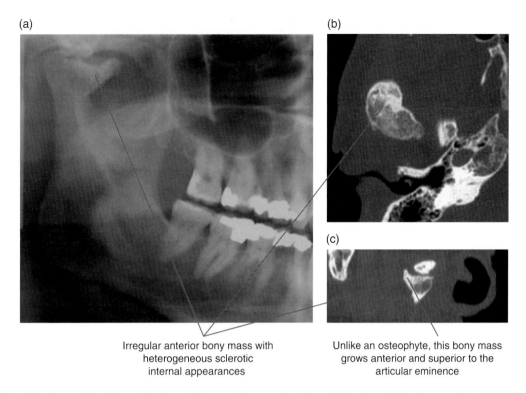

(a)

(b)

(c)

Irregular anterior bony mass with
heterogeneous sclerotic
internal appearances

Unlike an osteophyte, this bony mass
grows anterior and superior to the
articular eminence

Figure 18.35 Osteochondroma of the right mandibular condyle: cropped panoramic radiograph (a) with axial (b) and corrected sagittal (c) MDCT images.

18.11 Malignant tumours (Figures 18.36–18.38;
see also Figures 11.3 and 11.4)

- Rare. Examples include metastatic disease, synovial sarcoma, osteosarcoma, chondrosarcoma, lymphoma, multiple myeloma, malignant fibrous histiocytoma and Ewing sarcoma.

- Should be examined with MDCT initially when there is clinical suspicion for a malignant tumour. MRI is almost always necessary.
- Refer to Chapter 11 for malignant features.

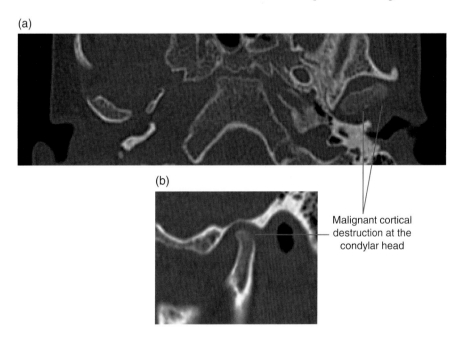

(a)

(b)

Malignant cortical
destruction at the
condylar head

Figure 18.36 Leukaemia involving the left condyle: axial (a) and corrected sagittal (b) MDCT images.

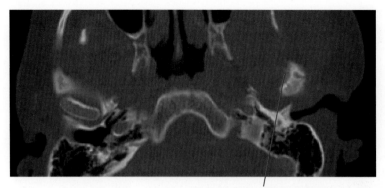

Spiculated periosteal response

Figure 18.37 Osteogenic sarcoma of the left condyle: axial MDCT image.

(a) (b)

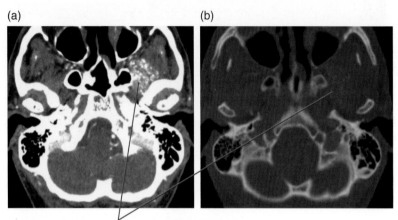

Contrast-enhanced muscle with multiple calcifications.
Note that a few demonstrate the ring/arc-like
appearance of cartilaginous calcifications

Figure 18.38 Chondrosarcoma from the skull base involving the left lateral pterygoid muscle: post-intravenous contrast axial soft tissue (a) and bone (b) MDCT images.

18.12 Synovial chondromatosis (Figure 18.39)

- *Synonyms*: synovial chondrometaplasia, synovial osteochondromatosis.
- Essentially a metaplastic condition where cartilaginous foci occur in the synovium. These may eventually detach into the joint space and calcify/ossify. Some consider these lesions to represent benign tumours which are self-limiting.
- Rare in the TMJ.
- Usually presents with pain, swelling, limited opening and crepitus.

Radiological features
- When calcification/ossification of the detached cartilaginous foci has occurred, a variable number of opacified loose bodies are seen within the joint space.
- MDCT is more sensitive in identifying small/subtle opacities and also demonstrates the soft tissue changes. CBCT may be sufficient for some cases. Small opacified loose joint bodies are often not identified on MRI although the soft tissue changes are best examined with this technique.

- Distension of the joint space with effusion and synovitis (MRI). MDCT may demonstrate severe distensions. MRI may demonstrate the synovial proliferation and larger loose joint bodies.
- The osseous structures of the TMJ may be normal or exhibit bony changes, usually degenerative in appearance.

Differential diagnosis

	Key radiological differences
Chondrocalcinosis (CPPD)	Can be difficult to differentiate radiologically. CPPD involving the TMJs classically presents with multiple small calcifications. Definite diagnosis is done via histological identification of calcium pyrophosphate crystals.
Synovial sarcoma	May be difficult to differentiate radiologically. Presence of a soft tissue mass and extension beyond the joint favour synovial chondrosarcoma.

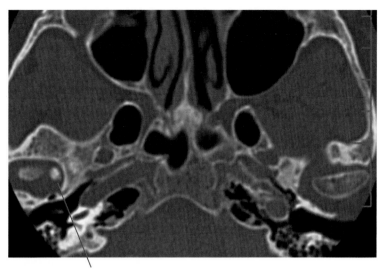

Focal ovoid opacity related to
ossification of a loose cartilaginous body

Figure 18.39 Synovial chondromatosis: axial MDCT image.

18.13 Calcium pyrophosphate deposition disease (Figure 18.40)

- *Synonyms*: CPPD, pseudogout, chondrocalcinosis, pyrophosphate arthropathy.
- Presence of calcium pyrophosphate dihydrate crystals in the joint space.
- Extremely rare in TMJs.
- Patients may be asymptomatic or present with pain, limited opening and crepitus.

Radiological features (temporomandibular joint)
- Usually presents with multiple small calcifications within the joint space.
- MDCT is more sensitive in identifying small/subtle opacities and also demonstrates the soft tissue changes. CBCT may be sufficient for some cases. Small opacified loose joint bodies are often not identified on MRI, although the soft tissue changes are best examined with this technique.

- Joint distension may be demonstrated (MRI). MDCT may demonstrate more substantial distensions. MRI may demonstrate effusion and synovitis.
- There may be associated bony changes, usually degenerative in appearance.

Differential diagnosis

	Key radiological differences
Synovial chondromatosis	Can be difficult to differentiate radiologically. CPPD classically presents with multiple small calcifications. Definite diagnosis is done via histological identification of calcium pyrophosphate crystals.
Synovial sarcoma	May be difficult to differentiate radiologically. Presence of a soft tissue mass and extension beyond the joint favour synovial chondrosarcoma.

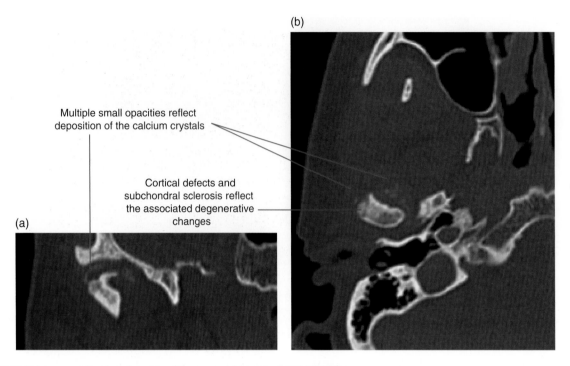

Multiple small opacities reflect deposition of the calcium crystals

Cortical defects and subchondral sclerosis reflect the associated degenerative changes

(a)

(b)

Figure 18.40 Calcium pyrophosphate deposition disease: coronal (a) and axial (b) MDCT images.

18.14 Ankylosis (Figures 18.41 and 18.42)

- Fibrous ankylosis of the TMJ is more commonly seen than bony ankylosis.
- May be unilateral or bilateral.
- Extremely limited mouth opening. Essentially only rotational movement of the condyle on opening and, occasionally, flexing of the condylar neck. There may be minimal translatory movement in fibrous ankylosis.
- Rare. Most commonly seen following surgery and erosive arthropathy.

Radiological features
- Fibrous ankyloses:
  - Extremely narrow joint space and 'parallel' appearance of the condylar cortex and the temporal bone cortex within the TMJ.
  - Imaging in the maximally opened position confirms primarily rotational movement with minimal or no translatory movement.
- Bony ankyloses:
  - Bony bridging between the condyle and temporal bone of the TMJ.
  - May present with one or a few focal small bridges, multiple bridges across the joint space or a continuity of the entire condyle with the glenoid fossa.

Multiple bony bridges connect the condyle to the articular eminence

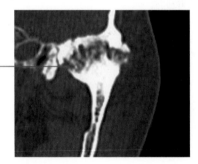

Figure 18.41 Bony ankylosis following the active phase of ankylosing spondylitis: corrected coronal MDCT image.

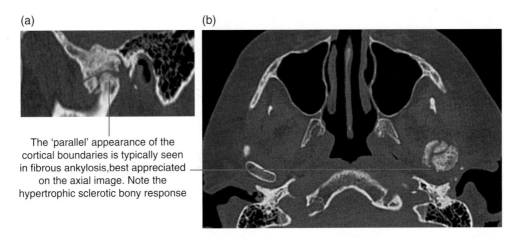

The 'parallel' appearance of the cortical boundaries is typically seen in fibrous ankylosis,best appreciated on the axial image. Note the hypertrophic sclerotic bony response

Figure 18.42 Postsurgical fibrous ankylosis of the left TMJ: corrected sagittal (a) and axial (b) MDCT images.

18.15 Other lesions affecting the temporomandibular joints

- Rare.
- Examples include the osteoma, osteoid osteoma, osteoblastoma, giant cell lesion, aneurysmal bone cyst, haemangioma, simple bone cyst, Langerhans cell histiocytosis and pigmented villonodular synovitis.
- MDCT demonstrates more of the radiological features, although CBCT may reveal sufficient key features of some of these conditions. MRI may be important.

18.16 Other non-temporomandibular joint conditions contributing to pain/dysfunction in the region of the temporomandibular joint and related structures (Figures 18.43 and 18.44; see also Figures 18.38 and 16.27)

- A large variety of other conditions can affect jaw function and/or contribute to pain related to the region of the TMJ and masticatory complex.
- Usually best examined with MDCT and/or MRI.
- Dentoalveolar inflammatory lesions (Chapter 5) can refer pain to the region of the TMJ and masticatory complex.

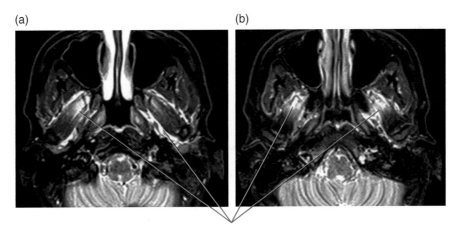

Linear pattern of increased signal

Figure 18.43 Bilateral lateral pterygoid strain: axial T2 MRI images (a,b).

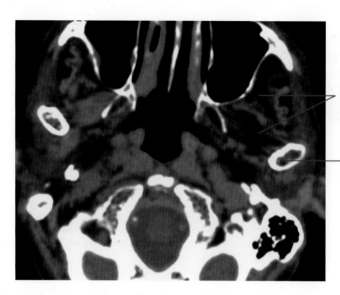

Low-density appearance of the left lateral pterygoid and temporalis muscles, related to fat-replaced atrophy

The left condyle demonstrates minimal translatory movement at maximal opening. Note the normal degree of translation on the right

Figure 18.44 Left-sided masticatory muscle atrophy (severe left TMJ hypomobility) related to a neuropathy: axial soft tissue MDCT image.

CHAPTER 19

Nasal Cavity, Paranasal Sinuses and Upper Aerodigestive Tract Impressions

Michael Bynevelt, Andrew Thompson and Bernard Koong

NASAL CAVITY AND PARANASAL SINUSES

19.1 Normal variations and developmental anomalies

There are numerous well-described nasal cavity and paranasal sinus anatomical variants. If present, they may predispose the patient to, and alter the appearance and significance of, pathological processes that affect this region.

Variations in pneumatisation (Figures 19.1–19.4)

- Constitutionally small or large sinuses.
- Arrested sphenoid pneumatisation.
- Variant intersinus septum position with resultant asymmetry of sinus size (frontal and sphenoid sinuses).
- Frontal sinus expansion, extending over the orbital roof.
- Sphenoid sinus expansion with pneumatisation of the anterior clinoid, pterygoid processes and greater sphenoid wing.
- Nasal turbinate pneumatisation; middle turbinate ('concha bullosa').
- Intersinus septum diverticula and air cells notably seen in the frontal sinus including the crista galli.
- Maxillary sinus palatal recesses.

Accessory ethmoid air cells (Figure 19.5)

- Agger nasi air cells: most anteroinferior of the accessory anterior ethmoid air cells, located in the lacrimal bone and sited anterior and inferior to the frontal recess.
- Kuhn cells: tiered anterior frontoethmoidal air cells superior to the agger nasi.

- Haller cells: inferolateral accessory ethmoid air cells sited below the medial orbital floor which may narrow the ostiomeatal complex.
- Onodi cell: a posterior ethmoid air cell pneumatised superolateral to the sphenoid sinus, and abutting the optic nerve canal. This anatomic proximity confers potential surgical risk to the optic nerve at endoscopic sinonasal surgery.

Aberrant transiting structures

- Internal carotid artery and optic nerve in the sphenoid sinus.
- Anterior ethmoid artery with an 'on mesentery' arrangement in the anterior ethmoidal air cells.
- Ectopic position of the infraorbital nerve and canal contained within an osseous maxillary sinus septation.

Accessory ostia (Figure 19.6)

- Maxillary sinus: medial wall draining into the hiatus semilunaris most commonly.

Aberrant anatomical position

- Deep olfactory fossa and low-lying cribriform plate.
- Cephalocele: meninges and/or brain parenchyma extending through a focal skull base dehiscence.

Others

- Nasal septum deviation and spurring.
- Variations of uncinate process attachment.
- Canalis sinuosus (anterosuperior alveolar nerve).

Atlas of Oral and Maxillofacial Radiology, First Edition. Bernard Koong.
© 2017 John Wiley & Sons Ltd. Published 2017 by John Wiley & Sons Ltd.

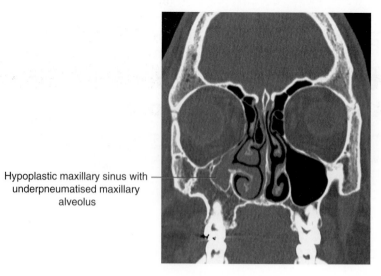

Figure 19.1 Maxillary sinus hypoplasia: coronal MDCT image.

Hypoplastic maxillary sinus with underpneumatised maxillary alveolus

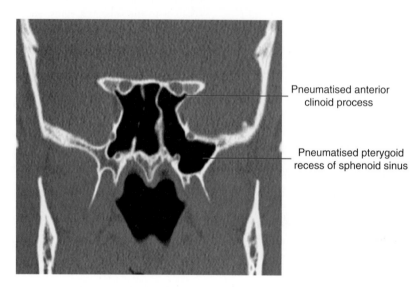

Figure 19.2 Sphenoid sinus variant pneumatisation: coronal MDCT image.

Pneumatised anterior clinoid process

Pneumatised pterygoid recess of sphenoid sinus

(a)

(b)

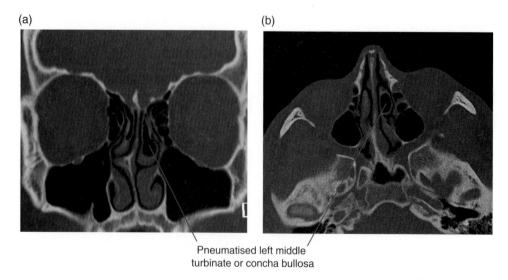

Pneumatised left middle turbinate or concha bullosa

Figure 19.3 Concha bullosa (pneumatised middle turbinate): coronal (a) and axial (b) MDCT images.

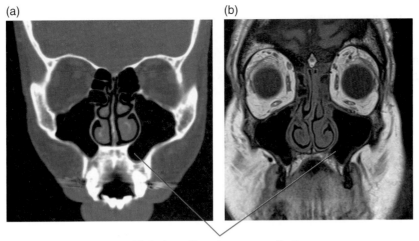

Variant maxillary sinus pneumatisation
inferomedially into the hard palate

Figure 19.4 Maxillary sinus palatal recesses: coronal MDCT (a) and coronal T1-weighted MRI (b) images.

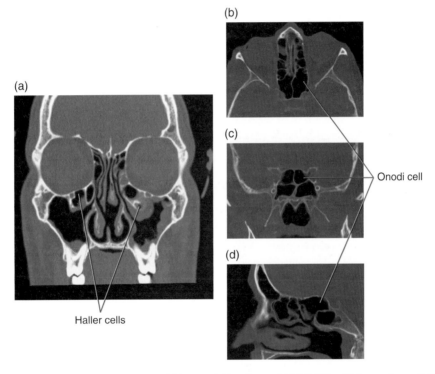

Onodi cell

Haller cells

Figure 19.5 Ethmoid air cell variations: coronal CT (a) and axial (b), coronal (c) and sagittal (d) MDCT multiplanar reformat (MPR) images.

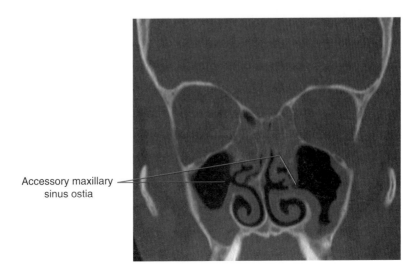

Accessory maxillary
sinus ostia

Figure 19.6 Accessory maxillary sinus ostia: coronal MDCT multiplanar reformat image.

19.2 Odontogenic conditions and dentoalveolar lesions

- Odontogenic conditions and alveolar lesions may:
  - Expand or extend into the nasal cavity or paranasal (usually maxillary) sinuses.
  - Cause/contribute to secondary inflammatory paranasal sinus disease, the maxillary sinus is most frequently involved.
- Includes odontogenic inflammatory disease, odontogenic cysts and cyst-like lesions, tumours, fibro-osseous lesions, hamartomas and other conditions that are discussed in other chapters.

19.3 Findings related to dental procedures

Oroantral communication (Figures 19.7–19.11)

- The osseous floor of the maxillary sinus is occasionally disrupted during extraction or other surgical procedures, resulting in a focal osseous defect in the maxillary floor. The mucoperiosteum at the antral floor may or may not remain intact.
- May contribute to acute or chronic sinusitis (also see Acute rhinosinusitis and Chronic rhinosinusitis, and refer to Chapter 5), usually ipsilateral, to varying extents. The maxillary sinuses are most commonly affected.
- Oroantral fistula may develop.
- Multidetector computed tomography (MDCT) or cone beam computed tomography (CBCT) are the imaging modalities of choice. MDCT is preferable if there are sinus symptoms.
- 2D radiography is not recommended as maxillary sinus cortical floor defect(s) cannot be excluded, even with multiple views.

Radiological features

- Focal discontinuity of the maxillary sinus cortical floor, usually over the apical aspect of a tooth socket.
- It may be radiologically difficult to identify whether the sinus mucoperiosteal lining over this cortical defect is preserved. Presence of an uninterrupted air channel extending from the oral cavity into the sinus air space through the cortical floor defect reflects an oroantral communication, but absence of this air channel does not exclude this entity.
- Longstanding oroantral communication may result in a chronic oroantral fistula. The established lining is not identified radiologically.
- If there is oroantral communication, there is often eventual secondary inflammatory disease affecting the maxillary sinus and, to a varying extent, the other ipsilateral paranasal sinuses.

Tooth displacement (Figures 19.10 and 19.11)

- During attempted removal of a tooth, a portion of the root may be displaced superiorly into the maxillary sinus, with associated oroantral communication (see Oroantral communication). Rarely, this is associated with trauma, usually severe.
- Tooth or root displacements into the nasal cavity are less common, and are more likely to be related to trauma (intrusive luxation) rather than to extractions.

Radiological features

- Imaging is employed to identify:
  - Presence of a root remnant within the sinus. The tooth root is occasionally displaced into the facial soft tissues rather than into the maxillary sinuses.
  - The precise location of the displaced tooth/root.
  - Location of the oroantral communication.
  - Presence and extent of related sinus disease.
- MDCT or CBCT are the imaging modalities of choice. MDCT is preferable if there are sinus symptoms.
- 2D radiography is not recommended as the presence of a root remnant cannot be fully excluded, the precise location is not well demonstrated, oroantral communication is usually not demonstrated and sinus disease is insufficiently well examined.
- The displaced tooth/root is most commonly seen within the inferior aspect of the maxillary sinus. It may remain submucoperiosteal or may be found freely within the sinus. Longstanding displaced roots are often associated with mucosal thickening.
- There may be associated maxillary sinus inflammatory disease with involvement, to a varying degrees, of the ipsilateral paranasal sinuses.

Differential diagnosis

	Key radiological differences
Any opaque structure within the maxillary sinuses may resemble a displaced tooth/root	The morphology, odontoid densities and presence of root canal(s)/pulp chamber usually clearly differentiate the tooth/root from other opacities. This is usually more difficult with 2D radiography. Examples include osteoma, exostosis, the base of antral septa and calcifications related to chronic inflammatory sinus disease.

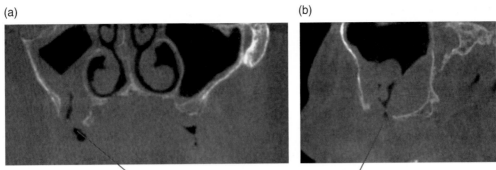

Focal discontinuity of the sinus cortical floor with an air track consistent with oroantral communication. Note the reactive sinus mucosal thickening

Figure 19.7 Postextraction right maxillary oroantral communication with associated reactive mucosal thickening at the sinus floor: coronal (a) and corrected sagittal (b) CBCT images.

Completely opacified sinus due to mucosal thickening and fluid. The ostiomeatal complex is opacified

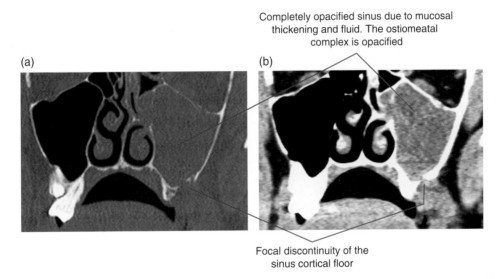

Focal discontinuity of the sinus cortical floor

Figure 19.8 Postextraction left oroantral communication with secondary left maxillary inflammatory disease: coronal bone (a) and soft tissue (b) MDCT images.

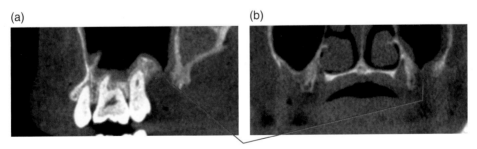

Focal discontinuity of the sinus cortical floor with minimal mucosal thickening. Absence of an air track does not exclude an oroantral communication

Figure 19.9 Postextraction left oroantral communication with minimal reactive mucosal thickening at the sinus base: corrected sagittal (a) and coronal (b) CBCT images.

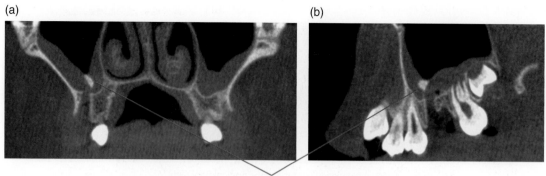

(a) (b)

Root fragment within the sinus, lying within the thickened sinus mucosa.
Note the associated sinus cortical defect at the socket apex

Figure 19.10 Recent displacement of the 16 mesiobuccal root apex into the right maxillary sinus with an associated oroantral defect at the socket apex: coronal (a) and corrected sagittal (b) CBCT images.

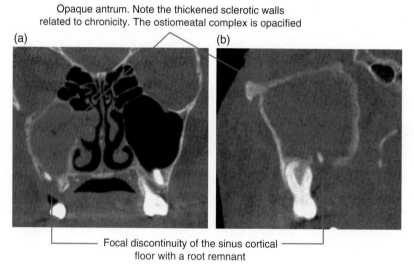

Opaque antrum. Note the thickened sclerotic walls
related to chronicity. The ostiomeatal complex is opacified

(a) (b)

Focal discontinuity of the sinus cortical
floor with a root remnant

Figure 19.11 Right maxillary oroantral communication with the 17 root remnant and associated secondary acute-on-chronic inflammatory sinus disease: coronal (a) and corrected sagittal (b) CBCT images.

Dental implants (Figures 19.12–19.15)

- Maxillary implants may extend through the maxillary sinus or nasal cortical floor and mucoperiosteum into the sinonasal airspace.
  - Often remain disease free, especially those extending into the maxillary sinuses. However, the potential for related sinonasal inflammatory disease requires consideration.
- Sinus floor lift procedures may be required for the placement of posterior maxillary implants. The radiological appearances vary substantially. The sinus lift usually results in a focal prominence(s) at the antral base of variable size, morphology and density depending on the type of procedure and the graft material used.
  - Following the procedure, there may be mild to moderate associated mucosal thickening, which is usually not of clinical significance. Occasionally, these lifts can be infected with associated variable ipsilateral sinus inflammatory changes.
- Severe inflammatory peri-implant bone loss in the posterior maxilla may approach the sinus floor. There is usually sinus reactive mucosal thickening. Occasionally, there is associated focal effacement of the sinus cortical floor.

Periapical osseous healing

- Post-treatment (extraction/enucleation or endodontic therapy) periapical osseous healing at the maxillary sinus floor may sometimes result in a bony prominence, of variable size and morphology, at the maxillary sinus floor. Most commonly seen following treatment for periapical inflammatory lesions (refer to Chapter 5) and radicular cysts (refer to Chapter 8).

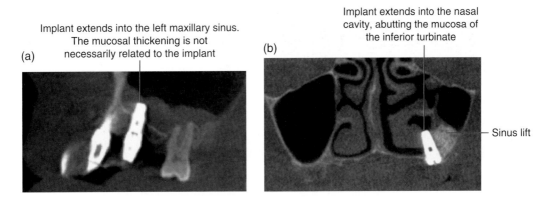

Implant extends into the left maxillary sinus. The mucosal thickening is not necessarily related to the implant

Implant extends into the nasal cavity, abutting the mucosa of the inferior turbinate

Sinus lift

Figure 19.12 Two different cases of an implant extending into the maxillary sinus (a) and nasal cavity (b): corrected sagittal (a) and coronal (b) CBCT images.

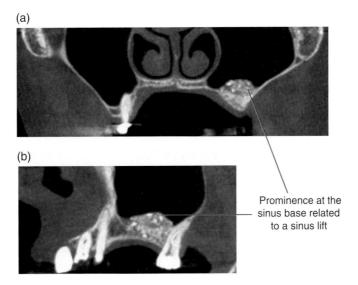

Prominence at the sinus base related to a sinus lift

Figure 19.13 Sinus lift for implant placement at the 26 site. No focal osseous abnormality and clear maxillary sinus: coronal (a) and corrected sagittal (b) CBCT images.

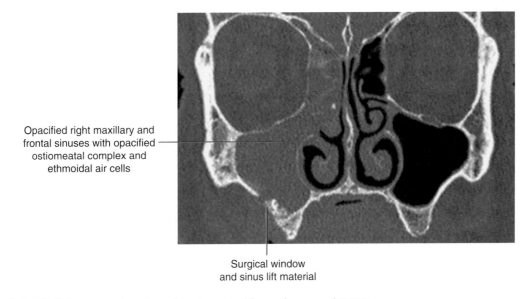

Opacified right maxillary and frontal sinuses with opacified ostiomeatal complex and ethmoidal air cells

Surgical window and sinus lift material

Figure 19.14 Right-sided inflammatory sinus disease following a sinus lift procedure: coronal CBCT image.

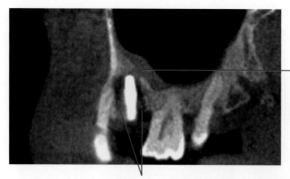

Associated inflammatory focal effacement of the sinus cortical floor with reactive mucosal thickening

Inflammatory mesial and distal peri-implant lucencies extending to the implant apex. Note that varying degrees of peri-implant artefactual lucent appearances are often seen with CBCT and also MDCT – the evaluation of the peri-implant bone may therefore not be possible in some cases. In many cases, it may be difficult to fully exclude peri-implant bone pathology with a width of 1 mm or less with CBCT and MDCT

Figure 19.15 Peri-implantitis of the left maxillary implant: corrected sagittal CBCT image.

19.4 Inflammatory paranasal sinus disease

Paranasal sinus inflammation is common and there are imaging findings that are apparent on dental and orofacial imaging. These may be important to recognise in order to expedite management. Inflammatory disease may be acute or chronic, and specific pathophysiological variants can be particularly virulent, requiring emergency care.

The clinical presentation of pain related to paranasal sinus and dentoalveolar disease may be similar, requiring radiological differentiation. In addition, inflammatory paranasal sinus disease may be secondary to dentoalveolar conditions and procedures (refer to Odontogenic conditions and dentoalveolar lesions and Findings related to dental procedures; also refer to Chapter 5).

Acute rhinosinusitis (Figures 19.16 and 19.17)

- An acute inflammatory condition of the nasal cavity and paranasal sinus mucosa.
- Ethmoid and maxillary sinuses are most commonly affected.
- Patterns of sinus involvement have been described: the infundibular type (isolated maxillary sinus), ostiomeatal complex type (involving the maxillary and ipsilateral adjacent frontal and ethmoid sinuses) and the sphenoethmoidal type (involving the sphenoid sinus, sphenoethmoidal recess and posterior ethmoid air cells). A significant percentage of patients with acute rhinosinusitis do not comfortably 'fit' into only one of these patterns of involvement.
- Viral, allergic or barotrauma-induced inflammation causing mucosal swelling results in ostial obstruction and causes increased mucus production. This may facilitate secondary

bacterial infection (*Streptococcus pneumoniae, Haemophilus influenzae, Moraxella catarrhalis*). Impaired mucociliary drainage is a significant aetiological factor resulting from both increased mucus production and decreased ciliary function.

- Predisposing conditions include structural anatomical alterations (congenital, post-traumatic, neoplastic), allergies, immunoglobulin deficiencies, cystic fibrosis and other conditions of impaired cilial function.
- Children and young adults are most commonly affected, presenting clinically with facial pain, headache, nasal discharge, localised facial swelling and fever.
- Complications reflect locoregional spread of infection, including orbital subperiosteal collection, orbital cellulitis, septic thrombophlebitis and abscess formation, myositis, optic neuritis and ischaemic neuropathy. Osteomyelitis, subdural empyema, meningitis, cerebritis, cerebral venous thrombosis and abscess formation in the brain, skull base or subgaleal (Pott's puffy tumour) tissues may occur.

Radiological features

- Plain radiographs, including panoramic radiographs, may reveal mucosal thickening, sinus opacification or air–fluid levels. However, the advent of low-dose MDCT has rendered plain films obsolete for the assessment of sinonasal disease.
- MDCT is excellent for defining sinus involvement, associated osseous changes and regional complications. The density of sinus content, drainage pathway patency and osseous integrity can be assessed. Contrast may be useful if complications are suspected. MDCT is often utilised in severe or refractory infections but may be used to exclude sinus involvement in assumed allergic rhinitis.

- CBCT may be sufficient in some less complex cases. However, the internal densities within the paranasal sinuses and soft tissue changes are not well demonstrated with CBCT. In addition, some CBCT units may not demonstrate fine bony structures or subtle osseous changes.
- Imaging assessment should always extend to include the maxillary dentition to exclude odontogenic-related sinusitis.
- Focal bone rarefaction or dehiscence may be evident.
- Magnetic resonance imaging (MRI) will optimally characterise suspected complications. Inflammatory secretions are usually of simple fluid signal, hypo- and hyperintense on T1- and T2-weighted imaging, respectively, but may present as the converse when secretions are inspissated and/or highly proteinaceous. Inflammatory mucosal thickening is T2 hyperintense and will show avid enhancement. If additional soft tissue components enhance, alternative inflammatory and neoplastic diseases should be considered.

Differential diagnosis

	Key radiological differences
Trauma	Associated bone fractures, evidence of surgery.

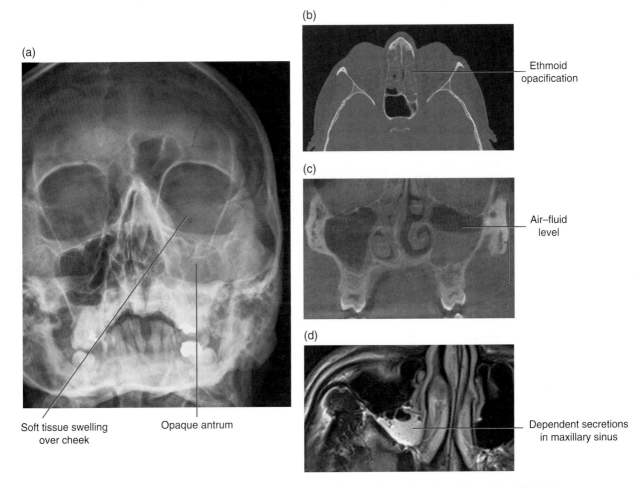

Figure 19.16 Acute inflammatory disease: frontal radiograph (a), axial MDCT (b), coronal CBCT (c) and axial T2-weighted MRI (d) images.

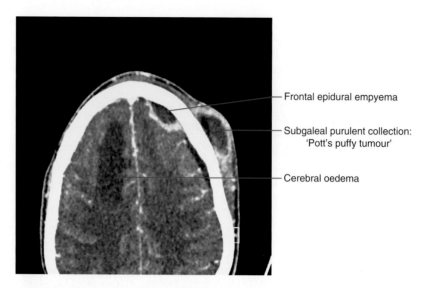

Frontal epidural empyema

Subgaleal purulent collection: 'Pott's puffy tumour'

Cerebral oedema

Figure 19.17 Acute frontal sinusitis – complications: axial contrast-enhanced MDCT image.

Chronic rhinosinusitis (Figure 19.18)

- An inflammatory condition of the paranasal sinuses and nasal cavity lasting 12 weeks or longer.
- May be categorised into several aetiological subtypes: infective, allergic and allergic fungal.
- Multiple pathophysiological factors play a role in this condition, including immunocompetence, pre-existing conditions such as cystic fibrosis, dental disease, sinonasal anatomical variations and environmental factors (microbiological and industrial).
- Nasal discharge and obstruction, anosmia, headache and facial pain are common clinical symptoms reflecting frequent ethmoid air-cell and maxillary sinus involvement.

Radiological features

- Imaging features are similar to those seen in acute rhinosinusitis. However, on plain radiography and MDCT/CBCT, the sinuses, particularly the maxillary sinus, may be reduced in size with associated marginal sclerosis and thickening of sinus walls.
- MDCT or CBCT may additionally reveal lobulated or polypoidal mucosa.

- MRI is usually only indicated for complicated disease, particularly if there is suspicion of an underlying obstructing mass lesion contributing to a recognisable pattern of sinus involvement.

Differential diagnosis

	Key radiological differences
Sinonasal mycetoma	Focal sinus changes, hyperdense low T2 signal sinus contents, no bone destruction.
Allergic fungal sinusitis	Multifocal sinus changes, hyperdense low T2 signal sinus contents, expansile, osseous remodelling.
Fungal sinusitis (invasive)	Bone destruction, hyperdense low T2 signal sinus contents, extrasinus involvement.
Sinonasal polyposis	Multifocal, lobulated mucosal thickening.
Granulomatous disease	Multifocal, lobulated mucosal thickening, septal loss.
Sinonasal tumour	Bone destruction, focal soft tissue lesion, sinus obstruction.

(a)

Retracted anterior and posterolateral maxillary sinus walls

Increased retroantral fat

Orbital floor depression, increased intraorbital fat, hypoglobus

(b)

Small, contracted sinus

Figure 19.18 Silent sinus syndrome: axial (a) and coronal (b) MDCT images.

Silent sinus syndrome (Figure 19.18)

- Painless volume reduction of the maxillary sinus, secondary to chronic infundibular obstruction.
- Mucus stagnation, wall thinning and negative internal pressure are postulated to cause antral wall retraction.
- Clinically there is enophthalmos, hypoglobus, diplopia and facial asymmetry.

Radiological features

- Unilateral completely opacified small maxillary sinus, with depression of the orbital floor, ipsilateral increased orbital volume, inward bowing of the posterolateral sinus wall and prominent retroantral fat pad can be seen on MDCT.
- The uncinate process, medial wall of the maxilla and the middle turbinate may be lateralised and there may be nasal septal bowing.
- CBCT usually demonstrates most of these bony changes.

Differential diagnosis

	Key radiological differences
Maxillary sinus hypoplasia	The antrum is incompletely pneumatised, and in particular the sinus has not pneumatised the maxillary alveolus, which will be asymmetrically increased in craniocaudal depth.
Iatrogenic/ post surgery	Relevant clinical history.
Trauma	Relevant clinical history, fractures.

Mucous retention cysts (Figure 19.19)

- The vast majority are postinflammatory lesions that arise secondary to sinomucinous gland obstruction within the paranasal sinuses. Often incidentally identified on dentofacial imaging, not requiring treatment. Occasionally they are reactive, related to a maxillary posterior dentoalveolar inflammatory lesion.
- Generally small, rounded and well circumscribed at the maxillary sinus floor.

Radiological features

- Typically dome shaped and usually uniformly low attenuating lesions on MDCT. Low T1 and high T2 signal on MRI. CBCT demonstrates the typical morphology.
- Longstanding lesions containing inspissated fluid may develop the converse in MRI signal characteristics.
- Osseous integrity of the sinus floor is preserved.

Differential diagnosis

	Key radiological differences
Sinonasal tumour (juvenile angiofibroma, inverting papilloma)	Bone destruction/remodelling, focal soft tissue mass lesion, sinus obstruction.
Sinonasal mucocele	Osseous expansion of an entire sinus cavity.
Small solitary polyps	Arising from the floor of the maxillary sinus; can be difficult to differentiate.
Odontogenic cyst from the maxillary alveolar process	Presence of a calcified rim superior to the antral opacification represents the elevated cortex of the maxillary dental arch, confirming the lytic expansile lesion to be of odontogenic aetiology.

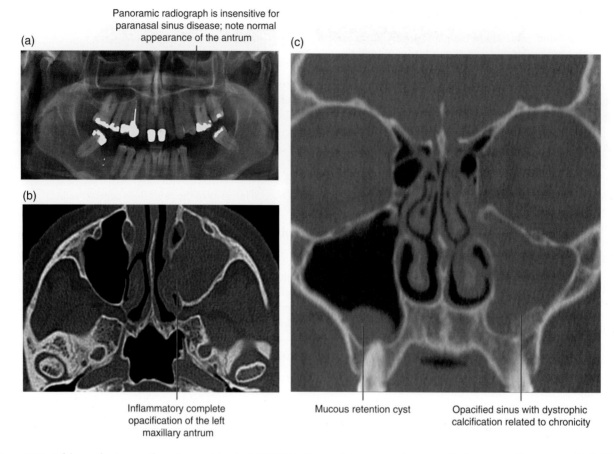

Figure 19.19 Left 'opaque' antrum: orthopantogram (a) and axial MDCT (b) images. Mucous retention cyst and inflammatory disease: coronal MDCT magnetic proton recoil image (c).

Sinonasal mucoceles (Figure 19.20)

- Expanded sinus cavity filled with accumulated mucus secondary to chronic major ostial obstruction.
- Approximately two-thirds of mucoceles arise in the frontal sinus with the remaining sinuses equally represented amongst the remaining one-third.
- Clinical presentation depends on the involved sinus, for example mucoceles of the frontal sinus commonly present with cosmetic deformity and orbital symptoms.
- Predisposing factors include previous trauma and sinus surgery, chronic rhinosinusitis, cranial dysplasias as well as sinonasal manifestations of systemic disease such as cystic fibrosis.
- Complications may arise secondary to regional mass effect on the brain or orbit.

Radiological features

- MDCT demonstrates the key feature of expansile remodelling of the osseous sinus walls: hypodense content (high attenuation if material is inspissated or superinfected with fungus), mild peripheral contrast enhancement unless infected when the marginal enhancement is usually thick. These features are not appreciated on CBCT.
- No central enhancement, which when present would raise the possibility of an underlying neoplasm.

- Lesions often bow into the orbit and cranial cavity, exhibiting variable mass effect.
- On MRI, mucoceles exhibit variable signal as a result of the protein content, hydration and degree of inspissation.

Differential diagnosis

	Key radiological differences
Sinonasal tumours (juvenile angiofibroma, inverting papilloma)	Bone destruction/moulding, focal soft tissue lesion, sinus obstruction.
Sinonasal lymphoma	Nasal location more common than sinus, diffusion restriction.
Retention cysts	Retention cysts, well defined, non-enhancing, isolated and confined to the sinus of origin.
Cephalocele	Communication with the subarachnoid space, may contain meninges or brain parenchyma.
Allergic fungal sinusitis	Multifocal sinus changes, hyperdense low T2 signal sinus contents, bone thinning with expansile, osseous remodelling.

(a)   (b)

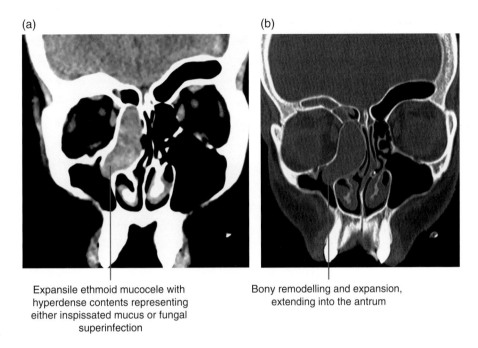

Expansile ethmoid mucocele with hyperdense contents representing either inspissated mucus or fungal superinfection

Bony remodelling and expansion, extending into the antrum

Figure 19.20 Ethmoid mucocele: coronal soft tissue (a) and bone (b) MDCT images.

Fungal rhinosinusitis

Infection of the nasal cavity and paranasal sinuses can take different forms (e.g. allergic and invasive), often on the basis of a pre-existing or coincidental condition.

Allergic fungal rhinosinusitis (Figure 19.21)

- Non-invasive chronic rhinosinusitis is caused by the presence of an infective fungal agent and a type 1 immunoglobulin E-mediated hypersensitivity reaction to fungal antigens.
- Multiple paranasal sinuses are usually involved bilaterally and asymmetrically, the ethmoid and maxillary sinuses most commonly.
- Patients present with symptoms of chronic rhinosinusitis, have an intact immune system but often an atopic history.
- Major diagnostic criteria (Bent and Kuhn) include eosinophilic mucin and a positive fungal stain as well as the imaging characteristics listed below.

Radiological features
- MDCT demonstrates centrally non-enhancing, hyperdense material within the sinus surrounded peripherally by thickened relatively low-attenuation, often polypoidal and contrast-enhancing mucosa. These features are usually not sufficiently well demonstrated with CBCT.
- Mucoperiosteal thickening, sinus expansion, bone attenuation and remodelling may be present.
- Low T2 and mixed T1 signal material is seen on MRI, located centrally in the sinus indicating relatively proteinaceous content, fungal elements and/or inspissated material.

Differential diagnosis

	Key radiological differences
Chronic rhinosinusitis	Mucoperiosteal thickening, no sinus expansion.
Sinonasal polyposis	Multifocal, lobulated mucosal thickening.
Sinonasal tumour	Bone destruction, focal soft tissue mass, sinus obstruction.
Sinonasal mycetoma	Hyperdense on computed tomography (CT); hypointense T2 signal on MRI.

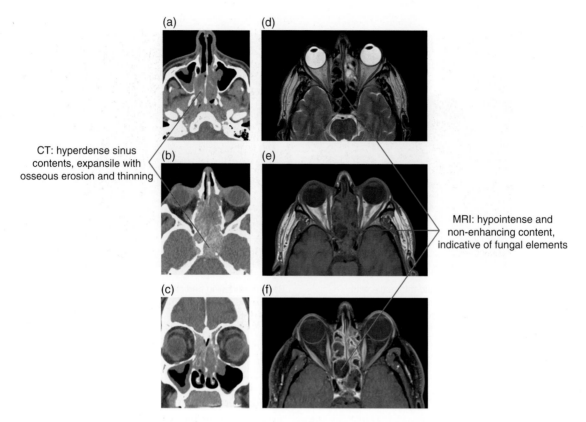

CT: hyperdense sinus contents, expansile with osseous erosion and thinning

MRI: hypointense and non-enhancing content, indicative of fungal elements

Figure 19.21 Allergic fungal sinusitis. Axial (a,b) and coronal (c) MDCT images; axial T2-weighted MRI (d), axial T1-weighted MRI (e) and fat-saturated gadolinium-enhanced axial T1-weighted MRI (f) images.

Sinonasal mycetoma (Figure 19.22)
- Non-invasive saprophytic fungal (usually *Aspergillus*) growth forming a 'ball' of tightly packed hyphae.
- More commonly seen in middle-aged women; patients are often immunocompetent and non-atopic.

Radiological features
- MDCT reveals a single sinus cavity (usually maxillary) filled with hyperdense material, with punctate or linear calcifications within the matrix. The variable attenuation characteristics of the sinus contents are not usually appreciated on CBCT and subtle calcifications may not be demonstrated.
- May be mildly expansile and co-exist within a mucocele. However, the osseous margins may be thinned, or sclerotic and thickened.

- MRI reveals a non-enhancing hypointense mass on both T1- and T2-weighted imaging; however, the signal characteristics may change depending on the water and protein content.

Differential diagnosis

	Key radiological differences
Chronic rhinosinusitis	Mucoperiosteal thickening, no sinus expansion.
Sinonasal polyposis	Multifocal, lobulated mucosal thickening.
Sinonasal tumour	Bone destruction, focal soft tissue mass, sinus obstruction.
Fungal sinusitis (allergic/invasive)	Bone destruction, hyperdense low T2 signal sinus contents, extrasinus involvement.

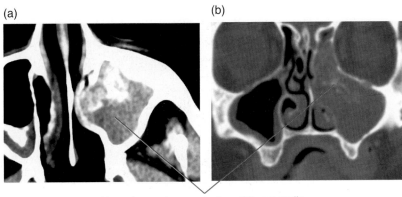

Hyperdense sinus contents, mildly expansile
with osseous erosion and thinning

Figure 19.22 Sinonasal mycetoma: axial soft tissue (a) and coronal bone (b) MDCT magnetic proton recoil images.

Invasive fungal rhinosinusitis (Figure 19.23)

- Aggressive and often rapidly fatal acute angioinvasive fungal infection usually presenting in an immunocompromised patient, although occasionally occurring in the immunocompetent.
- Patients at risk include those receiving chemotherapy or glucocorticoids; clinical scenarios include coexisting malignancy, post bone marrow transplantation, HIV infection and diabetes.
- Characteristic rapid locoregional spread, with angioinvasive pathophysiology, involving the sinonasal mucosa and bone, orbits, intracranial compartment, cavernous sinuses and deep spaces of the upper neck.
- Extensive trans-spatial phlegmon, necrosis and abscess formation results.
- Clinical presentation includes headache, pain, fever, orbital symptoms, cranial neuropathies and a destructive process arising from the paranasal sinuses.

Radiological features

- Identification of subtle early imaging findings is critical and potentially life-saving.
- Hallmark early features include:
  - Necrotic, non-enhancing sinonasal mucosa, with otherwise relatively benign-appearing inflammatory changes.
  - Inflammatory changes involving regional spaces, particularly the retroantral fat, orbits.
  - Early destructive bony changes involving the turbinates and sinus walls.
  - Hyperdense sinus material on CT and mixed signal T1/low T2 material on MRI.
- Late imaging findings include intracranial spread, with cerebritis, arterial infarction, arterial mycotic pseudo-aneurysm formation and septic thrombophlebitis.

Differential diagnosis

	Key radiological differences
Chronic rhinosinusitis	Mucoperiosteal thickening, no sinus expansion.
Sinonasal polyposis	Multifocal, lobulated mucosal thickening.
Sinonasal tumour	Bone destruction, focal soft tissue mass, sinus obstruction.
Allergic fungal sinusitis	Multifocal sinus changes, hyperdense low T2 signal sinus contents, no bone destruction but expansile, osseous remodelling.
Granulomatous disease	Multifocal, lobulated mucosal thickening, septal loss.
Sinonasal lymphoma	Nasal location more common than sinus, diffusion restriction.

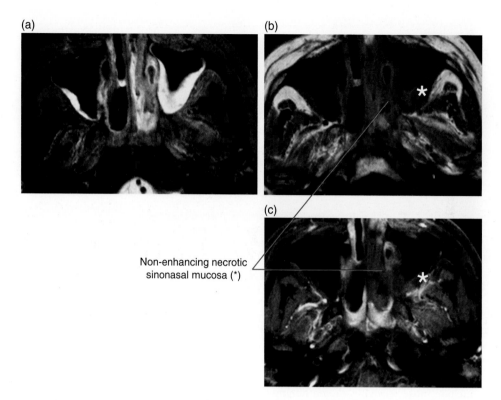

(a)

(b)

(c)

Non-enhancing necrotic
sinonasal mucosa (*)

Figure 19.23 Acute invasive fungal sinusitis: axial fat-saturated T2-weighted (a), axial T1-weighted (b) and axial fat-saturated gadolinium-enhanced T1-weighted MRI (c) images. Asterisks indicate abnormal signal and enhancement in the retroantral fat.

Sinonasal polyposis (Figure 19.24)

- A condition of multifocal inflammatory polypoid swellings of the paranasal sinus and nasal mucosa.
- Most commonly associated with allergic paranasal sinusitis but can result from localised chronic inflammatory mucosal hypertrophy and present as a solitary lesion.

Radiological features

- MDCT studies demonstrate mucoid or soft tissue attenuation mucosal lobulations, which can be associated with bony remodelling, mild erosion and rarefaction.
- Polypoid lesions may be hyperattenuating on MDCT, reflecting proteinaceous or inspissated content, or fungal superinfection. This is usually not appreciated on CBCT.
- Calcific bodies can be present.
- Following contrast administration, the polyps demonstrate only peripheral contrast enhancement.

- On MRI, the polypoid structures are of mixed signal, reflecting the protein content and degree of hydration.

Differential diagnosis

	Key radiological differences
Sinonasal tumour	Bone destruction, focal soft tissue lesion, sinus obstruction.
Allergic fungal sinusitis	Multifocal sinus changes, hyperdense low T2 signal sinus contents, no bone destruction but expansile, osseous remodelling.
Granulomatous disease	Multifocal, lobulated mucosal thickening, septal loss.
Retention cysts	Well defined, non-enhancing, isolated.
Topical decongestion use	Corrugated appearance of the nasal mucosa.

(a)   (b)   (c)

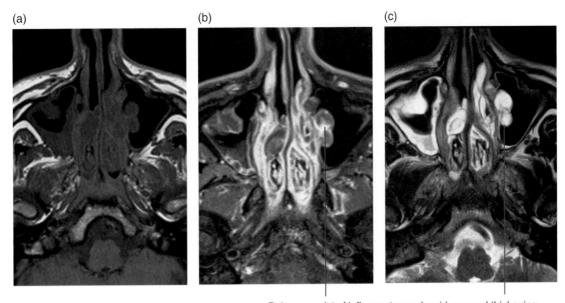

Polyps consist of inflammatory polypoid mucosal thickening,
with peripheral enhancement and hyperintense T2 signal

Figure 19.24 Sinonasal polyposis: axial T1-weighted (a), fat-saturated gadolinium-enhanced T1-weighted (b) and axial T2-weighted MRI (c) images.

Antrochoanal polyps (Figure 19.25)

- Inflammatory polyps which arise in the maxillary antrum but traverse and widen the maxillary or accessory ostium.
- Commonly extend through the posterior choanae to the naso-pharyngeal airway, presenting as a large dumbbell-shaped mass.

Radiological features

- May thin adjacent bone and demonstrate mild peripheral enhancement.
- No central enhancement; if so, a solid neoplasm should be considered.

Differential diagnosis

	Key radiological differences
Sinonasal tumour (juvenile angiofibroma, inverting papilloma)	Bone destruction/moulding, focal soft tissue lesion, sinus obstruction.
Sinonasal mucocele	Focal sinus changes, hyperdense low T2 signal sinus contents, bone expansion.
Granulomatous disease	Multifocal, lobulated mucosal thickening, septal loss.
Sinonasal lymphoma	Nasal location more common than sinus, diffusion restriction.
Retention cysts	Retention cysts, well defined, non-enhancing, isolated and confined to the sinus of origin.
Cephalocele	Communication with the subarachnoid space, may contain meninges or brain parenchyma.

Granulomatous sinonasal inflammatory disease

- Can have a number of different causes.

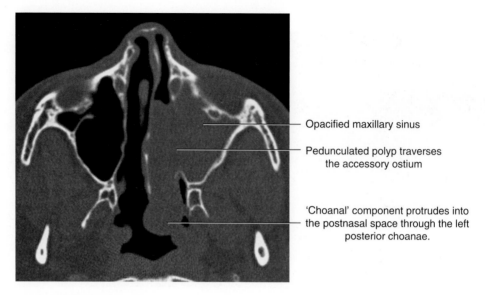

Opacified maxillary sinus

Pedunculated polyp traverses the accessory ostium

'Choanal' component protrudes into the postnasal space through the left posterior choanae.

Figure 19.25 Antrochoanal polyp: axial MDCT image.

Granulomatosis with polyangiitis (previously known as Wegener granulomatosis) (Figure 19.26)

- An idiopathic systemic necrotising vasculitis with granuloma formation.
- Particularly affects the upper and lower respiratory tracts, kidneys, skin and joints.
- Patients classically present with nodular nasal soft tissue with associated septal perforation.
- Non-septal sinonasal bone destruction (turbinates, lateral walls, sinuses) may be seen, with invasion into adjacent tissues, most commonly the orbit.
- Associated with chronic inflammatory sinus change.
- Additional satellite mucosal involvement can be seen in the nasopharynx, subglottic larynx, oral cavity, temporal bone and salivary glands.

Radiological features

- MDCT demonstrates nodular mucosa with extensive, usually bilaterally asymmetric, bone destruction/demineralisation including loss of the nasal septum, which may involve the hard palate (which may result in an oronasal or oroantral fistula).
- Associated infiltration of soft tissues in the periantral regions, orbits, deep spaces of the head and neck and also the cranial cavity.

- On MRI, T2 hypointense nodular masses within T2 hyperintense inflamed mucosa which avidly and homogeneously enhances with contrast administration.

Differential diagnosis

	Key radiological differences
Nasal cocaine necrosis	Social history, localised septal dehiscence without lobulated sinus mucosal thickening.
Allergic fungal sinusitis	Multifocal sinus changes, hyperdense low T2 signal sinus contents, no bone destruction but expansile, osseous remodelling.
Fungal sinusitis (invasive)	Bone destruction, hyperdense low T2 signal sinus contents, extrasinus involvement.
Malignancy	Bone destruction, focal soft tissue lesion, sinus obstruction.
Sinonasal lymphoma	Nasal location more common than sinus, diffusion restriction on MRI.

Sarcoidosis

- Has an identical appearance to granulomatosis with polyangiitis; however, the sinonasal region is less commonly involved.

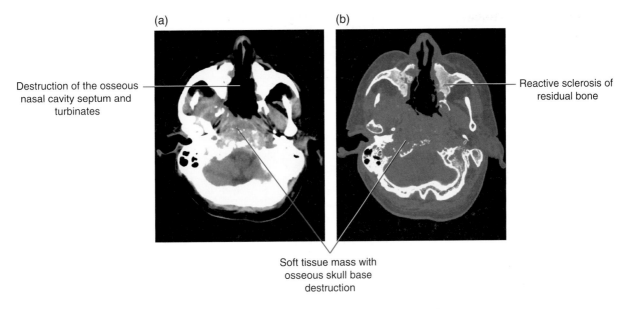

Destruction of the osseous nasal cavity septum and turbinates

Reactive sclerosis of residual bone

Soft tissue mass with osseous skull base destruction

Figure 19.26 Granulomatosis with polyangiitis (Wegener granulomatosis): axial soft tissue (a) and bone (b) MDCT images.

Nasal cocaine necrosis (Figure 19.27)

- Associated with cocaine misuse.

Radiological features

- A characteristic perforation of the osteocartilaginous nasal septum is present, which can involve the turbinates and palate without a significant soft tissue mass. This most frequently affects the quadrangular cartilage and, to a lesser extent, the vomer and perpendicular ethmoid lamina.

Differential diagnosis

Key radiological differences

Granulomatosis with polyangiitis	No social history, sinonasal polypoidal mucosal thickening with associated bone destruction.
Fungal sinusitis (invasive)	Bone destruction, hyperdense low T2 signal sinus contents, extrasinus involvement.
Malignancy	Bone destruction, focal soft tissue lesion, sinus obstruction.
Sinonasal lymphoma	Nasal location more common than sinus, diffusion restriction on MRI.

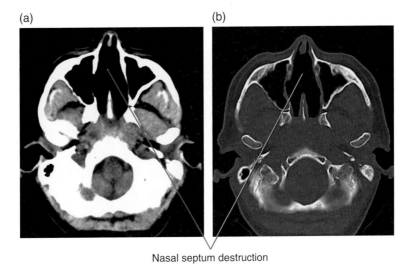

Nasal septum destruction

Figure 19.27 Nasal cocaine necrosis: axial soft tissue (a) and bone (b) MDCT images.

19.5 Neoplastic disease

Benign tumours

Juvenile angiofibroma (Figure 19.28)

- A benign highly vascular hamartoma arising from the posterior nasal cavity in the region of the sphenopalatine foramen, which is typically widened by the mass.
- Clinically, a lesion of adolescent males presenting with nasal obstruction and/or epistaxis.
- Morphologically usually a well circumscribed, moderately large mass at diagnosis within the posterior nasal cavity; with extension into the nasopharynx, pterygopalatine fossa, sphenoid and maxillary sinuses, infratemporal fossa/masticator space, inferior orbital fissure and middle cranial fossa.

Radiological features

- Lateral plain radiographs, including the panoramic radiograph, and CBCT demonstrate anterior displacement of the posterior maxillary antral wall, termed the 'bow sign', as well as sinus opacification.
- On MDCT, the juvenile angiofibroma is a diffuse, intensely contrast-enhancing soft tissue mass centred on the sphenopalatine foramen causing nasal and sinus obstruction and with associated bony erosion and remodelling.
- MRI reveals a mixed signal mass on T1- and T2-weighted imaging with avid contrast enhancement and associated intralesional signal voids.
- Angiography, including CT and magnetic resonance angiography, demonstrates enlargement of the ipsilateral internal maxillary and external carotid arteries. Catheter angiography reveals an intense tumour blush with supply from the internal maxillary and ascending pharyngeal branches of the external carotid artery, and is often performed prior to surgery with a view to preoperative embolisation.

Differential diagnosis

	Key radiological differences
Antrochoanal polyp	Homogeneous contiguous antronasal lesion, ostial expansion.
Inverting papilloma	Lateral nasal wall mass, cerebriform contrast-enhancing pattern, sinus obstruction.
Nasal haemangioma	Avidly enhancing nasal septal lesion.
Nasal haemangiopericytoma	Avidly enhancing, flow voids, bone destruction, nasal cavity.
Rhabdomyosarcoma	Destructive mass: orbit, paranasal sinuses, nasopharynx, parapharyngeal spaces.
Cephalocele	Communication with the subarachnoid space, may contain meninges or brain parenchyma.

Sinus osteoma (see Figure 10.28)

- Benign, slow-growing neoplasm consisting of new bone formation.
- Can obstruct the sinus and cause mucoceles, trans-spatial infections and fistulae to form.
- Subtypes include lesions composed of dense 'ivory' cortical bone or more lucent 'spongiose' cancellous (marrow containing) bone.
- Multiple osteomata are seen in Gardner syndrome.

Radiological features

- MDCT and CBCT: well-demarcated, homogeneous, rounded or sessile lesions, most commonly seen in the frontal and ethmoid sinuses.

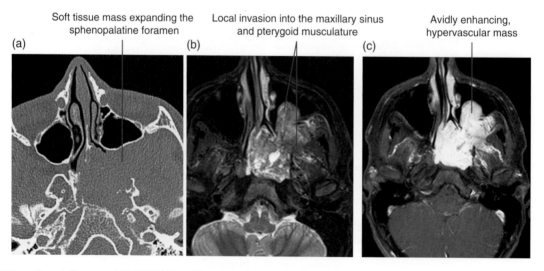

Soft tissue mass expanding the sphenopalatine foramen   (a)

Local invasion into the maxillary sinus and pterygoid musculature   (b)

Avidly enhancing, hypervascular mass   (c)

Figure 19.28 Juvenile angiofibroma: axial MDCT (a), axial fat-saturated T2-weighted (b) and axial fat-saturated gadolinium-enhanced T1-weighted MRI (c) images.

- Dense cortical bone or 'spongiform' cancellous bone.
- MRI signal and enhancement may be complex, and appear aggressive, depending on the relative component of cancellous, enhancing bone.

Differential diagnosis

	Key radiological differences
Fibrous dysplasia	Ground-glass matrix.
Exostosis	Ossified, cauliflower-like protuberant lesion.
Fungal sinusitis (allergic/invasive)	Bone destruction, hyperdense low T2 signal sinus contents, extrasinus involvement.
Ossifying fibroma	Calcified soft tissue mass encased by bony rim.
Osteosarcoma	Destructive soft tissue mass with ossified components.

Sinonasal inverting papilloma (Figure 19.29)

- A benign but locally aggressive squamous epithelial neoplasm.
- Arises from the region of the middle meatus and lateral wall of the nose.
- Affects middle-aged men with non-specific symptoms of nasal obstruction and discharge.
- May present as a small polypoid lesion or large destructive mass with extension into the maxillary antrum and nasal cavity, as well as other adjacent paranasal sinuses, the orbit and into the cranial cavity. An 'ostiomeatal unit' obstruction pattern secondary to middle meatus involvement may also be seen.
- 10% of lesions degenerate into a squamous cell carcinoma (SCCa) or have a coexisting intralesional SCCa.

Radiological features

- Presents as a soft tissue lobulated mass on MDCT.
- Focal hyperostosis/sclerosis may be seen at the point of osseous attachment, but often causes expansile bony remodelling.

- If aggressive bony destruction is present, an intrinsic SCCa should be considered.
- MRI sequences demonstrate a lesion of mixed signal.
- Contrast-enhanced studies help to define tumour from retained secretions secondary to ostial obstruction and the lesion itself may exhibit a characteristic folded ('cerebriform') appearance, although this is a non-specific finding.

Differential diagnosis

	Key radiological differences
Antrochoanal polyp	Homogeneous contiguous antronasal lesion, ostial expansion.
Sinonasal polyposis	Multifocal lobulated mucosal thickening.
Juvenile angiofibroma	Avidly enhancing, sphenopalatine foramen, flow voids.
Sinonasal malignancy	Bone destruction, focal soft tissue lesion, sinus obstruction.

Sinonasal cancers

These cancers comprise a range of malignant tumours that arise from the nasal cavity and paranasal sinuses. The clinical presentation is classically of indolent, chronic symptoms which may include nasal obstruction, localised pain and epistaxis. Histological subtypes include SCCa, adenocarcinoma, adenoid cystic carcinoma, esthesioneuroblastoma (olfactory neuroblastoma), sinonasal undifferentiated carcinoma, melanoma and lymphoma.

The radiological features of sinonasal malignancy on CT and MRI are non-specific and are those of an aggressive and expansile soft tissue mass, with locoregional invasion and sinus obstruction. Although there are imaging findings which may suggest a malignant subtype, there are no CT or MRI features which will reliably predict histology.

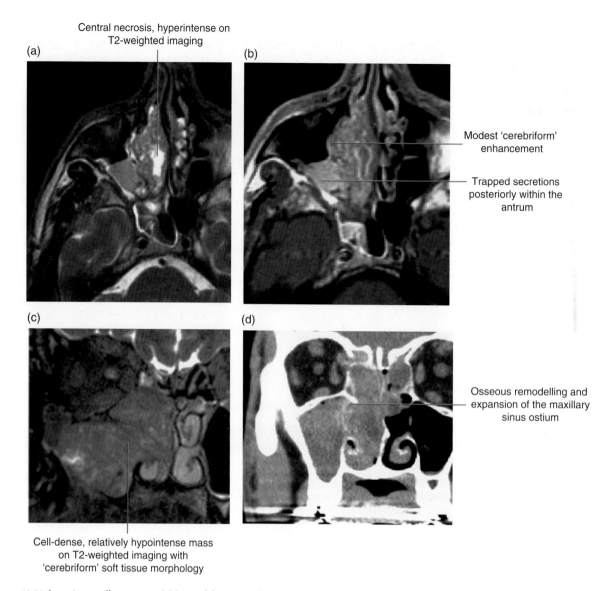

Figure 19.29 Inverting papilloma, *in situ* SCCa: axial fat-saturated T2-weighted MRI (a), axial fat-saturated gadolinium-enhanced T1-weighted MRI (b), coronal fat-saturated T2-weighted MRI (c) and coronal MDCT (d) images.

Sinonasal SCCa (Figures 19.30 and 19.31; see also Figure 11.1)

- The most common sinonasal cancer, constituting two-thirds of malignant lesions, with the majority arising from the maxillary sinus.

Radiological features

- MDCT demonstrates a solid contrast-enhancing mass with bone destruction. The bony destruction is demonstrated with CBCT.
- On MRI the lesion is intermediate to low T2-weighted signal intensity secondary to the relatively cell-dense neoplastic tissue with mild heterogeneous contrast enhancement.
- Approximately 10–20% of maxillary lesions have nodal involvement at diagnosis, mainly at the retropharyngeal and level 2 stations.

Differential diagnosis

	Key radiological differences
Fungal sinusitis (invasive)	Bone destruction, hyperdense low T2 signal sinus contents, extrasinus involvement.
Granulomatosis with polyangiitis	Multifocal lobulated mucosal thickening, septal loss.
Sinonasal lymphoma	Nasal location more common than sinus, diffusion restriction on MRI.
Melanoma	Variable T1, low T2 signal, may be haemorrhagic.

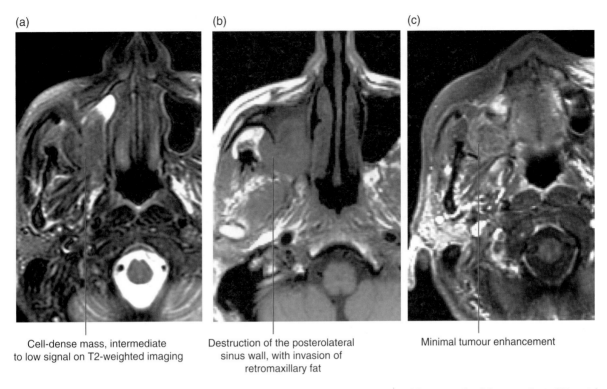

(a) Cell-dense mass, intermediate to low signal on T2-weighted imaging

(b) Destruction of the posterolateral sinus wall, with invasion of retromaxillary fat

(c) Minimal tumour enhancement

Figure 19.30 Maxillary sinus SCCa: axial fat-saturated T2-weighted (a), axial T1-weighted (b) and axial fat-saturated gadolinium-enhanced T1-weighted MRI (c) images.

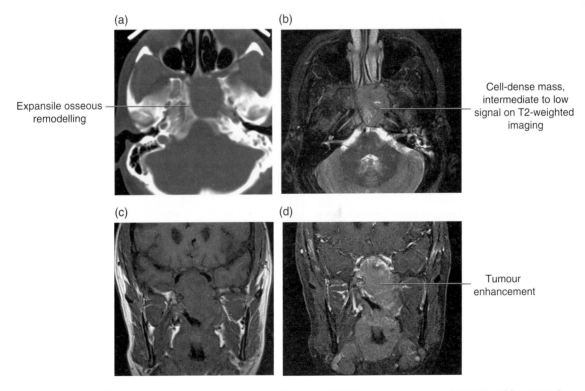

(a) Expansile osseous remodelling

(b) Cell-dense mass, intermediate to low signal on T2-weighted imaging

(c)

(d) Tumour enhancement

Figure 19.31 Sphenoid sinus SCCa: axial MDCT (a), axial fat-saturated T2-weighted MRI (b), coronal T1-weighted MRI (c) and fat-saturated gadolinium-enhanced coronal T1-weighted MRI (d) images.

Sinonasal adenocarcinoma (Figure 19.32)

- An epithelial neoplasm arising from the sinonasal mucosa.
- Most commonly seen in the ethmoid sinus, associated with industrial wood dust and leather exposure.

Radiological features

- With variable histology from well to poorly differentiated, the lesions are of mixed T2 signal and moderately enhance.
- Rarely involve lymph nodes at diagnosis.

Differential diagnosis

	Key radiological differences
SCCa	Destructive maxillary tumour.
Sinonasal undifferentiated carcinoma	Large destructive ethmoid and sphenoid mass, perineural spread.
Esthesioneuroblastoma	Enhancing, ethmoid/anterior cranial fossa mass, cysts at the tumour–brain interface.

Fungal sinusitis (invasive)	Bone destruction, hyperdense low T2 signal sinus contents, extrasinus involvement.

Minor salivary gland adenoid cystic carcinoma

- Grows insidiously.
- When small, this may be easily mistaken for benign inflammation of the sinuses and therefore often presents when advanced.
- With a propensity for perineural invasion, lesions often have positive surgical margins and are commonly recurrent.

Sinonasal undifferentiated carcinoma

- An aggressive and usually large paranasal sinus neoplasm.
- Rapidly progressive with extensive local, including bone, invasion, involving the orbits and intracranial structures, with perineural spread.
- High percentage of local and distant metastases at diagnosis.

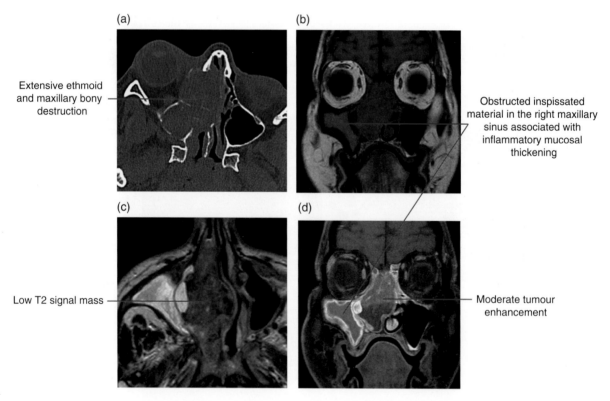

Extensive ethmoid and maxillary bony destruction

Obstructed inspissated material in the right maxillary sinus associated with inflammatory mucosal thickening

Low T2 signal mass

Moderate tumour enhancement

Figure 19.32 Ethmoid adenocarcinoma: axial MDCT (a), axial fat-saturated T2-weighted MRI (b), coronal T1-weighted MRI (c) and coronal fat-saturated gadolinium-enhanced T1-weighted MRI (d) images.

Esthesioneuroblastoma or olfactory neuroblastoma
(Figure 19.33)

- A malignant neuroectodermal tumour arising from the olfactory mucosa in the superior nasal cavity in the region of the cribriform plate.
- More commonly seen in males, the tumour has a bimodal age distribution at the second and sixth decades with epistaxis, anosmia and obstructive symptoms.
- Ectopic lesions can be found in the inferior meatus, intracranially and within the pituitary fossa.
- Metastatic spread is present in approximately one-third at diagnosis.
- Occasionally lesions are associated with paraneoplastic hyponatraemia (excessive antidiuretic hormone secretion) or Cushing syndrome (excessive adrenocorticotropic hormone secretion).

Radiological features
- Morphologically the lesion is dumbbell shaped as a result of 'waisting' at the cribriform plate, which is focally destroyed; well demonstrated on MDCT.
- MRI; intermediate to hypointense on T1-weighted imaging and hyperintense on T2, enhancing prominently following contrast administration.
- The lesion may contain haemorrhagic foci and demonstrate cysts at the tumour–brain interface.

Differential diagnosis

	Key radiological differences
Sinonasal malignancy	Bone destruction, focal soft tissue lesion, sinus obstruction.
Sinonasal lymphoma	Nasal location more common than sinus, diffusion restriction on MRI.
Meningioma	Transosseous, enhancing, osteodural thickening.
Olfactory schwannoma	Anterior cranial fossa, extending into ethmoid sinuses, contrast enhancing.
Melanoma	Variable T1, low T2 signal, may be haemorrhagic.

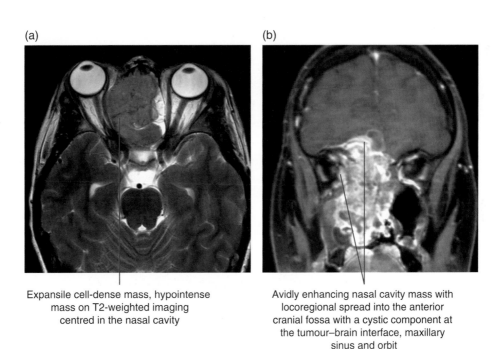

(a)

(b)

Expansile cell-dense mass, hypointense mass on T2-weighted imaging centred in the nasal cavity

Avidly enhancing nasal cavity mass with locoregional spread into the anterior cranial fossa with a cystic component at the tumour–brain interface, maxillary sinus and orbit

Figure 19.33 Esthesioneuroblastoma: axial T2-weighted (a) and coronal fat-saturated gadolinium-enhanced T1-weighted MRI (b) images.

Lymphoma (Figure 19.34)
- More common in the nasal cavity than in the sinuses.

Radiological features
- The appearance is similar to other neoplasms but hyperattenuating on MDCT and of low signal on T2-weighted imaging owing to the cellular high nuclear-to-cytoplasmic ratio.
- Homogeneous contrast enhancement is seen in the majority.
- May be associated with permeative bone infiltrative changes, remodelling and destruction, which can be demonstrated with CBCT.

Differential diagnosis

	Key radiological differences
Sinonasal granulomatous disease	Multifocal, lobulated mucosal thickening, septal loss.
SCCa	Destructive maxillary tumour.
Esthesioneuroblastoma	Enhancing, ethmoid/anterior cranial fossa mass, cysts at the tumour–brain interface.
Metastases	Destructive tumour, known primary.
Melanoma	Variable T1, low T2 signal, may be haemorrhagic.

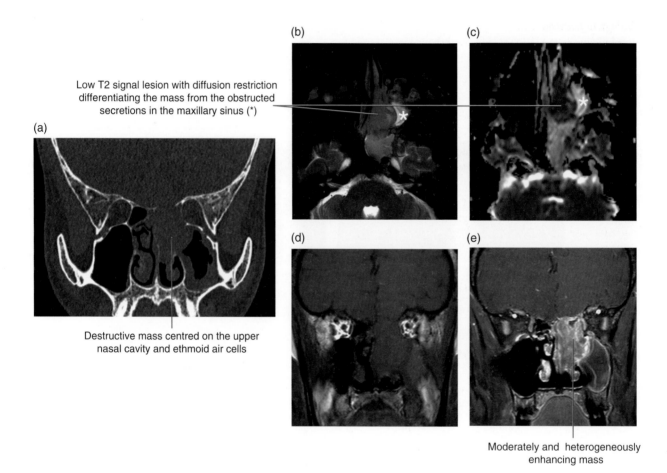

Low T2 signal lesion with diffusion restriction differentiating the mass from the obstructed secretions in the maxillary sinus (*)

Destructive mass centred on the upper nasal cavity and ethmoid air cells

Moderately and heterogeneously enhancing mass

Figure 19.34 Sinonasal lymphoma: coronal MDCT (a), axial T2-weighted MRI (b), apparent diffusion coefficient map (c), coronal T1-weighted MRI (d) and coronal fat-saturated gadolinium-enhanced T1-weighted MRI (e) images.

PHARYNGEAL AIRWAY IMPRESSIONS

There are a number of conditions that narrow or alter the pharyngeal aerodigestive tract outline can be seen on panoramic, cephalometric and other plain 2D radiographs and also CBCT. These can be grouped according to anatomical location and pathophysiological cause. Plain film radiographs and CBCT are suboptimal examinations for soft tissue characterisation. Enhanced MDCT and MRI will be necessary.

19.6 Summary of causes of nasopharyngeal narrowing

- Congenital: choanal atresia/stenosis, encephalocele.
- Inflammatory: adenoidal enlargement, polyps (solitary).
- Neoplastic: nasopharyngeal carcinoma, juvenile angiofibroma, rhabdomyosarcoma.
- Trauma: foreign body lodgement, haematoma.

19.7 Summary of causes of oropharyngeal narrowing

- Congenital: due to micrognathia and posterior positioning of the tongue base in conditions such as Pierre Robin and Treacher Collins syndrome; macroglossia in conditions such as cretinism; branchial cleft cysts.
- Inflammatory: tonsillar hyperplasia and associated abscess formation, cellulitis and abscess formation related to dental and/or oral infections
- Neoplastic:
  ○ Mucosal lesions: lingual tumour/cyst, tonsillar SCCa.
  ○ Parapharyngeal lesions: parotid gland (deep lobe) – minor salivary gland lesions, nerve sheath tumours, lymphoma.
- Trauma: foreign body lodgement, haematoma.

19.8 Malignant disease

Nasopharyngeal carcinoma (NPC) (Figure 19.35)

- A malignant tumour of the upper aerodigestive tract, distinct from other head and neck SCCa. Most commonly arising from the lateral recess of the nasopharyngeal mucosal space. Often clinically silent until large.

- Common in South-East Asia.
- Aetiological association with genetic factors, environmental factors and infection. Exposure to nitrosamines (dry salted fish), polycyclic hydrocarbons, chronic nasal infection, Epstein–Barr virus and smoking are all thought to play a role.
- Early spread laterally, via the foramen of Morgagni, to breach the pharyngobasilar fascia and involve the levator veli palatini muscle, may be seen, with resultant Eustachian tube dysfunction and serous otitis media.
- Direct spread is seen to the nasal cavity, pterygopalatine fossa, clivus, basisphenoid/occiput and temporal bones, oropharynx as well as the parapharyngeal and retropharyngeal spaces.
- Cervical lymph node involvement is very common at diagnosis, particularly involving the retropharyngeal, deep cervical and spinal accessory lymph node groups.

Radiological features

- MDCT demonstrates a lesion arising from the fossa of Rosenmüller. Bony erosion of the skull base is best illustrated with MDCT. The associated airway lumen outline alteration and skull base destruction may be incidentally identified on a dentofacial CBCT examination.
- Perineural infiltration and locoregional spread, initially to the parapharyngeal space, are best demonstrated with MRI.
- Involvement of the skull base marrow, often without frank erosion or destruction, is evident if the tumour replaces the normal T1 hyperintense fatty marrow, initially at the clivus.
- Lymph node involvement can be demonstrated with MDCT and MRI; ^{18}F-fludeoxyglucose (FDG) positron emission tomography (PET) is a useful adjunct to regional nodal staging.

Differential diagnosis

	Key radiological differences
Non-Hodgkin lymphoma	Homogeneously enhancing, diffusion restricting on MRI.
Tonsil (adenoid) hypertrophy	Non-infiltrating symmetric enlargement; preservation of normal lymphoid architecture.

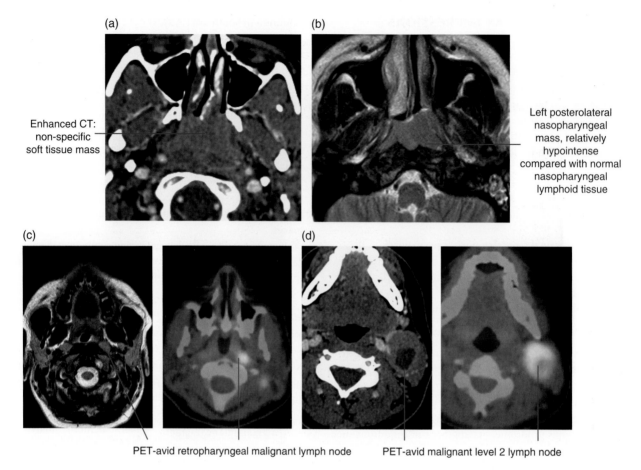

Figure 19.35 Nasopharyngeal SCCa: axial contrast-enhanced MDCT (a), axial T2-weighted MRI (b), axial T2-weighted MRI with positron emission tomography (PET)/CT (c) and axial contrast-enhanced MDCT with PET/CT (d) images.

Oropharyngeal squamous cell carcinoma
(Figure 19.36)

- May arise from several subsites in the oropharynx, including the base of the tongue, epiglottis, soft palate and pharyngeal walls.
- Non-keratinising subtype association with human papillomavirus type 16.
- Alcohol and smoking are risk factors.
- Clinically the lesions present as painless ulcerations or mucosal masses.

Radiological features
- CBCT may reveal a non-specific soft tissue mass, impinging upon the airway lumen. Small lesions will be occult on CBCT; MDCT will optimally demonstrate the varied appearances, including small enhancing mucosal lesions, extensive submucosal tumour spread and large necrotic masses.

- MRI characteristics are hypointense on T1-weighted imaging, hyperintense on T2-weighted imaging with contrast enhancement.
- 60% of patients have malignant cervical adenopathy at diagnosis.
- FDG PET can identify metastatic nodal disease and provide locoregional staging.

Differential diagnosis

	Key radiological differences
Alternative malignancy	Similar appearances but differing epicentre.
Non-Hodgkin lymphoma	Homogeneously enhancing, diffusion restricting on MRI.
Tonsil hypertrophy	Non-infiltrating symmetric enlargement.
Venolymphatic malformation	T2 hyperintensity, avid enhancement.

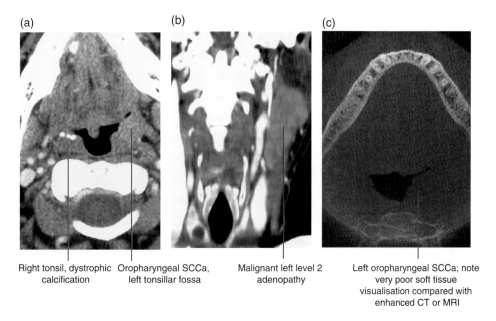

Right tonsil, dystrophic calcification | Oropharyngeal SCCa, left tonsillar fossa

Malignant left level 2 adenopathy

Left oropharyngeal SCCa; note very poor soft tissue visualisation compared with enhanced CT or MRI

Figure 19.36 Oropharyngeal SCCa: axial MDCT (a), coronal MDCT (b) and axial CBCT (c) images.

19.9 Benign entities

Tornwald cyst (Figure 19.37)

- A benign midline notochordal remnant sited at the midline posterior nasopharyngeal space.
- Commonly a well-defined ovoid lesion covered by mucosa, ventral to the longus colli muscle.

Radiological features
- MRI demonstrates an intermediate T1 signal, hyperintense T2-weighted signal lesion that may be hypointense if proteinaceous. Mild peripheral enhancement.
- MDCT may demonstrate low attenuation.
- CBCT may demonstrate a prominence at the posterior nasopharyngeal wall.

Differential diagnosis

	Key radiological differences
Postinfection retention cyst	Non-midline.
Cystic neoplasm	Contrast enhancing and irregular.

Tortuous carotid arteries (Figure 19.38)

- Medial, retropharyngeal tortuosity of the common or internal carotid arteries.
- May present clinically as a pulsatile mass.
- Potentially of surgical significance.

Radiological features
- Lateral radiographs are insensitive but may show widening of the prevertebral soft tissues.
- Enhanced cross-sectional imaging is necessary for characterisation, MDCT/MR angiography.
- CBCT may demonstrate the associated pharyngeal wall prominence.

Differential diagnosis

	Key radiological differences
Arterial dissection and pseudoaneurysm	Focal dilatation; possible trauma history.

Lingual thyroid (Figure 19.39)

- Ectopic thyroid tissue located at the tongue base, at the site of the foramen caecum; or located anywhere along the course of the embryological thyroglossal duct.

Radiological features
- The lesion will have identical imaging characteristics to the normal thyroid gland. If a lingual thyroid is suspected, preoperative confirmation of the presence of a normally sited thyroid gland is essential.
- Thyroid tissue is hyperdense on MDCT due to the presence of intrinsic iodine.
- Well defined, with avid homogeneous enhancement relative to the tongue.
- A radionuclide iodine scan may be helpful as a confirmatory study and also identify the presence of thyroid tissue elsewhere.

Differential diagnosis

Key radiological differences

Prominent lingual tonsil	Often associated with palatine tonsil and adenoid hypertrophy.
Neoplasm (SCCa, non-Hodgkin lymphoma)	Irregular mass, modest enhancement only.
Venolymphatic malformation	T2 hyperintensity, avid enhancement.

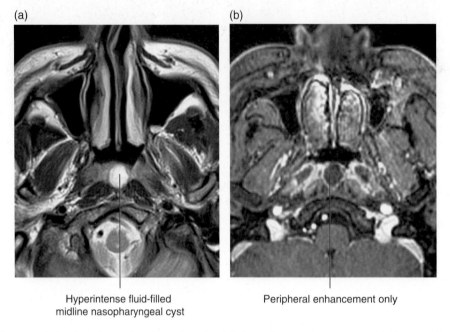

(a)   (b)

Hyperintense fluid-filled
midline nasopharyngeal cyst

Peripheral enhancement only

Figure 19.37 Tornwald cyst: axial T2-weighted (a) and axial fat-saturated gadolinium-enhanced T1-weighted MRI (b) images.

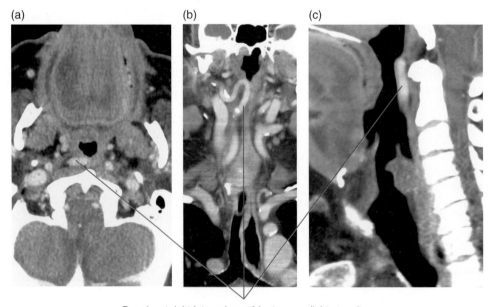

(a)   (b)   (c)

Prominent right internal carotid artery medial tortuosity
(tonsillar loop) – note the submucosal position in the oropharynx

Figure 19.38 Internal carotid artery, retropharyngeal loop: axial (a), coronal (b) and sagittal (c) contrast-enhanced MDCT images.

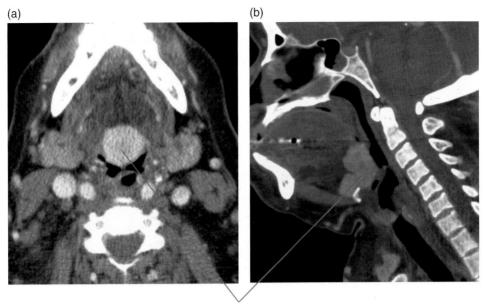

Ectopic thyroid gland at the base of the tongue, along
the course of the embryological thyroglossal duct

Figure 19.39 Lingual thyroid: axial (a) and sagittal (b) contrast-enhanced MDCT images.

Foreign body ingestion

- Can occur at any age, but more commonly in younger children.
- Objects get may get lodged proximally at the tonsillar fossae, the tongue base, piriform sinus, oesophagus or larynx.
- Fish bones are the most common foreign body in the adult population, and may cause viscus perforation with subsequent inflammation and abscess formation.

Radiological features

- Non-anatomical radio-opaque foreign material.
- Soft tissue swelling and oedema.

Differential diagnosis

	Key radiological differences
Abscess	Unwell patient, ring contrast enhancement.
Neoplasm	Large, associated soft tissue mass with destructive changes.

19.10 Inflammatory lesions

Tonsil hypertrophy and adenoid hypertrophy
(Figure 19.40)

- A condition of mainly younger children which occurs as a result of chronic inflammation of the tonsil and adenoidal lymphoid tissue on the basis of bacterial and viral infection. An example of the latter being the Epstein–Barr virus.
- Eustachian tube orifice obstruction may result, with subsequent otitis media.

Radiological features

- Lateral soft tissue neck radiograph, sagittal imaging or reconstructions: lobulated posterior nasopharyngeal thickening effacing the upper aerodigestive tract.
- CBCT will demonstrate the associated oropharyngeal airway outline changes.

Differential diagnosis

	Key radiological differences
Oro- or nasopharyngeal SCCa, non-Hodgkin lymphoma	Age, clinically not septic, local adenopathy.
Peritonsillar abscess	Septic patient, peripheral contrast enhancement at MDCT.

Retention cysts

- Mucosal retention cysts may be present in the oro- or nasopharynx, and are usually subcentimetre in size.

Radiological features

- Low attenuation on MDCT, fluid signal, hyperintense T2-weighted imaging, non-enhancing.
- Airway outline alteration may be appreciated with CBCT.

Differential diagnosis

	Key radiological differences
Tornwald cyst	Midline nasopharynx, dorsal submucosal location.
Cystic neoplasm	Contrast enhancing and irregular.
Thyroglossal duct remnant	Foramen caecum location.

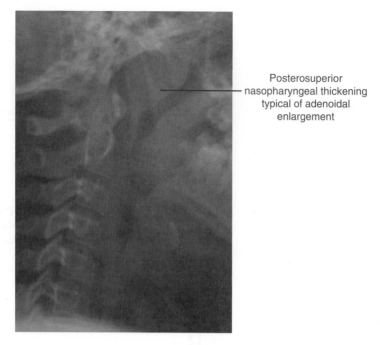

Posterosuperior nasopharyngeal thickening typical of adenoidal enlargement

Figure 19.40 Tonsil and adenoid hypertrophy: plain lateral neck radiograph.

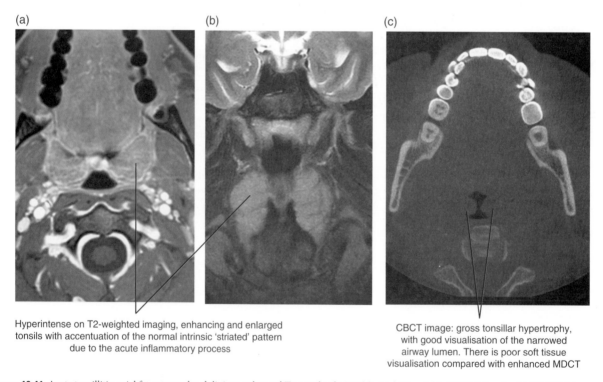

(a) (b) (c)

Hyperintense on T2-weighted imaging, enhancing and enlarged tonsils with accentuation of the normal intrinsic 'striated' pattern due to the acute inflammatory process

CBCT image: gross tonsillar hypertrophy, with good visualisation of the narrowed airway lumen. There is poor soft tissue visualisation compared with enhanced MDCT

Figure 19.41 Acute tonsillitis: axial fat-saturated gadolinium-enhanced T1-weighted MRI (a), axial T2-weighted MRI (b) and axial CBCT (c) images.

Tonsillitis (Figure 19.41)

- A common viral or bacterial inflammatory condition of the tonsils, which clinically presents with a sore throat, fever, dysphagia and trismus.

- The palatine tonsils are most commonly affected bilaterally; inflammation may involve the lingual and adenoid tonsillar tissue.

Radiological features

- See Tonsillar and peritonsillar abcess.

Tonsillar and peritonsillar abscess (Figure 19.42)

- Local complication of acute tonsillitis, with necrosis and suppuration resulting in a reactive inflammatory capsule, intra- or peritonsillar abscess.
- Necrotic material may rupture laterally through the superior constrictor muscle and extend into the parapharyngeal space, masticator and submandibular spaces (peritonsillar abscess).
- Clinical deterioration, with systemic sepsis, is often observed; airway compromise is possible with bilateral involvement.

Radiological features

- CBCT is insensitive for accurate soft tissue characterisation but will suggest airway compromise.
- MDCT appearance is variable but often there is hypoattenuation associated with enlarged tonsils.
- MRI demonstrates T2 hyperintensity with exaggerated striated enhancement which indicates that, even though inflamed, there is preservation of the native lymphoid architecture.
- Relatively non-enhancing areas within the tonsil or peritonsillar tissues suggest necrosis, suppuration and abscess formation.
- Reactive cervical lymph nodes are commonly evident.

Differential diagnosis

	Key radiological differences
Oropharyngeal tonsil SCCa, non-Hodgkin lymphoma	Age, clinically non-toxic, local adenopathy.
Retention cyst	Non-toxic, well defined, no marginal enhancement.

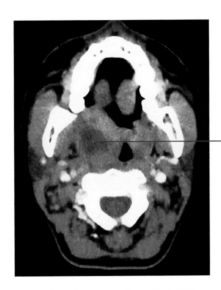

Fluid attenuation mass which is not enhancing, consistent with a peritonsillar abscess

Figure 19.42 Peritonsillar abscess, 'quinsy': axial contrast-enhanced MDCT image.

(a)   (b)

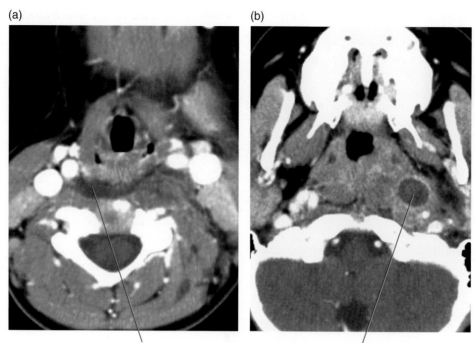

Retropharyngeal abscess (a) and sequela of suppurative retropharyngeal adenopathy (b) secondary to bacterial infection

Figure 19.43 Retropharyngeal abscess (a) and adenopathy (b): axial contrast-enhanced MDCT images.

Retropharyngeal space abscess (Figure 19.43)

- Consequence of suppurative retropharyngeal lymphadeno-pathy.
- Potential for spread to the skull base or mediastinum.
- Can result from foreign body perforation and contiguous cervical spine sepsis.
- Patients are usually extremely unwell and symptoms include sore throat, fever and neck pain.

Radiological features
- Lateral plain films may show prevertebral soft tissue thickening.
- Cross-sectional imaging demonstrates peripherally enhancing, centrally necrotic enlarged retropharyngeal lymph nodes and retropharyngeal space fluid collection; the latter may also show marginal enhancement.
- Mediastinal extension and airway compromise are important complications to exclude.
- Lateral trans-spatial spread to the carotid space, with result-ant internal jugular vein thrombosis, arterial narrowing and pseudoaneurysm formation, is possible.

Differential diagnosis

	Key radiological differences
Prevertebral haematoma	Trauma history, bony injury.
Simple retropharyngeal effusion (upper respiratory tract infection, venous thrombosis, longus colli tendinitis)	No enhancement.
Malignant or suppurative adenopathy	Ring enhancement and perinodal stranding.

Acute longus colli tendinitis (Figure 19.44)

- Self-limiting inflammatory condition in the prevertebral soft tissue secondary to calcium hydroxyapatite deposition in the longus colli muscle tendon; notably the superior oblique fibres as they insert into the C1 anterior tubercle.
- Clinically, patients complain of acute severe neck pain and odynophagia.

Radiological features
- MDCT demonstrates calcification in the prevertebral muscles at the C1/2 level, with surrounding hypodense inflammatory changes and a non-enhancing retropharyngeal space effusion.

Differential diagnosis

	Key radiological differences
Retropharyngeal abscess	Septic patient, with/ without marginal contrast enhancement.
Prevertebral haematoma	Relevant clinical history, bony injury.
Retropharyngeal effusion (upper respiratory tract infection, venous thrombosis)	No calcification.

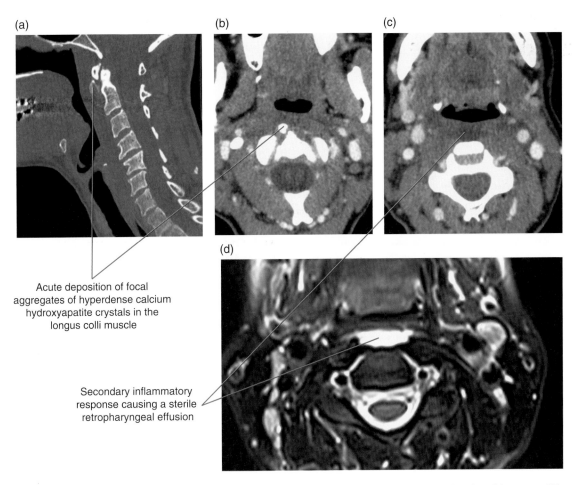

Acute deposition of focal aggregates of hyperdense calcium hydroxyapatite crystals in the longus colli muscle

Secondary inflammatory response causing a sterile retropharyngeal effusion

Figure 19.44 Acute longus colli tendinitis: sagittal bone MDCT multiplanar reformat (a), axial soft tissue MDCT (b,c) and axial fat-saturated T2-weighted MRI (d) images.

19.11 Retropharyngeal adenopathy

(Figures 19.35 and 19.43b)

- The retropharyngeal lymph nodes are located between the skull base and the level of the hyoid bone inferiorly, laterally in the retropharyngeal space and medial to the internal carotid artery.
- Reactive enlargement secondary to regional upper respiratory tract infections is common in the paediatric age group. Significant enlargement in adults is uncommon, in which case malignancy must be excluded.
- Malignant adenopathy occurs secondary to locoregional primary malignancy, including nasopharyngeal carcinoma, thyroid and sinonasal malignancies.

Radiological features

- Reactive lymph nodes are usually only mildly increased in diameter, ovoid in the craniocaudal dimension and the presence of a coincident pharyngeal inflammatory condition is noted.
- Necrotic or suppurative lymph nodes are enlarged but also demonstrate ring contrast enhancement and perinodal stranding.
- Malignant adenopathy can appear very similar to a necrotic inflammatory lymph node but is seen in association with a locoregional primary neoplasm.

CHAPTER 20
The Skull Base

Michael Bynevelt and Andrew Thompson

The base of the skull is a symmetric but irregular bony plate that supports and protects the brain and associated structures. It contains foramina which act as conduits, not only for transmitting blood vessels and nerves between the brain and the body but also for the regional spread of pathological processes. The base of the skull also provides housing for a number of special sensory mechanisms, the paranasal sinuses and components of the masticatory apparatus. A number of processes cause changes in the skull base that may be visualised on dental and orofacial imaging and may have important consequences for patient management.

Developmental variations in structure and lesions in the skull base are often incidentally noted on radiographs and cone beam computed tomography (CBCT). These are commonly incidental and require no clinical attention but can be confused with pathological entities. However, some lesions are important to identify, requiring intervention and/or monitoring. It should be noted that CBCT is not the imaging modality of choice for skull base lesions.

CONSTITUTIONAL AND DEVELOPMENTAL VARIATIONS

20.1 Ossification of the interclinoid ligaments (Figure 20.1)

- Ossification may occur in dura mater bands that bridge the anterior and posterior clinoid processes of the sphenoid.
- Close proximity to neurovascular structures may interfere with surgical procedures in this region.

Radiological features
- Well-corticated bony bridge extending between the anterior and posterior clinoid process.

Differential diagnosis

	Key radiological differences
Vascular calcification	Multifocal, incomplete.
Meningioma	Associated dural mass, bony hyperostosis.

Atlas of Oral and Maxillofacial Radiology, First Edition. Bernard Koong.
© 2017 John Wiley & Sons Ltd. Published 2017 by John Wiley & Sons Ltd.

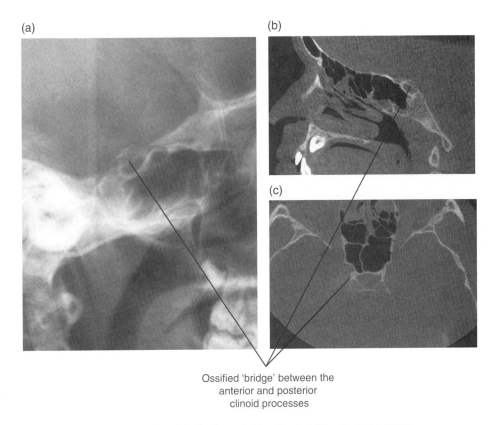

Ossified 'bridge' between the
anterior and posterior
clinoid processes

Figure 20.1 Ossification of the interclinoid ligament: lateral skull radiograph (a) and sagittal (b) and axial (c) CBCT images.

20.2 Benign notochordal cell tumour (ecchordosis physaliphora) (Figure 20.2)

- Hamartomatous and ectopically located midline remnant of the primitive notochord.
- Incidentally found in approximately 2% of autopsies.
- Can be located in tissues anywhere between the dorsum sellae and the coccyx.

Radiological features

- In the skull base, the lesion may involve the clivus as a non-aggressive-appearing, well-defined smoothly corticated scalloped bony lucency, particularly on multidetector computed tomography (MDCT). It may bear a pedicle (which itself is sometimes osseous) that is intradural.
- Low signal on T1-weighted MRI, but hyperintense on T2-weighted imaging and the intradural component may be outlined by the surrounding cerebrospinal fluid (CSF). This may be difficult to define due to CSF pulsation artefacts when sited at the prepontine cistern.

- Does not enhance, in contradistinction to the main differential diagnosis, chordoma, which exhibits prominent enhancement.

Differential diagnosis

	Key radiological differences
Chordoma	Destructive, calcification, enhancement.
Persistence of the craniopharyngeal canal	Transosseous linear/lobulated tract – sella to nasopharynx.
Dermoid/epidermoid	High T1 signal, diffusion restricting on MRI.
Arachnoid cyst	MRI signal equivalent to CSF, no diffusion restriction.
Metastases	Destructive tumour, primary known, multifocal.
Pituitary adenoma	Sella involvement, no normal pituitary visualised.

(a)

(b)

(c)

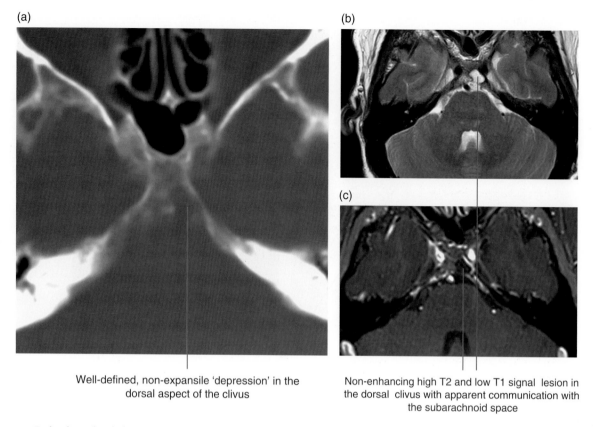

Well-defined, non-expansile 'depression' in the dorsal aspect of the clivus

Non-enhancing high T2 and low T1 signal lesion in the dorsal clivus with apparent communication with the subarachnoid space

Figure 20.2 Ecchordosis physaliphora: axial MDCT image (a), axial T2-weighted MRI (b) and axial fat-saturated gadolinium-enhanced T1-weighted MRI (c).

20.3 Persistence of the craniopharyngeal canal (Figure 20.3)

- Lack of involution of the embryological craniopharyngeal canal.
- Thought to result from incomplete closure of the anterior pituitary precursor, Rathke's pouch, and may contain rests of pituitary tissue.
- Rare but can be associated with ectopic anterior pituitary tissue, cephaloceles, tumours commonly found in this region, such as pituitary adenomas, craniopharyngioma and germ cell tumours. In this circumstance, the canal is usually larger in diameter, and may be associated with other midline anomalies of the brain.

Radiological features
- Well-corticated slightly oblique vertical tubular defect in the midline of the sphenoid body extending from the floor of the sella turcica, dorsal to the sphenoid sinus, to the naso-pharyngeal region.
- On MRI appears as a low T1 and high T2 signal tubular tract traversing the sphenoid body.

Differential diagnosis

	Key radiological differences
Encephalocele	Communication with subarachnoid space with/ without neural contents.
Synchondrosis and variants	Non tubular.

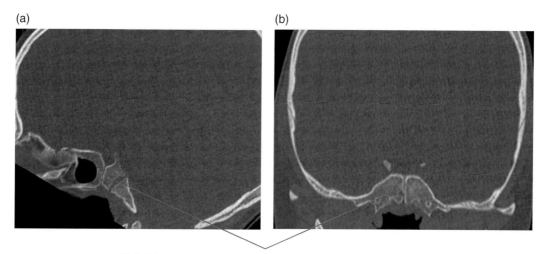

Well-defined midline craniocaudal canal extending from the sella turcica to the rostral sphenoid

Figure 20.3 Persistent craniopharyngeal canal: sagittal (a) and coronal (b) multiplanar reformatted MDCT images.

20.4 Arrested pneumatisation of the skull base (Figure 20.4)

- An asymptomatic abnormality which is most commonly discovered incidentally on cross-sectional imaging.
- Persistence of atypical fatty marrow in the central skull base, thought to result from arrested sphenoid sinus pneumatisation.

Radiological features
- Non-expansile on CBCT and MDCT and also well defined with a sclerotic margin and internal curvilinear opacities. Additionally, MDCT may demonstrate the internal fat attenuation.
- Bony trabeculation is a common feature, but the marginal cortical bony integrity is preserved.

- On MRI, lesions are of high and low signal on T1- and T2-weighted imaging, respectively.

Differential diagnosis

	Key radiological differences
Intraosseous lipoma	T1 hyperintense; low signal on fat-saturated sequences.
Haemangioma	Contrast enhancing, trabeculation, fatty T1 hyperintense.
Fibrous dysplasia	Ground-glass matrix.
Chordoma	Midline clival; T2 hyperintense, destructive, calcification.
Benign notochordal cell tumour	Midline clival; T2 hyperintense, corticated and pedunculated.

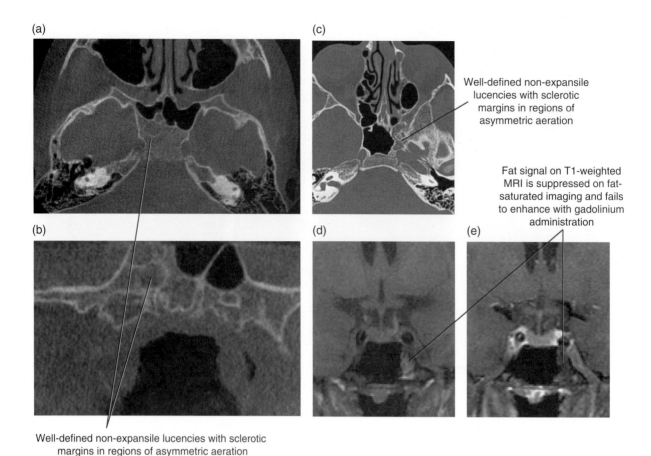

(a)

(c)

Well-defined non-expansile lucencies with sclerotic margins in regions of asymmetric aeration

Fat signal on T1-weighted MRI is suppressed on fat-saturated imaging and fails to enhance with gadolinium administration

(b)

(d)

(e)

Well-defined non-expansile lucencies with sclerotic margins in regions of asymmetric aeration

Figure 20.4 Arrested skull base pneumatisation: axial (a) and coronal multiplanar reformatted CBCT images (b), axial MDCT image (c), coronal T1-weighted MRI (d) and fat-saturated gadolinium-enhanced T1-weighted MRI (e).

20.5 Meningoencephaloceles (Figure 20.5)

- Herniations of meninges containing CSF (meningocele) and brain tissue (meningoencephalocele) through an osteodural defect in the skull base.
- May be congenital, which is more common in South-East Asian females, or acquired secondary to a focal pathological dehiscence in the integrity of the skull base.
- Primary lesions can arise anywhere, but are more common in the frontoethmoidal region, components of the sphenoid and petrous temporal bones.
- Heterogeneous in appearance depending on their underlying cause. There may be an associated CSF leak, which can be particularly seen in the setting of trauma.

Radiological features

- Heterogeneous on MDCT but contain CSF and a soft tissue mass that can be demonstrated to be in continuity with the brain through a dehiscent segment of the skull base. The osseous abnormality can be demonstrated on CBCT.
- High-resolution MRI, the soft tissue components may follow the signal of brain constituents on T1- and T2-weighted imaging,

but signal is often relatively low and high on T1- and T2-weighted imaging, respectively, due to gliosis from chronic injury.

- Contrast enhancement of the herniated meninges is seen, but usually not of the parenchymal component, unless complications such as infection occur.
- Cisternography may reveal the passage of contrast into the mass, to outline the soft tissue components, and is only performed if there is diagnostic uncertainty from other studies.

Differential diagnosis

	Key radiological differences
Trauma/iatrogenic	Relevant clinical history, associated fractures.
Anterior neuropore anomalies	Midline communication between the anterior cranial fossa and the nasal bridge region.
Sinonasal mucocele	Focal sinus changes, high-density/low T2 signal sinus contents, bone expansion.
Solitary polyposis	Homogeneous contiguous antronasal lesion, ostial expansion.

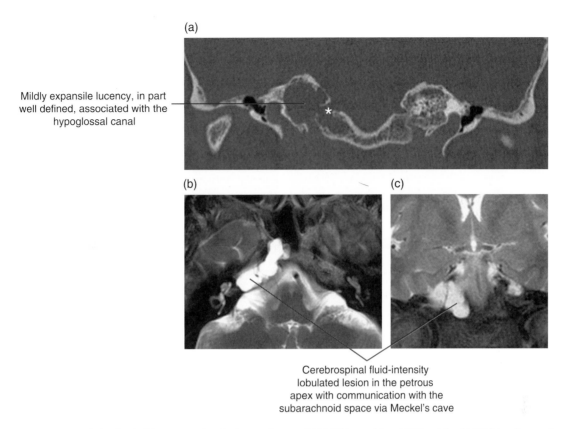

(a)

Mildly expansile lucency, in part well defined, associated with the hypoglossal canal

(b)   (c)

Cerebrospinal fluid-intensity lobulated lesion in the petrous apex with communication with the subarachnoid space via Meckel's cave

Figure 20.5 Petrous apex cephalocele: skull base coronal multiplanar reformatted MDCT image (a), axial T2-weighted MRI (b) and coronal T2-weighted MRI (c).

20.6 Nasolacrimal duct mucocele (dacryocystocele) (Figure 20.6)

- Small, round medial canthal mass usually presenting at birth with an associated submucosal nasal cavity mass at the inferior meatus.
- Results from nasolacrimal duct obstruction which may be primary or secondary to infection.
- Lesions expand into the orbit as well as the nasal cavity.

Radiological features
- CBCT and MDCT demonstrate smooth expansion of the bony nasolacrimal duct with usually low-attenuation material and mild peripheral contrast enhancement.
- Bone destruction is not a feature, and if present raises the possibility of a malignant neoplasm.
- On MRI there can be mixed signal, which is dependent on the protein concentration of the contents.

Differential diagnosis

Key radiological differences

Trauma/iatrogenic	Relevant clinical history, associated fractures.
Encephalocele	Communication with subarachnoid space with/ without neural contents.
Anterior neuropore anomalies	Midline communication between the anterior cranial fossa and the nasal bridge region.
Solitary polyposis	Homogeneous contiguous antronasal lesion, ostial expansion.
Dermoid	High T1 signal, fat saturation positive, diffusion restricting on MRI.

(a)   (b)

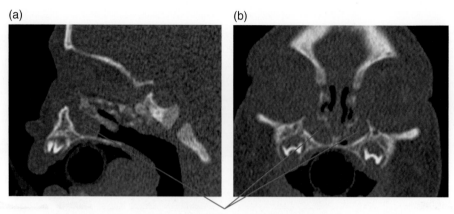

Enlarged nasolacrimal ducts bilaterally secondary to congenitally obstructed
collecting systems and associated cystic masses extending into the nasal cavity

Figure 20.6 Nasolacrimal duct mucocele (dacryocystocele) empty sella syndrome: sagittal (a) and coronal (b) multiplanar reformatted MDCT images.

20.7 Empty sella syndrome (Figure 20.7)

- A diagnosis made when the pituitary fossa, which may be expanded, is nearly completely filled with CSF, compressing the normal pituitary glandular tissue against the sellar floor.
- The pituitary stalk and infundibulum assume normal positions and enhance appropriately following the administration of contrast.
- May be primary when there is a dehiscence in the diaphragma turcica in a scenario that may or may not be associated with raised intracranial pressure. Empty sella syndrome is a feature of idiopathic intracranial hypertension syndrome.
- Secondary empty sella syndrome may also result from historical pituitary damage, such as with haemorrhage into a pituitary macroadenoma, or the consequence of surgical or radiation treatment.
- In adults, empty sella syndrome is not an uncommon finding and is usually asymptomatic, but in the paediatric setting the finding is more likely to be clinically relevant.

Radiological features

- Moderately enlarged sella containing CSF with a midline, normal positioned pituitary stalk.
- Rind of pituitary tissue lining the floor of the sella.
- No bone destruction.
- Well demonstrated on MDCT and MRI, bony changes can be seen on CBCT.

Differential diagnosis

	Key radiological differences
Intrasellar arachnoid cyst	Signal and attenuation equal to CSF, no diffusion restriction on MRI.
Rathke's cleft cyst	Signal and attenuation different from CSF, no diffusion restriction.
Intrasellar epidermoid cyst	Signal and attenuation equal to CSF, diffusion restriction on MRI.
Intracranial hypertension	Optic nerve sheath patulous, dural venous outflow obstruction.
Prior pituitary apoplexy	Clinical history, enlarged sella, abnormal pituitary tissue, with/without evidence of previous haemorrhage.

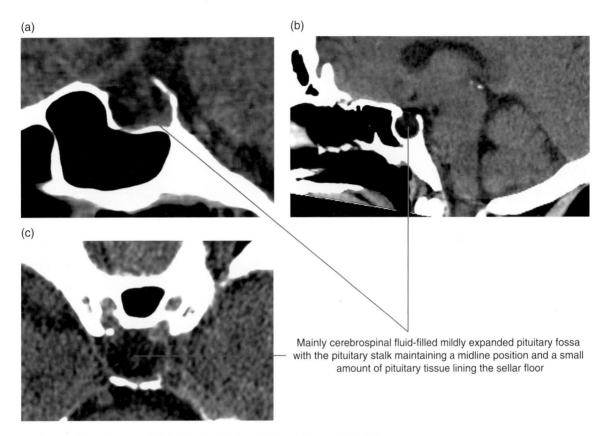

(a)

(b)

(c)

Mainly cerebrospinal fluid-filled mildly expanded pituitary fossa with the pituitary stalk maintaining a midline position and a small amount of pituitary tissue lining the sellar floor

Figure 20.7 Empty sella syndrome: sagittal (a,b) and axial (c) multiplanar reformatted MDCT images.

LESIONS OF THE SKULL BASE

There are a number of lesions, mainly neoplastic, that can arise in the skull base resulting in bony deformity and/or destruction. These changes can be visualised on dental radiographs and CBCT.

20.8 Pituitary macroadenoma (Figure 20.8)

- A benign tumour composed of glandular tissue originating from the anterior lobe of the pituitary. If greater than 1 cm in size, it is classified as a macroadenoma; if smaller, a micro-adenoma. Given the scope of this chapter, macroadenoma will only be described.
- Usually grow beyond the sella turcica, which houses the normal gland, extending superiorly into the suprasellar cistern and laterally bowing, and less frequently invading into the cavernous sinus.
- Occasionally infiltrates towards the basisphenoid or basi-occiput inferiorly, but is contiguous with a soft tissue mass in an eroded sella.

Radiological features
- A critical differentiating observation is the absence of a normal pituitary gland when assessing lesions that involve the sellar contents. Rarely an adenoma can arise from a craniopharyngeal

duct remnant and a normal pituitary can be seen in the sella distinct from a lesion within the sphenoid bone.
- On cross-sectional imaging, the mass is lobular in outline but infiltrating/bowing/scalloping the basisphenoid/occipital bone through the sellar floor. The bony changes are demonstrated on CBCT.
- The matrix of the mass on MDCT is relatively homogeneous but can be variable due to cysts, haemorrhage and/or necrosis. Calcification is rare but may help in distinguishing from other lesions in this location. Enhancement patterns are extremely variable.
- On MRI, the signal on T1-weighted imaging is typically isointense to grey matter and seen to replace the normal high-signal fatty marrow of the bony base of skull. The signal on T2-weighted imaging is variable, particularly in the setting of cystic change and intratumoral haemorrhage. With intravenous contrast there is intense, heterogeneous enhancement, and, where components are in contact with the dura, a dural 'tail' may be seen, mimicking a meningioma.
- Macroadenomas can encase the cavernous and petrous internal carotid arteries; however, the vessel is not narrowed as a consequence.

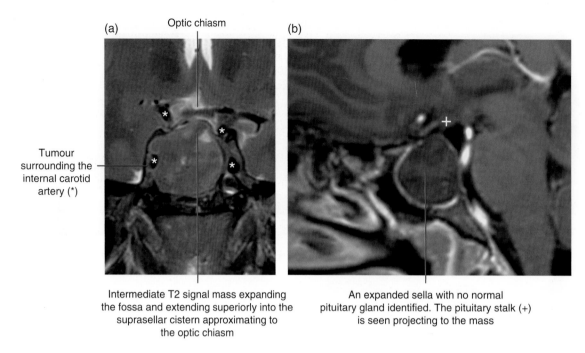

(a)   Optic chiasm   (b)

Tumour
surrounding the
internal carotid
artery (*)

Intermediate T2 signal mass expanding
the fossa and extending superiorly into the
suprasellar cistern approximating to
the optic chiasm

An expanded sella with no normal
pituitary gland identified. The pituitary stalk (+)
is seen projecting to the mass

Figure 20.8 Invasive pituitary macroadenoma: coronal T2-weighted (a) and sagittal gadolinium-enhanced T1 (b) images.

Differential diagnosis

Key radiological differences

Metastases	Destructive tumour, primary known, multiple.
Plasmacytoma	Well-marginated lytic, T2 hypointense homogeneously contrast enhanced.
Chordoma	Midline clival, T2 hyperintense, destructive, calcification.
Chondrosarcoma	Parasagittal, based on petroclival suture, T2 hyperintense, destructive, calcification.
Meningioma	Transosseous, enhancing dural thickening, extra-axial.
Nasopharyngeal carcinoma	Mass centred on, and extending from, the lateral nasopharynx.

20.9 Clival chordoma (Figure 20.9)

- Midline clival mass arising from malignant transformation of notochordal remnants.
- Can occur in the midline, from the skull base to the sacrum.
- Slow growing but locally invasive, often with infiltrative margins and a high rate of recurrence following resection.

Radiological features
- On MDCT, an infiltrative or well-circumscribed lytic midline clival mass. Foci of intralesional calcification are thought to represent fragments of clivus rather than neoplastic calcification, the latter seen in chondrosarcoma and chondroid variants

of chordoma. Only the bony changes are demonstrated with CBCT.
- On MRI, the tumour is isointense on T1-weighted imaging but may contain cystic, proteinaceous and haemorrhagic foci, resulting in an increased T1 signal. High signal on T2-weighted imaging is characteristic for chordoma; however, poorly differentiated lesions can be predominantly of low signal.
- Variable contrast enhancement profiles are seen.
- The lesion may displace the pituitary gland, particularly superiorly, and project dorsally, where it may invaginate into the pons.

Differential diagnosis

Key radiological differences

Metastases	Destructive tumour, primary known, multiple.
Non-Hodgkin lymphoma	Homogeneously enhancing, diffusion restricting on MRI, bone infiltration.
Plasmacytoma	Well-marginated lytic, T2 hypointense, homogeneously contrast enhancing.
Invasive pituitary macroadenoma	Sphenoid mass, no normal pituitary, sellar involvement.
Chondrosarcoma	Parasagittal, based on petroclival synchondrosis, T2 hyperintense, destructive, calcification.
Meningioma	Transosseous, enhancing dural thickening, extra-axial.

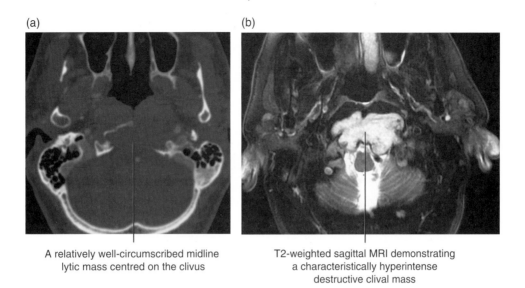

(a)   (b)

A relatively well-circumscribed midline
lytic mass centred on the clivus

T2-weighted sagittal MRI demonstrating
a characteristically hyperintense
destructive clival mass

Figure 20.9 Clival chordoma: axial MDCT image (a) and axial fat-saturated T2-weighted MRI (b).

20.10 Skull base meningioma (Figures 20.10 and 20.11)

- The most common intracranial neoplasm, which can take a number of distinct morphological forms.
- Most often presents as a dural-based extra-axial mass, but may be pedunculated or osteodurally invasive as an 'en-plaque' lesion, which causes bony thickening.
- Usually slow growing; however, occasionally atypical and anaplastic subtypes exhibit an aggressive pattern of growth.
- Common sites in the skull base are the olfactory groove, tuberculum sellae, sphenoid wing (anterior cranial fossa), cavernous sinus, petroclival junction (middle cranial fossa), petrous temporal bone (cerebellopontine angle) and jugular foramen/foramen magnum (posterior cranial fossa).
- Associated with a graduated margin of dural thickening ('dural tail'), which may be secondary to infiltration and/or a reactive change.

Radiological features

- MDCT most commonly demonstrates a hyperattenuating mass, with variable (nil to dense) calcification and avid contrast enhancement.
- The variety of associated bony changes are well illustrated on MDCT but also on CBCT, including hyperostosis (thickening of the cortex and marrow space), frank invasion with permeative lytic change and buckling resulting in expansion of an underlying sinus (pneumosinus dilatans).
- On MRI, isointense to grey matter on both T1- and T2-weighted imaging, avidly contrast enhancing often illustrating a 'sunburst' appearance and the characteristic marginal 'dural tail'.

- Vasogenic oedema can be seen in the adjacent brain depending on histological subtypes or degree of parenchymal invasion.
- Demonstrate relative restriction on diffusion MRI.
- Branches of the external carotid artery, particularly from meningeal vessels, mainly supply the lesions but also draw supply from superficial adjacent pial arteries.
- Meningiomas can also spread along neurovascular structures and extend through the skull base foramina, giving rise to an associated neuropathy.

Differential diagnosis

	Key radiological differences
Metastases	Destructive tumour, primary known, multiple.
Plasmacytoma	Well-marginated lytic, T2 hypointense.
Chordoma	Midline clival, T2 hyperintense, destructive, calcification.
Chondrosarcoma	Parasagittal, based on the petroclival suture, T2 hyperintense, destructive, calcification.
Invasive pituitary macroadenoma	Sphenoid mass, no normal pituitary, sellar involvement.
Sarcoidosis	Dural thickening, chest radiograph – enlarged lymph nodes.
Tuberculosis	Dural thickening, chest radiograph – abnormal.
Schwannoma	Perineural location, bony scalloping.
Nasopharyngeal carcinoma	Mass centred on the lateral nasopharynx.

(a) (b)

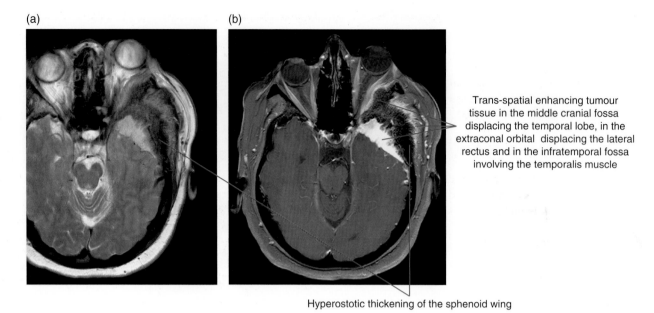

Trans-spatial enhancing tumour tissue in the middle cranial fossa displacing the temporal lobe, in the extraconal orbital displacing the lateral rectus and in the infratemporal fossa involving the temporalis muscle

Hyperostotic thickening of the sphenoid wing

Figure 20.10 Base of skull meningioma: axial T2 turbo spin echo (a) and axial fat-saturated gadolinium-enhanced T1-weighted (b) MRI.

(a) (b)

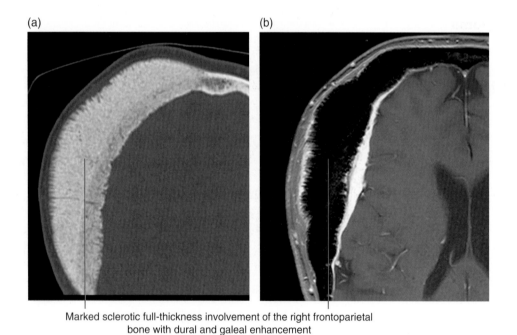

Marked sclerotic full-thickness involvement of the right frontoparietal bone with dural and galeal enhancement

Figure 20.11 Calvarial meningioma: axial bone MDCT image (a) and axial fat-saturated gadolinium-enhanced T1-weighted MRI (b).

20.11 Skull base metastasis (Figure 20.12)

- Metastases present mainly in the clinical setting of a known malignancy and/or metastases.
- Can be solitary or multiple to the skull base but usually reminiscent of metastases seen elsewhere in the bony skeleton.
- Common primaries include breast, lung, prostate, thyroid, hepatocellular carcinoma.
- Metastatic disease may take the form of perineural infiltration, when the tumour spreads along nerves. Squamous cell carcinoma is the most common tumour type. On imaging, there is tubular neural thickening, enhancement and occasionally expansion of bony foramina.

Radiological features

- Most commonly seen as a destructive or infiltrating mass on MDCT, CBCT and on MRI, replacing the T1 hyperintense fatty marrow.
- Exhibits low T2 intensity, diffusion restriction owing to hypercellularity, and geographic or permeative margins.

Differential diagnosis

Key radiological differences

Invasive pituitary macroadenoma	Sphenoid mass, no normal pituitary, sellar involvement.
Plasmacytoma	Well-marginated lytic, T2 hypointense.
Chordoma	Midline clival, T2 hyperintense, destructive, calcification.
Chondrosarcoma	Parasagittal, based on the petroclival suture, T2 hyperintense, destructive, calcification.
Meningioma	Transosseous, enhancing dural thickening.
Non-Hodgkin lymphoma	Homogeneously enhancing, diffusion restricting on MRI, bone infiltration.
Nasopharyngeal carcinoma	Mass centred on the lateral nasopharynx.

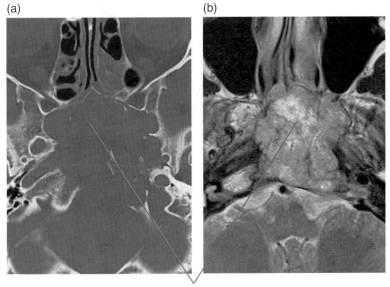

(a)   (b)

A locally destructive lesion in the central skull base eroding and destroying bone and consisting of heterogeneous signal on T2-weighted imaging

Figure 20.12 Skull base metastasis from renal cell carcinoma: axial MDCT image (a) and axial fat-saturated T2-weighted MRI (b).

20.12 Chondrosarcoma (Figure 20.13; see also Figure 11.12)

- Slow-growing yet malignant bone tumour with a matrix consisting of primitive mesenchymal cells and chondroid elements.
- May arise from a pre-existing benign chondroid or fibro-osseus lesion.
- Typically paramedian, centred at the petroclival fissure, differentiating the mass from the main differential diagnosis, chordoma.

Radiological features
- On MDCT, the paramedian mass appears lytic with distinct 'ring and arc' calcifications in the majority: the lower the grade, the more calcifications. A degree of bony scalloping may also be evident. The bony changes and calcifications are often seen on CBCT.

- Hypoisointense on T1-weighted MRI with very high T2 signal and variable contrast enhancement, the latter more prominent in higher grades.

Differential diagnosis

	Key radiological differences
Metastases	Destructive tumour, primary known, multiple.
Invasive pituitary macroadenoma	Sphenoid mass, no normal pituitary, sellar involvement.
Plasmacytoma	Well-marginated lytic, T2 hypointense.
Chordoma	Midline clival, high T2 signal, destructive, calcification.
Meningioma	Transosseous, enhancing dural thickening.
Non-Hodgkin lymphoma	Homogeneously enhancing, diffusion restricting on MRI, bone infiltration.
Nasopharyngeal carcinoma	Mass centred on the lateral nasopharynx.

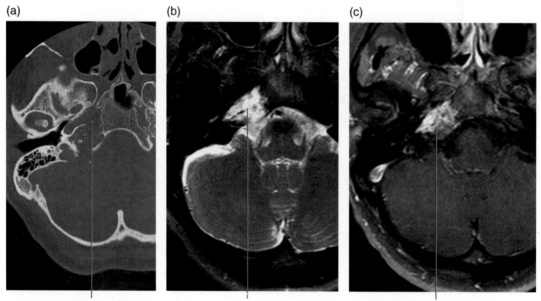

(a) (b) (c)

A lytic lesion is demonstrated centred on the petroclival synchondrosis involving the petrous apex and lateral clivus. Calcifications are seen within the lytic lesion

The irregular mass is of T2 hyperintensity and avidly contrast enhances. The low-signal areas are the result of matrix calcifications

Figure 20.13 Base of skull chondrosarcoma: axial MDCT image (a), axial fat-saturated T2-weighted MRI (b) and axial fat-saturated gadolinium-enhanced T1-weighted MRI (c).

20.13 Lymphoma (Figure 20.14)

Refer to section 11.3.

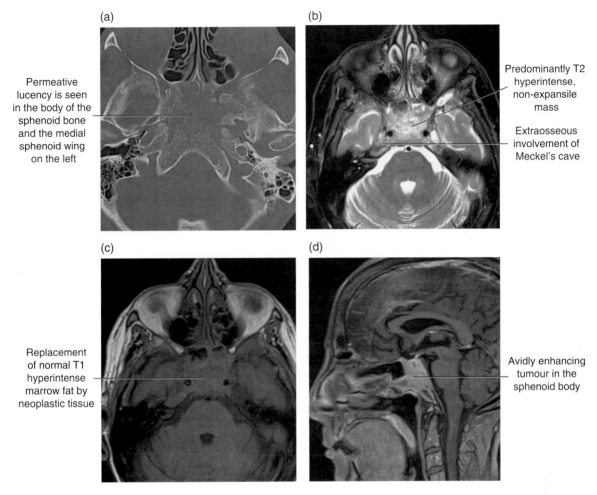

(a)

Permeative
lucency is seen
in the body of the
sphenoid bone
and the medial
sphenoid wing
on the left

(b)

Predominantly T2
hyperintense,
non-expansile
mass

Extraosseous
involvement of
Meckel's cave

(c)

Replacement
of normal T1
hyperintense
marrow fat by
neoplastic tissue

(d)

Avidly enhancing
tumour in the
sphenoid body

Figure 20.14 Lymphoma: axial MDCT image (a), axial fat-saturated T2-weighted MRI (b), axial T1-weighted MRI (c) and axial fat-saturated gadolinium-enhanced T1-weighted MRI (d).

20.14 Skull base plasmacytoma/multiple myeloma (Figure 20.15)

- Monoclonal plasma cell proliferation located anywhere in the skull base marrow.

Radiological features

- Well-marginated lytic lesion with a narrow transition zone on plain radiography.
- Appear as an invasive mass in the skull base on MDCT/CBCT as well as isointense and moderately hypointense on T1- and T2-weighted imaging respectively, with homogeneous contrast enhancement.
- More than half of patients with plasmacytoma have multiple lesions elsewhere and, therefore, multiple myeloma.

Differential diagnosis

	Key radiological differences
Metastases	Focally destructive, known primary.
Chordoma	Midline, calcifications, T2 hyperintense.
Non-Hodgkin lymphoma	Homogeneously enhancing, diffusion restricting on MRI, bone infiltration.
Invasive pituitary macroadenoma	Sphenoid mass, no normal pituitary, sellar involvement.
Nasopharyngeal carcinoma	Nasopharyngeal epicentre/origin.
Primary bone tumour, e.g. osteosarcoma	Focally destructive, calcifications.

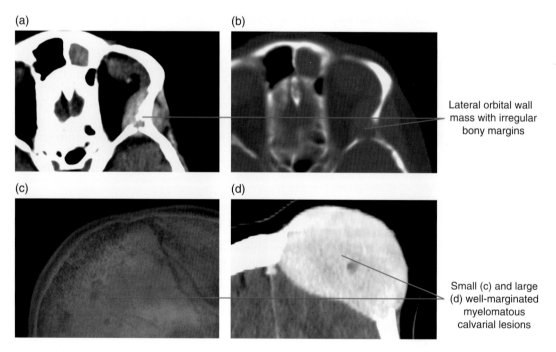

Lateral orbital wall mass with irregular bony margins

Small (c) and large (d) well-marginated myelomatous calvarial lesions

Figure 20.15 Base of skull and calvarial plasmacytoma/myeloma: axial contrast-enhanced soft tissue MDCT (a), bone MDCT (b), lateral skull radiograph (c) and coronal multiplanar reformatted contrast-enhanced MDCT (d) images.

20.15 Langerhans cell histiocytosis (Figure 20.16)

Refer to section 13.4.

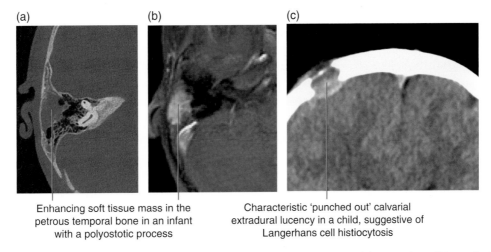

(a)   (b)   (c)

Enhancing soft tissue mass in the
petrous temporal bone in an infant
with a polyostotic process

Characteristic 'punched out' calvarial
extradural lucency in a child, suggestive of
Langerhans cell histiocytosis

Figure 20.16 Langerhans cell histiocytosis: axial skull base bone MDCT image (a), axial fat-saturated gadolinium-enhanced T1-weighted MRI (b) and axial calvarium soft tissue MDCT image (c).

20.16 Fibrous dysplasia (Figure 20.17)

- A benign fibro-osseous lesion that is caused by an abnormal proliferation of fibroblasts resulting in abnormal remodelling with zones of immature trabecular bone and dysplastic fibrous tissue.
- Can occur at one site (mono-ostotic) or at multiple sites (polyostotic); when the latter is associated with precocious puberty it is termed McCune–Albright syndrome.

Radiological features
- MDCT and/or CBCT demonstrates a characteristic low-attenuation, ground-glass appearance which may be associated with cystic change and thinning or thickening of the bone.
- On MRI, lesions are generally of T1 and T2 hypointensity but vary as a function of bony spicules, fibrous tissue content, haemorrhage, cystic change and complicating factors such as fracture.
- Internal septations can be present and the contrast enhancement can be heterogeneous, marginal and/or central.
- Malignant sarcomatous degeneration can occur in a small number of cases.

Differential diagnosis

	Key radiological differences
Paget disease	'Cotton-wool' mixed lysis and sclerosis, expansion.
Meningioma	Transosseous, enhancing dural thickening.
Skull base metastases	Osteosclerotic/osteolytic, destructive tumour, primary known, multiple.
Chronic infection	Osteosclerotic/osteolytic, dehiscence, periostitis.
Osteitis fibrosa cystica	Associated with tuberous sclerosis and neurofibromatosis.
Chronic renal failure	'Salt and pepper' skull, signs of bone softening, mandible brown tumours.
Extramedullary haematopoiesis	Calvarial and skull base thickening, dural, parasellar soft tissue lesions.

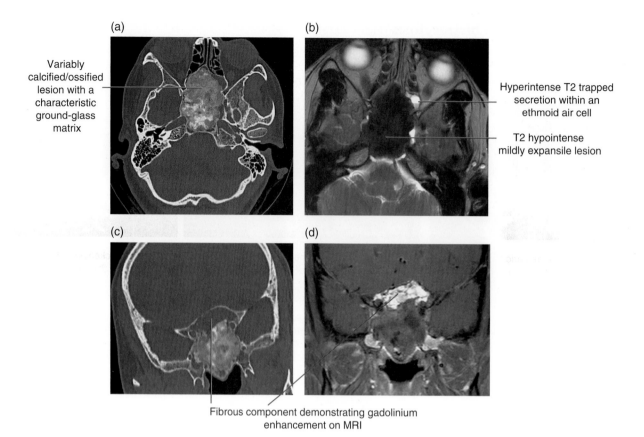

Variably calcified/ossified lesion with a characteristic ground-glass matrix

Hyperintense T2 trapped secretion within an ethmoid air cell

T2 hypointense mildly expansile lesion

Fibrous component demonstrating gadolinium enhancement on MRI

Figure 20.17 Skull base fibrous dysplasia: axial MDCT image (a), axial fat-saturated T2-weighted MRI (b), coronal multiplanar reformatted MDCT image (c) and coronal fat-saturated gadolinium-enhanced T1-weighted MRI (d).

20.17 Paget disease (Figure 20.18)

- Chronic disorder of aberrant osseous remodelling resulting in bone expansion and deformity, most commonly in the elderly.
- Exact cause is unknown, but genetic as well as environmental causes such as viruses are implicated.
- The skull vault and to a lesser extent skull base can be involved.
- Osteosarcoma and other tumours can arise in a small percentage.

Radiological features

- Radiographically three phases: lysis (radiolucent), lysis and sclerosis, and sclerosis.
- MDCT and CBCT can demonstrate geographically lytic regions in the early phase which progress to a 'cotton-wool'-appearing sclerosis with moderate expansion.

- On MRI, the affected bones are usually T1 hypointense with some increased signal foci due to factors such as haemorrhage. On T2-weighted and T1 postcontrast imaging, the bone is heterogeneous in signal and enhancement, respectively.

Differential diagnosis

	Key radiological differences
Fibrous dysplasia	Ground-glass matrix on CT.
Skull base metastases	Osteosclerotic/osteolytic, destructive tumour, primary known, multiple.
Osteopetrosis	Diffuse sclerosis, young.
Meningioma	Transosseous, enhancing dural thickening.
Hyperostosis frontalis interna	Symmetric frontal calvarial thickening.

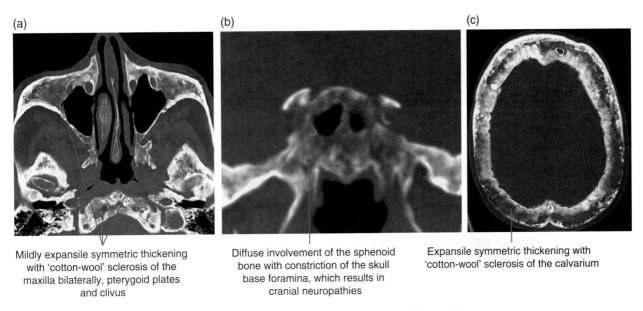

(a)

(b)

(c)

Mildly expansile symmetric thickening with 'cotton-wool' sclerosis of the maxilla bilaterally, pterygoid plates and clivus

Diffuse involvement of the sphenoid bone with constriction of the skull base foramina, which results in cranial neuropathies

Expansile symmetric thickening with 'cotton-wool' sclerosis of the calvarium

Figure 20.18 Paget disease: axial skull base (a), coronal multiplanar reformatted (b) and axial skull (c) MDCT images.

20.18 Petrous apex lesions (Figures 20.5 and 20.19–20.22)

- Lesions presenting in the petrous apex may be evident on dental imaging, particularly CBCT.
- Developmental asymmetric fatty marrow or pneumatisation may be mistaken for pathology.
- Potentially pneumatised, communicating with the middle ear cleft, inflammatory lesions can arise in the petrous apex. These can be categorised as non-expansile or expansile.
  - Non-expansile lesions include simple or complex proteinaceous effusions.
  - Expansile lesions and petrous apicitis may demonstrate coalescence of air cells, frank destruction and/or erosion of the petrous apex margin or labyrinth. These inflammatory lesions in general will require specialist referral and include mucocele, cholesteatoma and cholesterol granuloma.

  - Petrous apicitis can present with the triad of retro-orbital pain, otitis media and a palsy of the sixth cranial nerve. On cross-sectional imaging findings include a permeative process associated with an effusion as well as mucosal and adjacent dural contrast enhancement. There is often coexistent otomastoiditis and the possibility of intracranial complications requires attention.
  - MRI signal of complex effusions and expansile lesions is variable.
- Other lesions that may be seen at the petrous apex include aneurysms (uncommon complex mixed MRI signal demonstrating flow characteristics) and a range of neoplastic lesions including chondrosarcoma, chordoma, meningioma, metastatic disease, plasmacytoma and paraganglioma. Cephaloceles can be seen in this region and often communicate with the subarachnoid space via the posterolateral aspect of Meckel's cave.

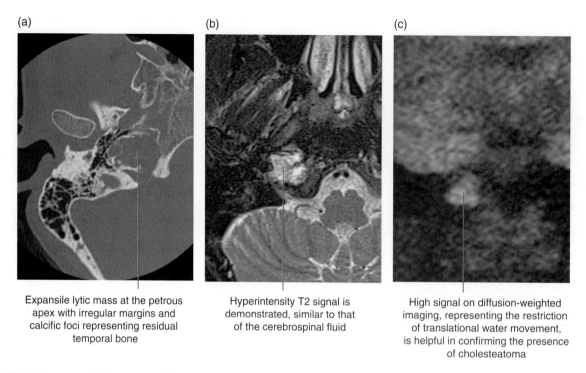

(a)

(b)

(c)

Expansile lytic mass at the petrous apex with irregular margins and calcific foci representing residual temporal bone

Hyperintensity T2 signal is demonstrated, similar to that of the cerebrospinal fluid

High signal on diffusion-weighted imaging, representing the restriction of translational water movement, is helpful in confirming the presence of cholesteatoma

Figure 20.19 Petrous apex cholesteatoma: axial MDCT image (a), axial fat-saturated T2-weighted MRI (b) and coronal diffusion-weighted MRI (c).

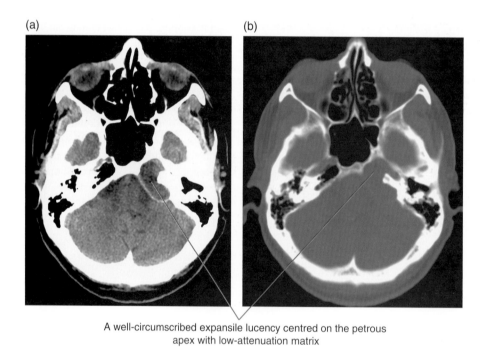

(a)

(b)

A well-circumscribed expansile lucency centred on the petrous apex with low-attenuation matrix

Figure 20.20 Petrous apex mucocele: axial skull base soft tissue (a) and bone window (b) MDCT images.

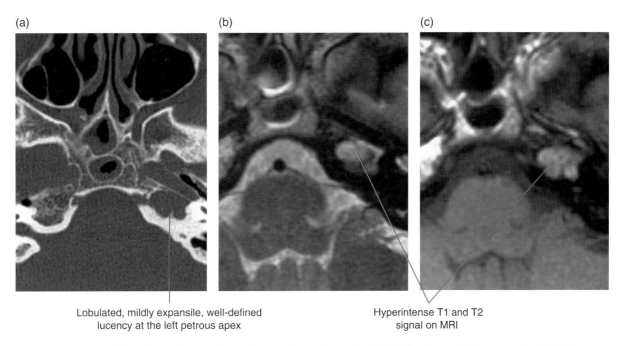

Lobulated, mildly expansile, well-defined
lucency at the left petrous apex

Hyperintense T1 and T2
signal on MRI

Figure 20.21 Petrous apex cholesterol granuloma: axial MDCT image (a), axial T2-weighted MRI (b) and coronal diffusion-weighted MRI (c).

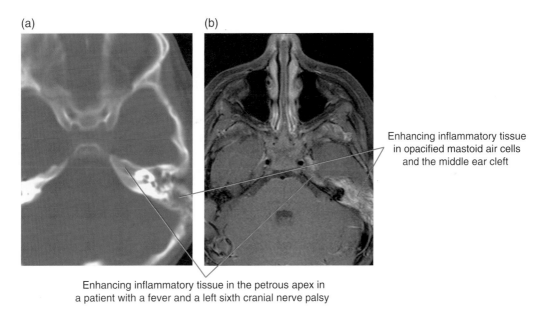

Enhancing inflammatory tissue
in opacified mastoid air cells
and the middle ear cleft

Enhancing inflammatory tissue in the petrous apex in
a patient with a fever and a left sixth cranial nerve palsy

Figure 20.22 Petrous apicitis: axial skull base MDCT image (a) and axial fat-saturated gadolinium-enhanced T1-weighted MRI (b).

EXPANSION OF SKULL BASE FORAMINA

Lesions that arise in the foraminae or in structures that pass through them should be considered when, on plain radiographs and CBCT, well-defined or irregular widening is identified.

20.19 Nerve sheath tumours (Figure 20.23)

- Benign, slow-growing lesions that, in the region of the skull base, arise from the cranial nerves and include schwannomas and neurofibromas.
- Lesions can arise in a variety of compartments – intracranially, extracranially in the upper neck spaces and traversing the skull

(a)

(b)

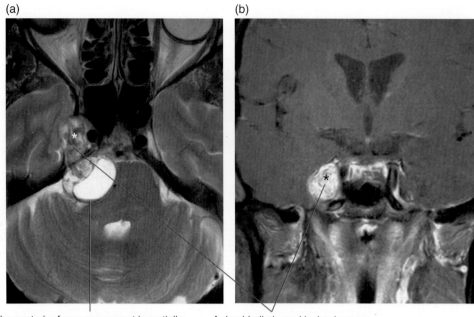

The posterior fossa component is partially
cystic, as illustrated by a shallow
dependent fluid–fluid level

A dumbbell-shaped lesion is seen
expanding Meckel's cave (*) and
filling the superior cerebellopontine angle

Figure 20.23 Nerve sheath tumour: axial T2-weighted (a) and coronal fat-saturated gadolinium-enhanced T1-weighted (b) MRI.

base foraminae – and are 'waisted' by the foramina, becoming 'bilobed' or 'dumbbell' shaped.

- Most commonly arise from the vestibular, trigeminal, oculomotor and hypoglossal nerves as well as in the region of the jugular foramen.
- Multiple lesions can be seen in the setting of neuro-fibromatosis.

Radiological features

- On MDCT, these are iso- to slightly hyperattenuating with brain, and may scallop the adjacent bone and enlarge the traversed foramina. The latter are usually demonstrated on CBCT.
- May be cystic and/or calcified.
- On MRI lesions are isointense on T1-weighted imaging and hyperintense on T2 with homogeneous contrast enhancement.

Differential diagnosis

	Key radiological differences
Metastases	Destructive tumour, primary known, multiple.
Aneurysm	Ring calcification, defined, avid enhancement, vessel associated.
Meningioma	Transosseous, enhancing dural thickening.
Inflammatory	Ill defined, enhancing, associated systemic features/encephalopathy.

20.20 Perineural metastatic disease

- Malignant tumours may invade and spread to regional sites via the perineural space.
- The commonest primary malignancies include: squamous cell carcinoma and salivary gland tumours, notably adenoid cystic carcinoma as well as lymphoma and melanoma.
- Commonly involved nerves include: the trigeminal and facial cranial nerves.

Radiological features

- On CBCT and MDCT scans, advanced perineural infiltration may be reflected in bony foraminal widening and marginal erosions.
- On MRI, nerve thickening, displacement of the perineural fat, foraminal and canalicular widening are also demonstrated with abnormal neural signal and contrast enhancement.

CHAPTER 21
The Cervical Spine

Michael Bynevelt and Andrew Thompson

The cervical vertebral column is included in many head and neck radiographs and is variably demonstrated on dental cone beam computed tomography (CBCT). A variety of degenerative conditions are very common, and some have clinical significance. Congenital variations, inflammatory and neoplastic conditions may also be encountered.

CONGENITAL VARIATIONS (Figures 21.1–21.5)

Asymmetric C1/C2 articulation. Asymmetry of the C1 lateral mass positioning with respect to the odontoid can be visualised on the anteroposterior C1/C2 radiograph, cone beam computed tomography (CBCT) or multidetector computed tomography (MDCT) reformats. This very common normal variant can be problematic in assessing trauma on plain radiographs.

Atlanto-occipital assimilation. This term covers fusion anomalies of all or part of the C1 segment with the basiocciput and is associated with basilar invagination.

Basilar invagination. Describes the inward and upward translation of the cervical spine in relation to the skull base, resulting in telescoping of the craniocervical junction into the cranial cavity. The odontoid is positioned more than 5 mm above the level of the Chamberlain line, drawn between the hard palate and posterior foramen magnum. This can result in compression of the brainstem and upper cervical cord, which may be symptomatic.

Cervicovertebral pseudosubluxation. A normal variant resulting from flexion mobility at C2/C3 and to a lesser extent C3/C4 levels in children. Less than or equal to 2 mm anterolisthesis is considered within normal limits.

Condylus tertius/basilar process. A 'third occipital condyle' can project from the base of the clivus, articulating with the tip of the odontoid. This is commonly associated with accessory ossicles.

Incompletely fused C1 ring. Posterior arch defects are more common than those of the anterior arch and can be midline or paramedian. Anterior arch defects on sagittal magnetic resonance imaging (MRI) appear as a fibrous pseudotumour with associated thickening of the adjacent bony elements.

Limbus vertebrae. A triangular fragment of bone, most commonly at the anterosuperior corner of a vertebral body associated with sclerotic margins: inferior and posterior margins less commonly. The cause is herniation of a portion of the nucleus pulposus underneath the ring apophysis before its fusion to the body, which may be caused by trauma. The ring apophysis remains separate from the main vertebral body.

Odontoid variations. Backward tilt, hypoplasia, aplasia, os odontoideum (an ossific body associated with a foreshortened C2 odontoid), ossiculum terminale (terminal odontoid ossification centre) are all developmental variations of the odontoid or dens of C2.

Platybasia. Abnormal flattening of the skull base, which occurs in a number of congenital conditions such as osteogenesis imperfecta and craniocleidodysostosis. Also can be a complication of trauma and bone-softening disorders such as Paget disease. On a lateral skull radiograph, MDCT, CBCT or MRI, there is an abnormally obtuse basal angle constructed by the plane of the anterior cranial fossa and the dorsum of the clivus. Platybasia can be associated with basilar invagination.

Ponticulus posticus or arcuate foramen. Anomalous bony bridge covering the vertebral artery groove of the atlas resulting from ossification of the posterior atlanto-occipital ligament.

Segmentation anomalies. Can be associated with more generalised disorders such as Klippel–Feil syndrome.

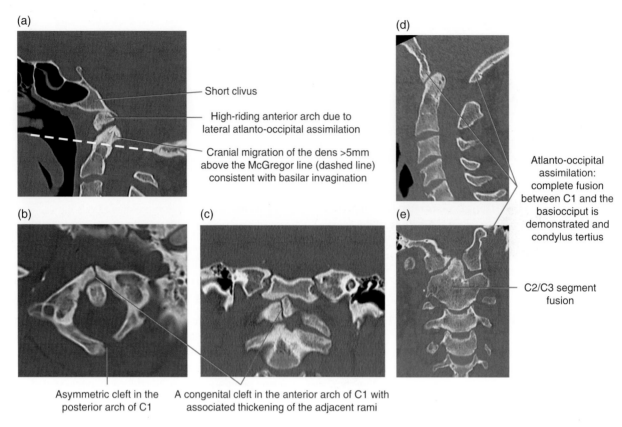

(a)

Short clivus

High-riding anterior arch due to lateral atlanto-occipital assimilation

Cranial migration of the dens >5mm above the McGregor line (dashed line) consistent with basilar invagination

(d)

Atlanto-occipital assimilation: complete fusion between C1 and the basiocciput is demonstrated and condylus tertius

(b)

(c)

(e)

C2/C3 segment fusion

Asymmetric cleft in the posterior arch of C1

A congenital cleft in the anterior arch of C1 with associated thickening of the adjacent rami

Figure 21.1 Atlanto-occipital assimilation and fusion defects: (a–e) MDCT multiplanar reformatted images.

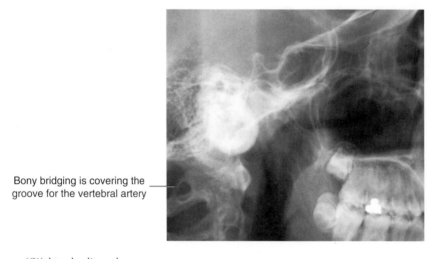

Bony bridging is covering the groove for the vertebral artery

Figure 21.2 Arcuate foramen (C1): lateral radiograph.

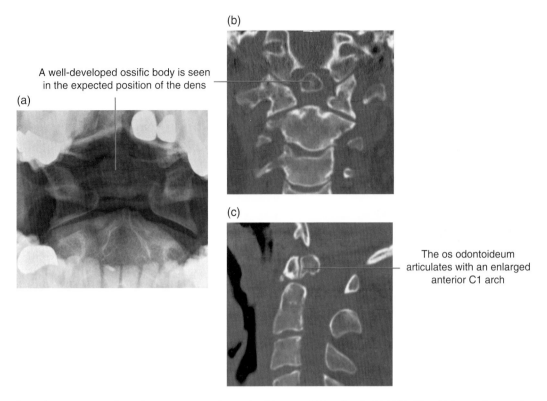

A well-developed ossific body is seen in the expected position of the dens

The os odontoideum articulates with an enlarged anterior C1 arch

Figure 21.3 Odontoid variations: os odontoideum – open mouth peg view (a), coronal (b) and sagittal (c) MDCT multiplanar reformatted upper cervical spine images.

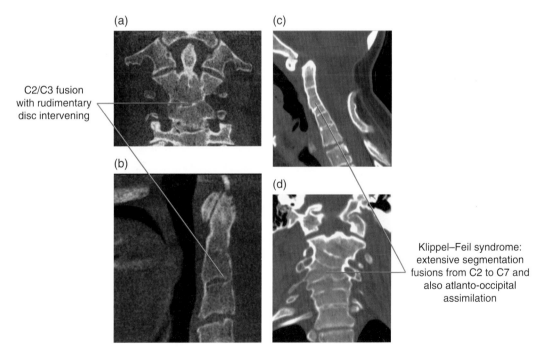

C2/C3 fusion with rudimentary disc intervening

Klippel–Feil syndrome: extensive segmentation fusions from C2 to C7 and also atlanto-occipital assimilation

Figure 21.4 Segmentation anomalies: CBCT reformatted (a,b) and MDCT reformatted (c,d) images.

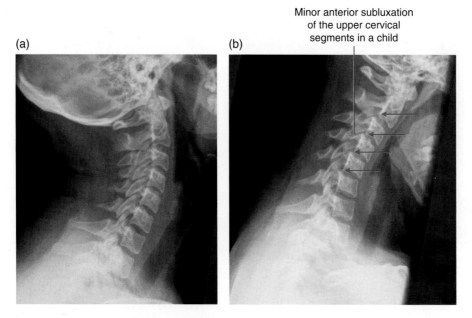

Figure 21.5 Cervicovertebral pseudosubluxation: extension (a) and (b) flexion lateral radiographs.

DEGENERATIVE DISEASE

21.1 Cervical spondylosis (Figure 21.6)

- A collective term describing chronic degenerative disease of the cervical spine.
- A common condition seen with advancing age, which affects the intervertebral discs and adjacent vertebral bodies, and may result in impingement upon the spinal cord and exiting nerve roots.
- Pathophysiological changes include:
  - Disc dehydration with loss of elasticity, eventually becoming fissured and collapsed.
  - Degenerative osteoarthritic changes also occur in the facet joints and uncovertebral articulations with laxity of the longitudinal ligaments and ligamentum flava.
  - Bony relationships are altered, the biomechanical unit is compromised and a 'spiralling' course of degenerative changes result.
  - Soft disc material may escape from the confines of the parent disc; however, herniation in this region is commonly accompanied by marginal osteophytes, which is an attempt to stabilise the degenerating biomechanical unit.
  - Arthritic changes in the facet joints result in hypertrophy of the joints themselves, synovial thickening and sometimes cyst formation. Ligamentum flavum thickening and infolding is seen in addition. These and productive degenerative changes arising from the uncovertebral joint can result in foraminal narrowing.
- Degenerative disc osteophytic complexes can result in partial or complete effacement of the cerebrospinal fluid around the spinal cord at the disc levels and can progress to compress the cord to varying degrees.
- Lower cervical disc levels are more commonly affected, particularly C5/C6.

Radiological features

- On MDCT, as well as CBCT, the disc degeneration is reflected in the loss of disc space height, endplate irregularity/sclerosis and marginal bony osteophytic ridging, sometimes with intradiscal gas. The uncovertebral joints similarly develop osteophytes. The facet joints demonstrate joint space narrowing with sclerosis and bone eburnation, intra-articular gas and osteophyte formation.
- On MRI, degenerative discs are of reduced signal and the osteophytic bony components are of low signal on all sequences. The impingement on the thecal contents is well characterised, as is the degree of foraminal compromise on oblique sagittal T2-weighted imaging. Effusions in the facet joints may be seen, particularly on T2-weighted imaging.

Differential diagnosis

	Key radiological differences
Ossification of the posterior longitudinal ligament	Flowing, contiguous thickening of posterior longitudinal ligament.
Inflammatory and depositional arthropathies	Erosive changes, subluxation.

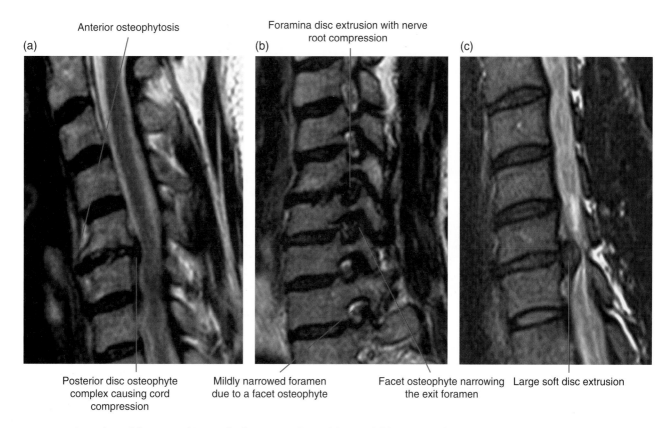

Anterior osteophytosis

Foramina disc extrusion with nerve root compression

(a)   (b)   (c)

Posterior disc osteophyte complex causing cord compression

Mildly narrowed foramen due to a facet osteophyte

Facet osteophyte narrowing the exit foramen   Large soft disc extrusion

Figure 21.6 Cervical spondylosis: sagittal T2-weighted MRI cervical spine (a), sagittal oblique T2-weighted MRI cervical spine foramina (b) and sagittal T2-weighted MRI cervical spine (c) images.

21.2 Diffuse idiopathic hyperostosis
(Figure 21.7)

- Associated with flowing ossification of the anterior longitudinal ligament along the anterior aspects of the vertebral bodies and adjacent annulus of the disc as well as the paraspinal tissues. There is often little or no associated degenerative change.
- Cervical changes may accompany the condition in the thoracic region, where it is most commonly found.

Radiological features
- Often incidentally detected on lateral chest radiographs as 'flowing-wax'-like bridging ossification extending over the anterior aspects of four or more contiguous vertebral segments.

- More accurately demonstrated and portrayed on MDCT.
- On MRI, the hypertrophic ligaments are of reduced signal on all sequences.

Differential diagnosis

	Key radiological differences
Degenerative disease	Multifocal disc and facet degenerative change.
Seronegative spondyloarthropathies	Sacroiliac joint involvement.

(a)   (b)

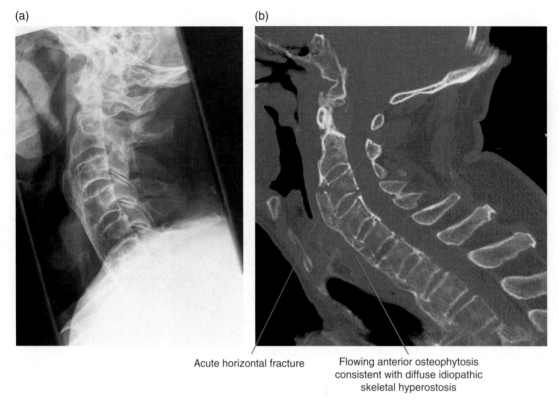

Acute horizontal fracture   Flowing anterior osteophytosis
consistent with diffuse idiopathic
skeletal hyperostosis

Figure 21.7 Diffuse idiopathic skeletal hyperostosis: lateral cervical spine radiograph (a) and sagittal multiplanar reformatted MDCT image (b).

21.3 Ossification of the posterior longitudinal ligament (Figure 21.8)

- Ossified islands of fatty marrow in the posterior longitudinal ligament, most commonly in the cervical region, that may be segmental, continuous or mixed. May cause spinal canal narrowing to an extent that precipitates a myelopathy.
- Many associated conditions are listed including diffuse idiopathic hyperostosis and ankylosing spondylitis.

Radiological features

- On cross-sectional imaging the lesions appear as multilevel contiguous 'T'- or 'mushroom'-shaped ossified bodies that may contain marrow (T1 hyperintense) signal projecting in the anterior epidural compartment to compress the thecal sac and contents.

Differential diagnosis

	Key radiological differences
Degeneration, disc herniation	Disc centric, non-continuous.
Meningioma	Dural based, enhancing.

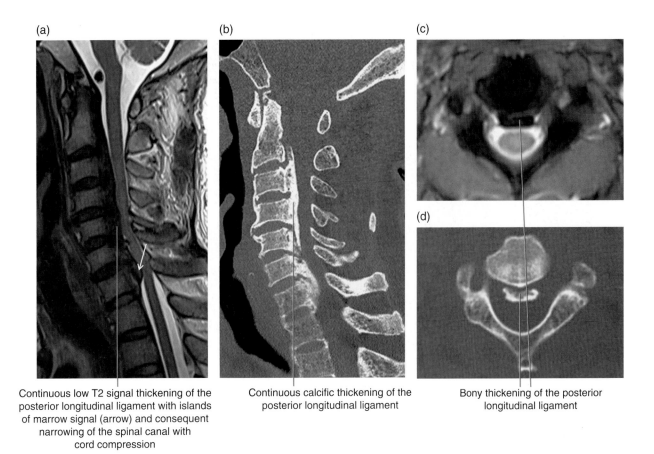

(a)

(b)

(c)

(d)

Continuous low T2 signal thickening of the posterior longitudinal ligament with islands of marrow signal (arrow) and consequent narrowing of the spinal canal with cord compression

Continuous calcific thickening of the posterior longitudinal ligament

Bony thickening of the posterior longitudinal ligament

Figure 21.8 Ossification of the posterior longitudinal ligament: sagittal T2-weighted cervical spine MRI (a), sagittal multiplanar reformatted MDCT image (b), axial T2-weighted cervical spine MRI (c) and axial cervical spine MDCT image (d).

INFLAMMATORY AND DEPOSITIONAL CONDITIONS

21.4 Rheumatoid arthritis (Figure 21.9)

- An erosive inflammatory arthritis that preferentially affects the cervical spine, particularly the atlantoaxial articulations.
- Pannus (inflamed thickened synovium) is seen about the odontoid process, resulting in bony erosion and destruction.
- Also affects the ligaments in this region, causing laxity, insufficiency and instability (anterior, lateral, rotatory, vertical) and neural impingement.

Radiological features
- Plain radiographs and cross-sectional imaging demonstrate a diffuse spondyloarthropathy featuring erosions, malalignment including atlantoaxial and subaxial subluxation, soft tissue and calcified inflammatory tissue (pannus) formation and osteopenia.

- Dynamic (active) views using a variety of imaging modalities can demonstrate instability, which is noted to be significant when the atlantodental interval is wider than 3 mm, the resultant spinal canal narrowing is <14 mm or lateral mass translation/rotation is more than 2 mm.
- Posterior subluxation is evident when the anterior arch of the atlas presents over the apex of the dens.
- Vertical instability is represented by basilar invagination, atlantoaxial impaction and cranial settling, which are the result of bony softening. This can be diagnosed when the apex of the dens is positioned more than 4.5 mm above McGregor's line (drawn between the posterior tip of the hard palate and the inferior opisthion).
- Below the C2 level (subaxial), changes are centred on the facet and uncovertebral joints causing joint space narrowing with erosions as well as instability, which is evident by anterior, but also posterior, subluxation (more than 2 mm is significant).
- Often CT and MRI are complementary in the evaluation of this condition, demonstrating the specific bony changes and consequent soft tissue changes, respectively.

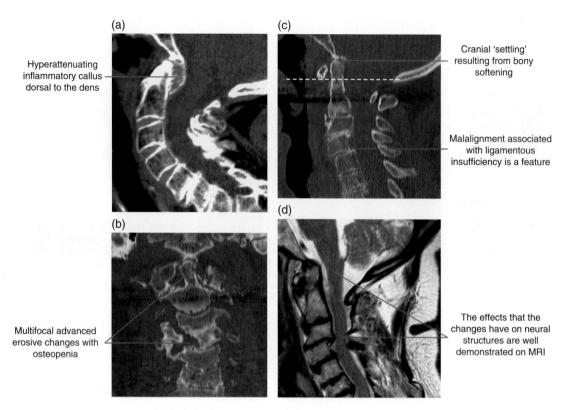

Figure 21.9 Rheumatoid arthritis: sagittal multiplanar reformatted (MPR) MDCT image (a), coronal multiplanar reformatted MDCT image (b), sagittal multiplanar reformatted MDCT image with the McGregor line indicated by the dashed line (c) and sagittal T2-weighted cervical spine MRI (d).

Differential diagnosis

	Key radiological differences
Seronegative spondyloarthropathies	Sacroiliac joint involvement.
Gout and calcium pyrophosphate deposition	Calcified foci, erosions.
Degenerative disease	Disc and facet degenerative change.
Infection	Disc involved, collections, paravertebral phlegmon.
Haemodialysis	History, endplate sclerosis/erosive, destructive.

21.5 Ankylosing spondylitis (Figure 21.10)

- An example of a chronic seronegative spondyloarthropathy with a predisposition for young adults with HLA B27 class I surface antigens.
- Presents initially as a sacroiliitis and erosions at the vertebral body corners (enthesitis of the annular fibre insertions), termed the Romanus lesion. There is progressive syndesmophyte formation of the vertebral segments moving cranially, resulting in complete fusion of the spinal skeleton.

Radiological features

- The Romanus lesion is seen as reactive endplate sclerosis ('shining corners') with squaring of the vertebral body and progressive ossification of the annular fibres, forming syndesmophytes, until there is complete spinal fusion progressing cranially over time.
- Facet joints also fuse and the completely fused vertebral column has been termed 'bamboo spine'; a complex with increased susceptibility to fracture.

Differential diagnosis

	Key radiological differences
Other seronegative spondyloarthropathies	Patterns of involvement, associated conditions.
Diffuse idiopathic hyperostosis	Anterior bridging osteophytes.
Ossification of the posterior longitudinal ligament	Continuous calcific thickening of the posterior longitudinal ligament.
Rheumatoid arthritis	Erosive disease more prominent, particularly the cervical spine.

(a) (b)

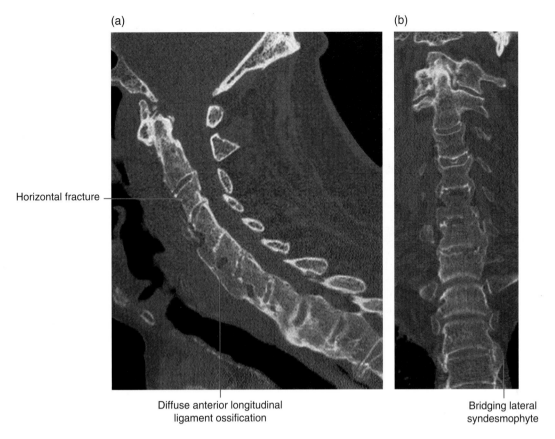

Horizontal fracture ⎯

Diffuse anterior longitudinal
ligament ossification

Bridging lateral
syndesmophyte

Figure 21.10 Ankylosing spondylitis: sagittal cervical spine multiplanar reformatted MDCT (a) and coronal multiplanar reformatted (b) images.

21.6 Osteomyelitis/discitis/facetal septic arthritis, including tuberculosis (Figure 21.11)

- Infection of the components of the spinal column result from haematogenous (transarterial and transvenous) or direct inoculation (adjacent infection, trauma, surgery).
- The cervical region is least commonly affected and intravenous drug users, the immunocompromised and those with diabetes are susceptible.
- Responsible organisms include *Staphylococcus aureus* and other pyogenic bacteria but also granulomatous, fungal and parasitic agents.
- With pyogenic infections, the vertebral endplates are commonly affected and, in the cervical region, the atlantodental joint and other articulations in the craniocervical junction region can be uniquely involved.
- There may be inflammatory phlegmon and/or abscess in the paravertebral and epidural spaces.

Radiological features
- Plain radiographs are not sensitive and the findings generally appear late in the clinical course, revealing disc space narrowing, prevertebral soft tissue thickening, demineralisation and erosive (particularly endplate) changes with possible progression to vertebral body collapse and deformity. Sclerosis and ankylosis can be seen in chronic or burnt-out disease.
- MDCT will define the bony changes with more clarity and also associated soft tissue changes, such as paraspinal including epidural collections. Bone changes can be visualised on CBCT.
- MRI is the modality of choice to characterise and stage the extent of the inflammatory process. Replacement of the fatty marrow signal with low-signal tissue on T1-weighted imaging with high T2 signal material present in the bone, discs and/or facet joints. Avid contrast enhancement is seen in the inflamed tissue outlining collections or abscesses.
- Bone scintigraphy will reveal increased activity in the endplates about the disc.

Differential diagnosis

	Key radiological differences
Metastases	Multifocally destructive, pedicle involvement.
Haemodialysis	Relevant clinical history, endplate sclerosis/ erosive, destructive.
Neuropathic spine	Relevant clinical history, endplate sclerosis/ erosive, destructive.

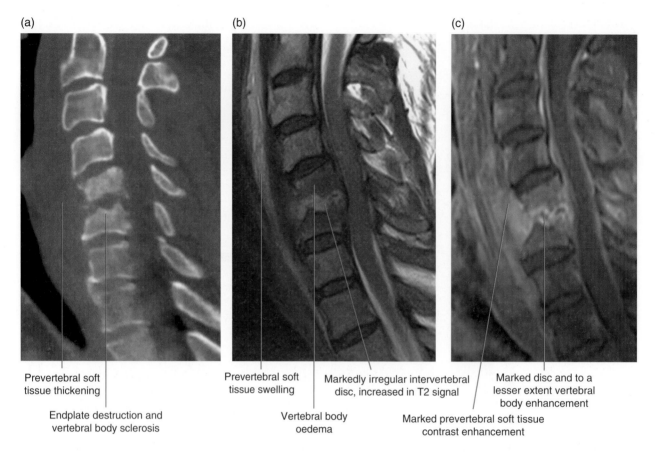

(a)   (b)   (c)

Prevertebral soft
tissue thickening

Endplate destruction and
vertebral body sclerosis

Prevertebral soft
tissue swelling

Vertebral body
oedema

Markedly irregular intervertebral
disc, increased in T2 signal

Marked disc and to a
lesser extent vertebral
body enhancement

Marked prevertebral soft tissue
contrast enhancement

Figure 21.11 C5/C6 infective discitis and osteomyelitis: sagittal cervical spine multiplanar reformatted MDCT image (a), sagittal T2-weighted MRI (b) and sagittal fat-saturated gadolinium-enhanced T1-weighted cervical spine MRI (c).

TUMOURS AND TUMOUR-LIKE LESIONS

21.7 Metastatic tumours (Figure 21.12)

- Most common neoplastic lesion affecting the vertebral column and may cause spinal cord compression.
- Commonest primary lesion locations are breast, lung, prostate and the kidneys.
- The posterior aspect of the vertebral body is the most common location with the epidural space and pedicles being secondarily involved. Often there is more than one deposit, and diffuse involvement may occur.
- Most commonly the deposits cause bone destruction extending into the paravertebral tissue causing nerve and cord compression, pathological vertebral fracturing and collapse, and instability when the posterior elements are invaded.
- Some metastatic tumours increase the mineralisation of the affected bone (sclerotic metastases); these include prostate, breast, carcinoid and medulloblastoma.

Radiological features
- Plain radiography sensitivity in detecting metastatic disease is low.
- On MRI have a variety of appearances depending on their histological subtype. Most commonly they are relatively well-defined, low-T1-weighted lesions relative to the fatty marrow with variable increased T2 signal, best identified on fat-saturated T2 sequences.
- Sclerotic, cell dense or lesions with high nuclear to cytoplasmic ratios demonstrate reduced T2 signal.
- Most metastases enhance, and pathological fracturing can complicate the signal characteristics.
- Restriction on diffusion MRI is suggestive of an underlying metastatic deposit in the setting of a fracture when an insufficiency injury is the main differential diagnosis.
- MDCT demonstrates a destructive process that is often multifocal and an associated soft tissue mass. CBCT demonstrates the bone destruction.

Differential diagnosis

	Key radiological differences
Multiple myeloma	Pedicle involvement, diffusion restriction.
Lymphoma, leukaemia	Permeative, non-expansile, diffusion restriction on MRI.
Myelofibrosis	Diffuse sclerosis/marrow replacement (low T1 signal).
Osteoporosis	No diffusion restriction or associated mass.

Infection	Disc centric.
Primary bone tumours	Younger patient.
Haemangioma	Vertical trabeculation. T1 hyperintensity.
Degenerative disease	Disc centric.
Paget disease	Expansion, trabecular prominence.
Renal osteodystrophy	'Rugger jersey' appearance.
Schmorl's node	Endplate related.

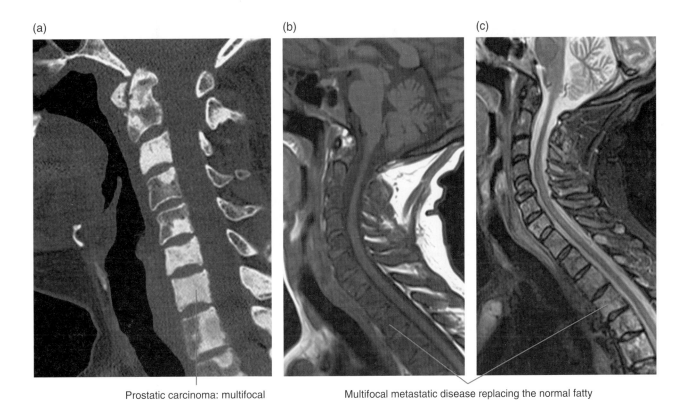

(a)

(b)

(c)

Prostatic carcinoma: multifocal sclerotic metastatic deposits

Multifocal metastatic disease replacing the normal fatty marrow signal on T1-weighted imaging is evident with fat-suppressed T2-weighted imaging

Figure 21.12 Metastatic spinal tumour: sagittal cervical spine multiplanar reformatted MDCT image (a), sagittal T1-weighted MRI (b) and sagittal cervical spine fat-saturated T2-weighted MRI (c).

21.8 Multiple myeloma

- Most common primary malignant bone neoplasm in adults, which is caused by a monoclonal proliferation of the plasma cells.
- Arising in the bone marrow, the disease can be multifocal/diffuse or solitary and focal in the form known as plasmacytoma.

Radiological features

- Multiple myeloma characteristically radiographically exhibits multiple well-defined 'punched-out' lytic lesions ('pepperpot' skull) with endosteal scalloping and can present with diffuse osteopenia.
- Lesions are limited to the distribution of red marrow in the older adult.
- Plasmacytoma presents as a single, large, usually expansile lesion, very commonly in a vertebral body.
- A skeletal survey is used to stage the disease, estimate the response to therapy and assess for complicating events.
- MDCT is used to assess aspects of complicated disease, in particular assessing the osseous changes and fractures, the latter for preoperative planning. CBCT demonstrates most of the bony changes.
- The infiltration and replacement of bone marrow is well demonstrated on T1 and fat-saturated T2 MRI sequences and lesions demonstrate variable contrast enhancement; however, given the risk of contrast nephropathy in these patients, administration of contrast should be considered in light of the patient's renal function and current guidelines.
- MRI can reveal several patterns of marrow involvement. Despite containing an infiltrate of plasma cells, the bone marrow can be normal. They can be focal or diffuse (homogeneous or inhomogeneous) and may have a distinct salt and pepper appearance. Focal lesions are well highlighted on the fat-saturated T2 sequences, whereas the diffuse disease is better illustrated on T1-weighted imaging.
- Whole-body short tau inversion–recovery (STIR) imaging is becoming a standard-of-care examination, replacing the skeletal survey in some centres.
- Nuclear medicine bone scintigraphy has limited utility in myeloma management as osteoblastic activity may not be increased; however, ^{18}F-fludeoxyglucose positron emission tomography demonstrates lesions of increased metabolism that correspond well to skeletal survey lesion load.

Differential diagnosis

	Key radiological differences
Metastases	Pedicle involvement, diffusion restriction.
Lymphoma, leukaemia	Permeative, non-expansile, diffusion restriction on MRI.
Osteoporosis	No diffusion restriction.
Hypercellular marrow	Organised diffuse marrow reconversion.

21.9 Aneurysmal bone cysts (Figure 21.13)

- Benign, highly vascular osseous non-neoplastic lesions of unknown origin.
- Spinal lesions occur in approximately 20% of cases and tend to arise from the posterior elements.

Radiological features

- On MDCT, the lesion comprises multiple cysts with internal septation and fluid–fluid levels. The bony and soft tissue components are well marginated. CBCT would only demonstrate the bony changes.
- On MRI, the lesions generally are hyperintense on T2-weighted images with multiloculated cystic areas with fluid–fluid levels being characteristic, but not specific for aneurysmal bone cysts.

Differential diagnosis

	Key radiological differences
Osteoblastoma	Well-defined lytic, expansible neural arch.
Osteosarcoma	Destructive in part sclerotic mass with/without fluid–fluid levels (telangiectatic type).
Chondroblastoma	Chondroid matrix calcifications.
Giant cell tumour	Lytic, lacking sclerotic margin, mixed signal/enhancing matrix.
Malignant nerve sheath tumour	Rapid growth, perineural with/without destruction with/without intradural involvement.
Plasmacytoma	Well-marginated lytic, T2 hypointense.

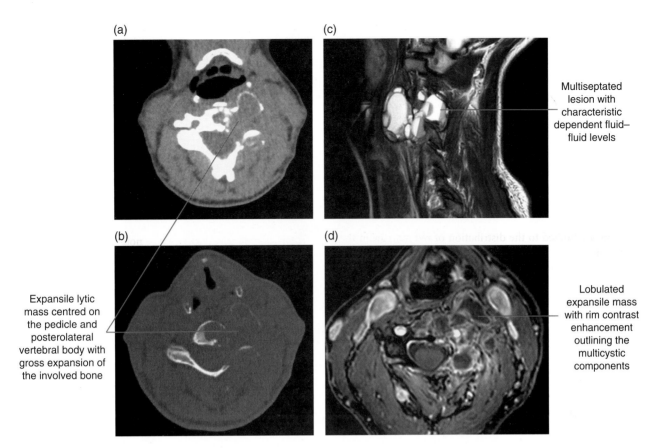

(a)

(c)

Multiseptated lesion with characteristic dependent fluid–fluid levels

Expansile lytic mass centred on the pedicle and posterolateral vertebral body with gross expansion of the involved bone

(b)

(d)

Lobulated expansile mass with rim contrast enhancement outlining the multicystic components

Figure 21.13 Aneurysmal bone cyst: axial cervical spine soft tissue (a) and bone (b) MDCT images; sagittal cervical spine T2-weighted (c) and axial fat-saturated T1-weighted (d) MRI.

21.10 Peripheral nerve sheath tumours
(Figure 21.14)

- Divided into two major benign categories – neurofibroma and schwannoma – and a malignant peripheral nerve sheath tumour thought to arise from transformation of plexiform neurofibromas.
- Spinal lesions originate from and grow along the spinal nerve root; the vast majority cause spinal neural foraminal widening and dumbbell-shaped tumours.
- Pathologically, neurofibromas can be divided into different types: localised, plexiform and diffuse:
  - Localised neurofibromas are identical to solitary neurofibromas; however, in the setting of *NF1*, they tend to be larger, multiple, unencapsulated, slow growing and, more commonly, deep in location.
  - Plexiform neurofibromas are pathognomonic for *NF1*, usually involve a long segment of a major nerve trunk, grow slowly and extend into the nerve branches and may undergo malignant degeneration.
  - Diffuse neurofibroma is uncommon, seen in the young, less frequently associated with neurofibromatosis type 1 and

involves the head and neck skin and subcutaneous tissues. Presents as a poorly defined process that spreads along connective tissue septa surrounding rather than destroying neighbouring structures.

Radiological features
- Schwannomas and neurofibromas are very similar in imaging appearance: well circumscribed, fusiform, dumbbell-shaped.
- Typically, the schwannoma is eccentrically located with respect to the nerve and the neurofibroma centrally located.
- Cystic degeneration, haemorrhage and cavitation are much more common in schwannomas.
- MDCT of plexiform neurofibromas shows large multilobulated low-attenuation masses, usually within a major nerve distribution. MRI reveals large elongate conglomerate masses. CBCT would demonstrate the bony changes in most cases.
- Findings suggestive of malignancy include tumours that are heterogeneous, are larger than 5 cm, are calcified, have ill-defined borders, prominent vascularity or enhancement, and have rapid growth.

Differential diagnosis

	Key radiological differences
Vascular malformations/ haemangioma	Flow on ultrasound, phleboliths, flow voids.
Inflammatory	Acute/subacute presentation, more symptomatic.
Metastases	Multiple, known primary.

Lymphoma	'Moulding configuration', diffusion restricting on MRI, homogeneous enhancement.
Haemangiopericytoma	Flow voids, heterogeneous matrix.
Fibrous histiocytoma	Similar appearances.
Sarcoma	Bone destruction.

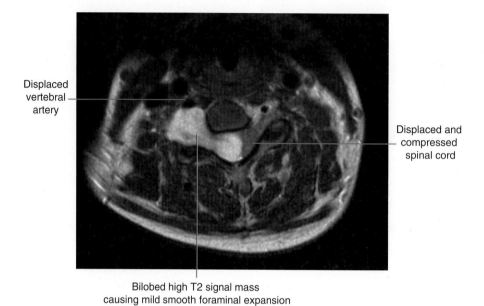

Displaced vertebral artery

Displaced and compressed spinal cord

Bilobed high T2 signal mass causing mild smooth foraminal expansion

Figure 21.14 Peripheral nerve sheath tumour: axial cervical spine T2-weighted MRI.

Index

Atlas of Oral and Maxillofacial Radiology, First Edition. Bernard Koong.
© 2017 John Wiley & Sons Ltd. Published 2017 by John Wiley & Sons Ltd.